Mental Health at Crossroads

Challenges and Solutions

1ˢᵗ Edition

Mental Health at Crossroads
Challenges and Solutions

Editors:

Rakesh Kumar Chadda, MD, FAMS, FRCPsych, DIFAPA
Professor & Head, Department of Psychiatry
Chief, National Drug Dependence Treatment Centre

Pratap Sharan, MD, PhD
Professor, Department of Psychiatry

Mamta Sood, MD, DPM
Professor, Department of Psychiatry

Koushik Sinha Deb, MD
Additional Professor, Department of Psychiatry

All India Institute of Medical Sciences, New Delhi 110029, India

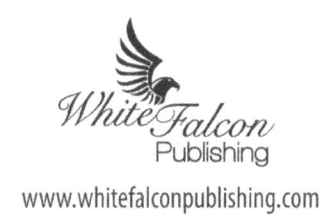

WhiteFalcon
Publishing

www.whitefalconpublishing.com

Mental Health at Crossroads - Challenges and Solutions
Rakesh Kumar Chadda, Pratap Sharan, Mamta Sood, Koushik Sinha Deb

www.whitefalconpublishing.com

ISBN - 978-1-63640-731-9

Contents

List of Contributors

Abhijit R. Rozatkar

Additional Professor, Department of Psychiatry, All India Institute of Medical Sciences Bhopal, Madhya Pradesh, India – 462020. E-mail: abhijitrozatkar@gmail.com

Amrita Roy

Ph.D. Scholar (Mental Health Rehabilitation), National Institute of Mental Health and Neuro Sciences (NIMHANS), Bengaluru, Karnataka, India – 560030. E-mail: pimmipal@gmail.com

Andrew Molodynski

Consultant Psychiatrist, Oxford Health NHS Foundation Trust; Honorary Senior Clinical Lecturer, Oxford University. E-mail: Andrew.Molodynski@oxfordhealth.nhs.uk

Aniruddha Basu

Associate Professor, Department of Psychiatry, All India Institute of Medical Sciences Kalyani, West Bengal, India – 741245. E-mail: draniruddhabasu@gmail.com

Anju Dhawan

Professor, National Drug Dependence Treatment Centre and Department of Psychiatry, All India Institute of Medical Sciences, New Delhi, India – 110029. E-mail: dranjudhawan@gmail.com

Atul Ambekar

Professor, National Drug Dependence Treatment Centre and Department of Psychiatry, All India Institute of Medical Sciences, New Delhi, India – 110029. E-mail: atul.ambekar@gmail.com

Bettina Sara Mathew

Senior Resident, Department of Psychiatry, Government Medical College, Kottayam, Kerala, India – 686008. E-mail: bettinamathew09@gmail.com

Bichitra Nanda Patra

Additional Professor, Department of Psychiatry, All India Institute of Medical Sciences, New Delhi, India – 110029. E-mail: patrab.aiims@gmail.com

Dhandapani Nandakumar

Research Officer, Department of Psychiatry, All India Institute of Medical Sciences, New Delhi, India – 110029. E-mail: dhandapaniashwin@gmail.com

Gagan Hans

Associate Professor, Department of Psychiatry, All India Institute of Medical Sciences, New Delhi, India – 110029. E-mail: gaganhans23@gmail.com

Gauri Shanker Kaloiya

Additional Professor of Clinical Psychology, National Drug Dependence Treatment Centre and Department of Psychiatry, All India Institute of Medical Sciences, New Delhi, India – 110029. E-mail: gkaloiya@gmail.com

Geetesh Kumar Singh

Research Officer (Clinical Psychologist), Department of Psychiatry, All India Institute of Medical Sciences Bhopal, Madhya Pradesh, India – 462020. E-mail: g_ksingh007@yahoo.com

Kashypi Garg
Senior Resident, Department of Psychiatry, SN Medical College, Agra, Uttar Pradesh, India – 282003. E-mail: gargkashypi@gmail.com

Koushik Sinha Deb
Additional Professor, Department of Psychiatry, All India Institute of Medical Sciences, New Delhi, India – 110029. E-mail: koushik.sinha.deb@gmail.com

Lini Philip
Clinical Psychologist, Department of Psychiatry & National Drug Dependence Treatment Centre, All India Institute of Medical Sciences, New Delhi, India – 110029. E-mail: lini.philip.30@gmail.com

Louise Penzenstadler
Consultant Psychiatrist, Addictology Division, Geneva University Hospital, Geneva, Switzerland. E-mail: louise.e.penzenstadler@hcuge.ch

Mamta Sood
Professor, Department of Psychiatry, All India Institute of Medical Sciences, New Delhi, India – 110029. E-mail: soodmamta@gmail.com

Mandeep Kaur
Senior Research Fellow, Department of Psychiatry, All India Institute of Medical Sciences, New Delhi, India – 110029. E-mail: deepnagpal28@gmail.com

Naveen Anand
Senior Resident, Department of Psychiatry, North Eastern Indira Gandhi Regional Institute of Health and Medical Sciences, Shillong, Meghalaya, India – 793018. E-mail: naveen.1489@gmail.com

Nileswar Das
Senior Resident, Department of Psychiatry, All India Institute of Medical Sciences, Ansari Nagar, New Delhi, India – 110029. E-mail: dr.nileswar@gmail.com

Pawan Sharma
Assistant Professor of Psychiatry, Patan Academy of Health Sciences, School of Medicine, Lalitpur, Nepal. E-mail: pawan60@gmail.com

Pratap Sharan
Professor, Department of Psychiatry, All India Institute of Medical Sciences, New Delhi, India – 110029. E-mail: pratapsharan@gmail.com

Preethy Kathiresan
Assistant Professor, Department of Psychiatry, All India Institute of Medical Sciences Jodhpur, Rajasthan, India – 342005. E-mail: princyaiims@gmail.com

Prioma Das
Psychiatric Social Worker, Department of Psychiatry, All India Institute of Medical Sciences Kalyani, West Bengal, India – 741245. E-mail: priomadas000@gmail.com

Priyanka Saha
Senior Resident, National Drug Dependence Treatment Centre and Department of Psychiatry, All India Institute of Medical Sciences, New Delhi, India – 110029. E-mail: drpriyanka614@gmail.com

Rachna Bhargava
Additional Professor (Clinical Psychology), National Drug Dependence Treatment Centre and Department of Psychiatry, All India Institute of Medical Sciences, New Delhi, India – 110029. E-mail: rachnabhargava@gmail.com

Rahul Mathur
Senior Resident, National Drug Dependence Treatment Centre and Department of Psychiatry, All India Institute of Medical Sciences, New Delhi, India – 110029. E-mail: jammyrahul17@gmail.com

Rajesh Sagar

Professor, Department of Psychiatry, All India Institute of Medical Sciences, New Delhi, India – 110029. E-mail: rsagar29@gmail.com

Rakesh Kumar Chadda

Professor & Head, Department of Psychiatry, and Chief, National Drug Dependence Treatment Centre, All India Institute of Medical Sciences, New Delhi, India – 110029. E-mail: drrakeshchadda@gmail.com

Raman Deep

Additional Professor, Department of Psychiatry, All India Institute of Medical Sciences, New Delhi, India – 110029. E-mail: drramandeep@gmail.com

Raveena Saroye

Consultant Psychiatrist, Vardaan Neuropsychiatry Clinic and De-Addiction Hospital, Patiala, Punjab, India – 147001. E-mail: saroyeraveena93@gmail.com

Ravi Gupta

Additional Professor, Division of Sleep Medicine, Department of Psychiatry, All India Institute of Medical Sciences, Rishikesh, Uttarakhand, India – 249203. E-mail: ravi.psyc@aiimsrishikesh.edu.in

Rohit Verma

Additional Professor, Department of Psychiatry, All India Institute of Medical Sciences, New Delhi, India – 110029. E-mail: rohit.aiims@gmail.com

Roy Abraham Kallivayalil

Professor & Head, Department of Psychiatry, Pushpagiri Institute of Medical Sciences, Tiruvalla, Kerala, India – 689101. E-mail: roykalli@gmail.com

Sathya Prakash

Consultant Psychiatrist, Institute of Brain and Spine & Holy Family Hospital, New Delhi, India. E-mail: dr.sathyaprakashtbts@gmail.com

Sayani Samanta

Nursing Officer, Department of Psychiatry, All India Institute of Medical Sciences Kalyani, West Bengal, India – 741245. E-mail: ssamanta011@gmail.com

Shalini Singh

Assistant Professor, Department of Psychiatry and National Drug Dependence Treatment Centre, All India Institute of Medical Sciences, New Delhi, India – 110029. E-mail: shalin.achra@gmail.com

Siddharth Sarkar

Additional Professor, Department of Psychiatry and National Drug Dependence Treatment Centre, All India Institute of Medical Sciences, New Delhi, India – 110029. E-mail: sidsarkar22@gmail.com

Sivakumar Thanapal

Additional Professor, Psychiatric Rehabilitation Services, Department of Psychiatry, National Institute of Mental Health and Neurosciences (NIMHANS), Bangalore, Karnataka, India – 560029, India. E-mail: drt.sivakumar@yahoo.co.in

Sumegha Mittal

Senior Resident, Department of Psychiatry, All India Institute of Medical Sciences, New Delhi, India – 110029. E-mail: mittalsumegha19@gmail.com

Swarndeep Singh

Assistant Professor, Department of Psychiatry, Government Medical College and Hospital, Chandigarh –160047. E-mail: sevisingh@gmail.com

UC Garg

Consultant Psychiatrist, Garg Medical Complex, M G Road, Agra, Uttar Pradesh, India – 282010. E-mail: uttamcgarg@gmail.com

Vaibhav Patil

Assistant Professor, Department of Psychiatry, All India Institute of Medical Sciences, New Delhi, India – 110029. E-mail: drvaibhavp317@gmail.com

Vijay Krishnan

Assistant Professor, Department of Psychiatry, All India Institute of Medical Sciences Rishikesh, Uttarakhand, India – 249203. E-mail: mail.vijay.krishnan@gmail.com

Yasser Khazaal

Professor of Psychiatry, Department of Psychiatry Lausanne University Hospital and Lausanne University, Switzerland. E-mail: yasserk1000@gmail.com

Yatan Pal Singh Balhara

Additional Professor, National Drug Dependence Treatment Centre and Department of Psychiatry, All India Institute of Medical Sciences, New Delhi, India – 110029. E-mail: ypsbalhara@gmail.com

List of Illustrators

Koushik Sinha Deb[1] and Abhishek Chakladar[2], Anuranjan Vishwakarma[2], Deeksha Kalra[2], Nileswar Das[2], Pallavi Rajhans[2], Rahul Mathur[2], Romil Saini[2], Shubham Narnoli[2]

[1.] Additional Professor, Department of Psychiatry, All India Institute of Medical Sciences, New Delhi, India – 110029.

[2.] Senior Resident, Department of Psychiatry, All India Institute of Medical Sciences, New Delhi, India – 110029.

All stock illustrations, icons and digital resources were licensed from www.freepik.com for commercial use.

Preface

The word "mental" often brings many stray feelings whenever it enters the thought process. The word has often been associated with mental illnesses, like schizophrenia, and mental hospitals. On the contrary, the World Health Organization (WHO), when it came into being, very clearly defined "Health" as not just the absence of illness, but a state of physical, mental and social well-being.

The book "Mental Health at Crossroads: Challenges and Solutions" is an attempt to familiarize the readers with the concepts of mental health, mental illness and how to help a person with mental illness. Why the title "Mental Health at Cross Roads" was chosen? Mental health is an aspect of health that we often neglect. It is not just a layperson and the society who ignore mental health, but the health professionals also tend to ignore this vital component of health, which is essential for the wellbeing and normal functioning of an individual. Here, it is important to state that we may also ignore physical health and indulge in unhealthy habits, but mental health gets much lower priority. The recent Covid-19 pandemic has brought a much-needed focus on mental health. This was recognized not only by health workers and the general population but also by policy-makers, political leadership, and the media. Stress and mental health issues were faced by most of the population, including those who were infected, their family members, the health care professionals and the frontline workers. Strategies like lockdown, quarantine and social distancing, which were used to control the spread of infection, further added to the mental health problems. Thus, the pandemic brought the much-needed focus on mental health, which was earlier considered a completely ignored component of health, often put into the backyards. Mental health emerged as equally important as physical health and crossed the barrier between mental and physical health, and hence, the title of the book – "Mental Health at Cross Roads".

The book comprises 34 chapters covering various aspects of mental health and illness, contributed by leading experts in the field. The book begins with a chapter discussing the concept of mental health, factors contributing to mental health and how a person can keep oneself in optimum mental health. This is followed by chapters on recognizing mental illness, mental ill health and disease burden, and myths and misconceptions associated with mental health and illness. Then, there are chapters detailing various kinds of mental illnesses, including severe mental illnesses, common mental illnesses, compulsive spectrum disorders, personality disorders and drug addiction. Behavioral addictions, a new emerging mental health issue with serious social ramifications, have been discussed in a separate chapter. The book includes dedicated chapters on suicide prevention and stigma due to mental ill health. Persons suffering from physical health problems often have coexisting mental health issues, which are often missed and interfere with the improvement in the primary physical illness. This book has an exclusive chapter discussing these issues.

Man has three biological needs – food, sleep and sex – and disturbances in either of these have mental health consequences, and therefore, we have included one chapter each deliberating on these topics. Similarly, the book includes chapters on mental health issues in different age groups, including children and the elderly, and special subsets of populations, like students and women. Mental health at the workplace is another important topic, which often does not receive adequate attention. Hence, we have included a chapter discussing this too.

How a person with mental illness can be helped has been comprehensively covered in chapters on treatments for mental ill health, psychotherapy and counseling, therapeutic communities, and family and mental health. Long-term care of persons with mental illness, disability benefits and rights of persons with mental illness have been discussed as separate chapters. We have also included chapters on spirituality and mental health, the role of resilience in mental health and the role of ancient Indian knowledge in mental health. Coercion in mental health, a debatable subject,

has been discussed in an exclusive chapter. In the 21st century, there has been a lot of emphasis on health promotion, including mental health promotion. In this background as well as considering the public health significance of mental disorders, this book has included chapters on prevention of mental disorders and promotion of mental health. The last chapter deliberates on how advances in information technology can be effectively used in the mental health sector.

The target readership for this book is intended to be general readers, individuals with mental illnesses and their family members, who need to understand the basic principles of mental health and how to help themselves or the person with mental illness. We earnestly hope that this book will also be useful for social scientists, educationists and health professionals.

Rakesh Kumar Chadda, Pratap Sharan
Mamta Sood, Koushik Sinha Deb

CHAPTER 1

Mental Health: Concept and Relevance

Rakesh K Chadda

Introduction

World Health Organization (WHO), when it came into being in 1948, defined health as 'a state of complete physical, mental and social well-being, and not merely the absence of disease or infirmity'. Mental health has thus been recognized as an integral part of our health. Taking care of mental health is as important as of physical health since the two are interlinked. Mental health is important for healthy living and contributes to a sense of satisfaction with life and reaching the desired goals.

What Constitutes Mental Health?

Mental health refers to a state of mental well-being and not just the absence of mental illness (Box 1). It may be considered a state of well-being with the ability to realize one's own strengths, cope with the normal stresses of life, work productively and contribute to one's community.

Further expanding the concept, mental health comprises awareness of one's potential and ability to utilize one's resources for the betterment of humanity, cope with life's stresses and adversities, and to realize a sense of contentment with life. Technically, mental health refers to cognitive, behavioral and emotional well-being, thus including how we think, act and feel. Any aberration in these components leads to disturbance in the mental health and constitutes mental ill-health.

It is important to understand here: When does a person cross the boundary between mental health and ill health? Or what happens when a person becomes mentally unwell? Our mind performs several functions, such as making decisions and judgments based on compiling and interpreting the information received by listening, reading and watching. Similarly, it determines how we behave and react in different situations. Our emotional reactions to various events and happenings in our day-to-day life are also determined by the mind. Our brain, being the controlling and coordinating authority of all the body systems, performs several other functions too. In simple words, mental ill-health can be conceptualized as an unhealthy state

---

Box 1. Health and Mental Health

Health:
'A state of complete physical, mental and social well-being and not merely the absence of disease or infirmity.' - World Health Organization, 1948

Mental health
'A state of mental well-being and not just absence of mental illness.'
A state of well-being with the ability to
- Realize one's own abilities
- Cope with the normal stresses of life
- Work productively
- Contribute to one's community

of the mind, the thinking part of the brain. If the mind is not able to perform its functions adequately and satisfactorily, it may lead to mental ill-health. Mental ill-health or illness is characterized by disturbances in thinking, perception, emotions or behavior leading to continued distress to the individual self or others, or inability to meet one's responsibilities in personal, familial, social or vocational spheres.

Factors Affecting Mental Health

Mental health is influenced by several factors spread across the biopsychosocial sphere, including physical, psychological and social influences. (**Table 1**)

Physical aspects of an individual comprise facial features, complexion, body constitution, height, weight, physical health or absence of physical illness, physical possessions and the physical environment. A healthy and balanced diet contributes to mental health, whereas nutritional deficiencies can put a person at risk of not only physical but also mental ill-health. Pollution of any kind, including air or noise pollution, noisy neighborhood, and extremes of weather and homelessness can have an adverse impact on mental health. Unhealthy lifestyles, such as erratic sleep patterns, erratic eating habits, physical inactivity and absence of physical exercise,

have a negative influence on mental health. In addition, genetic and familial factors also affect mental health, being associated with an increased risk of many mental illnesses, such as schizophrenia, depression, bipolar disorder and others. Resorting to alcohol, smoking or any other drug due to stress or as a leisure activity also affects mental health and increases the risk of mental ill-health.

Psychological factors, understandably, play a predominant role in determining mental health. The way one thinks, behaves, or interacts with others and copes with day-to-day stresses, affects one's mental health. Some of these behaviors would be determined by a person's personality. Personality is what makes a person unique and comprises various attributes, including physical characteristics or features, behavior, ways of reacting to different situations, personal qualities, interests and hobbies, and habits. Personality contributes to mental health since it relates to how a person copes with various day-to-day stresses, in a healthy or an unhealthy way. This topic is discussed in more detail in the chapter on 'Personality Disorders'.

Social factors also have a significant influence on mental health, since man is a social animal. A large range of social factors can affect mental health, including economic status, education, employment, work atmosphere, housing, home atmosphere, family, neighborhood, political

Table 1. *Biopsychosocial Determinants of Mental Health*

Biological	Psychological	Social
Genetic factors	Personality	Poverty
Physical health	Coping styles	Education
Nutrition		Rapid social change
Physical environment		Stress at work
Unhealthy lifestyle		Gender discrimination
		Social exclusion
		Exposure to violence
		Human rights violation
		Housing

stability and so on. A decent level of education, employment, stable family and reasonable housing do contribute to good mental health. Some common social influences that affect mental health adversely include social exclusion, discrimination on account of gender, caste, race or religion and violation of human rights. Exposure to violence and being victims of crime, a rapid social change, the emergence of pandemics and natural or manmade disasters, like earthquakes, floods, bomb blasts, landslides, and wars negatively affect mental health, whereas social and political stability has a positive impact on mental health.

Mental Health Across Lifespan

As a person grows from prenatal state to infancy, childhood, adolescence, adulthood and senescence, multiple factors affect one's mental health. Figure 1 summarizes how mental health is influenced during the growing years.

It is important to note here that maternal health during pregnancy, including the use of tobacco or alcohol by the mother during pregnancy and improper nutrition, can affect the mental health of the growing fetus, and later, the baby in the coming years. Fetal programming, along with a genetic endowment, governs fetal growth and aberrations during this period, and has the potential to affect mental health in further life. Thus, proper pregnancy care with balanced nutrition and all necessary precautions does have a role in maintaining the mental health of the child throughout life.

After birth and during the growing years, parenting plays an important role in inculcating the mental health of the child, and seeds for mental health in the future are sown during this period.

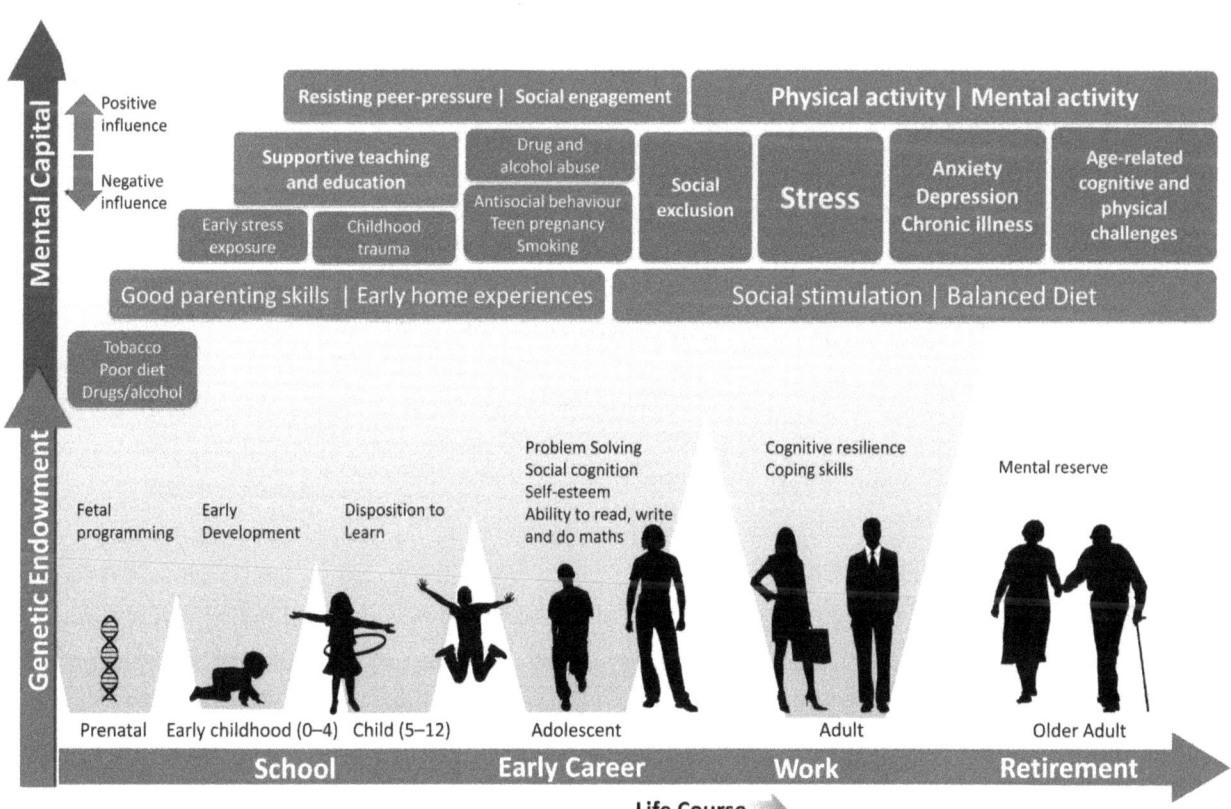

*Adapted from Beddington et al, 2008

Figure 1. *Influences on Mental Health Throughout Life**

Conflict amongst the parents, absence or death of one or both parents, divorce and separation of the parents all have adverse effects on the mental health of the growing child. Similarly, any major physical illness in the child and the parents can impact the mental health of the growing child. The presence of siblings or other children in the family may be beneficial for a child's mental health, as it helps in developing companionship as well as facilitates learning and coping. Thus, early home experiences have an important role to play in the mental health development of the child.

As the child grows further and reaches school, the school environment influences the child's mental health. Schools provide great scope for learning from the teachers and peers besides the formal education in form of social skills and also maturity. Bullying at school can have adverse effects on mental health. Regular parent-teacher meetings are helpful in identifying mental health issues in the child and finding an appropriate solution. Children at this age are also vulnerable to substance use, especially under peer pressure. The parents as well as the teachers need to be vigilant about this issue. Examination and study related stress needs to be dealt with in a constructive manner, and the child needs to be provided due support, help and care. Parents also need to ensure that the child is not missing school without their information. Resisting peer pressure and social engagement can help maintain sound mental health during this age. The growing child is also at risk of abuse and neglect, and parents need to take care of it.

A growing child's sexuality-related issues should also be taken care of by the parents without any hesitation or reservation since it goes a long way in the prevention of the development of sexual misconceptions affecting mental health. Parents also need to be careful about the issues of teenage pregnancy and provide adequate information to their children to enable them to behave responsibly.

As a child grows into adolescence and young adulthood, further education, career choice and sexuality become important factors affecting mental health and need to be taken care of by the parents along with teachers and counselors. The growing child should be provided all guidance and support to make a choice as per his/her liking, disposition, capabilities and options available.

Further, in adult life, as a person grows through adulthood, middle age and old age, the kind of stresses would keep on changing. Stress is going to be a part of life at all ages, but one needs to learn how to effectively cope with stress. As one grows older, one is likely to develop physical or mental health issues, along with age-related cognitive and physical challenges in old age. Maintaining a regular schedule of physical as well as mental activity accompanied by social stimulation (in form of communication with family, friends and society) helps oneself in managing stress and keeping oneself in good mental health.

Relation between Mental and Physical Health

As we discussed at the beginning of this chapter, health is a state of physical, mental and social well-being. Moreover, physical health and mental health are closely linked. An optimum level of mental health is essential for keeping oneself in optimum physical health. One very simple example is when a person gets tense and stressed, there are changes in the body in form of increased heart rate, increased respiratory rate, increase in muscle tone, sweating, dryness of mouth, etc.

Continued stress also lowers immunity and hence increases the risk of infections. Longstanding stress is also associated with increased muscle tone and may lead to chronic headache, backache and musculoskeletal pain in different body parts. Physical ill-health is also associated with secondary psychological reactions. Chronic and serious physical illnesses are likely to lead to more psychological reactions and hence mental ill-health.

Basic principles of keeping oneself mentally healthy are also applicable to keeping oneself physically healthy, which are discussed below.

Basic Principles for Maintaining Optimal Mental Health

How one can keep oneself mentally healthy is not difficult. There are some basic rules that, if followed properly, will keep one mentally healthy (**Box 2**).

Taking adequate sleep for 7-8 hours at night and having regular hours of sleep is the first step towards keeping oneself mentally healthy. One needs to control temptations to browse the attractive virtual media while going to bed, which may delay the time for going to bed and then delay one's time of getting up the next day and affect one's next day's functioning.

A regular schedule of physical exercise for 40-45 minutes at least 5-6 days a week is also an essential component for maintaining good mental health. The exercise may include brisk walks, stretching exercises or spending time at a gym depending on age, physical fitness, resources available and individual preference. It is important to mention here that exercise also helps in fighting depression and anxiety. Deep breathing exercises or some form of meditation can add to strengthening the stress coping ability and mental health.

Staying away from alcohol and psychoactive drugs is another key factor crucial for maintaining good mental health.

One also needs to socialize and communicate within one's family and social network. A trusting and supportive relationship is always helpful in

---

Box 2. Basic Principles of Maintaining Good Mental Health

- Regular physical exercise
- Adequate sleep
- Adequate diet
- Regularity of daily routine
- Communication, socialization, sharing of experiences
- Stay away from drugs, smoking and alcohol
- Learning stress management
- Yoga
- Meditation of any kind

---

coping with stress and keeps oneself in good mental health, whereas social isolation affects mental health adversely.

Religious practices depending on one's beliefs are also comforting and add to mental health.

These basic principles of mental health, if followed diligently, would help in keeping a person in good mental health and strengthen one's stress coping ability and help in fighting various lifestyle diseases. Figure 2 summarizes the road to mental health.

Conclusion

Mental health is one of the three integral components of health along with physical and social well-being. Mental health is not just the absence of mental illness, but a state of subjective well-being with an ability to cope with day-to-day stresses and to utilize one's potential to an optimum level. It is not difficult to keep oneself in optimum mental health. One needs to follow basic principles of the regularity of daily schedule, exercise and staying away from tobacco, drugs and alcohol.

Road to Mental Health

In India, about 1% people suffer from severe and about 5-10 % of suffer from common mental disorders.

There are many types of mental diseases, with many differing symptoms.

Signs of mental illness

Gradual or sudden change in thoughts, feelings or behavior

Continuation over long time

Affecting a person's daily routine, work, & interpersonal relationships

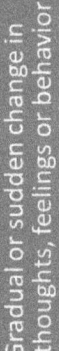

The contribution of family members is important in the treatment of mental illnesses

Maintaining a healthy & conducive environment and assigning light responsibilities.

Like diabetes & high blood pressure, mental diseases are caused by a combination of genetic, environmental, social & psychological factors.

Mental diseases are not caused by ghosts, witchcraft, evil spirits, bad karma, sins of past lives & lack of will power

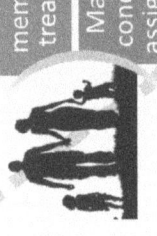

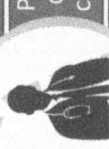

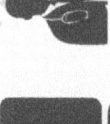

Treatment starts with one or two medicines & takes a few weeks to show effect.

Medicine should be continued even after recovery, till the doctor advises

Effective treatment of mental disorders is possible in less money

Medicines & psychotherapy are available for treatment.

Medicines side effects are generally mild & subside within the first few weeks.

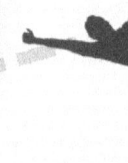

Mental illnesses can be successfully treated by doctors

Psychiatrists are available in district hospitals, medical colleges and private clinics

Government & voluntary organizations have opened addiction treatment centers at many places

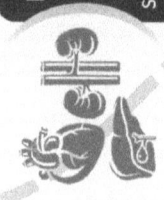

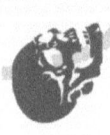

Towards Mental health

Figure 2. *Road to Mental Health*

KEY POINTS

➢ Health is a state of physical, mental and social well-being and not just the absence of illness.

➢ Mental health is a state of subjective well-being with an ability to cope with day-to-day stresses and contribute to society.

➢ Mental health and physical health are closely linked.

➢ Some basic principles, if regularly followed, can keep a person in perfect mental health.

REFERENCES

1. Beddington J, Cooper CL, Field J, Goswami U, Huppert FA, Jenkins R, Jones HS, Kirkwood TB, Sahakian BJ, Thomas SM. The mental wealth of nations. Nature. 2008 Oct 23;455(7216):1057-60

2. Mental health: strengthening our response. https://www.who.int/news-room/fact-sheets/detail/mental-health-strengthening-our-response. Accessed on 4th January 2022.

CHAPTER 2

Recognizing Mental Illnesses

Mamta Sood

Introduction

In the previous chapter, you became acquainted with the concept of mental health. Mental health is an integral part of overall health and as important as physical health.

It is easy to understand the meaning of physical health as we can see our bodies and different body parts. We can examine the functioning of our body and inner organs via visualization, touch, palpation or auscultation. This is further aided by different blood or other laboratory investigations or imaging modalities, like X-rays, CT or MRI scans. For example, hemoglobin levels of 12 g/dL in women and 15 g/dL in men imply that all the processes involved in hemoglobin synthesis in the body are intact and functioning well. In contrast, it is not possible to visualize or touch the processes associated with mental health, such as thinking, perception, emotions, understanding, problem solving, etc.

Similarly, the boundary between physical health and illness may not be difficult to discern. For example, a temperature of more than 98.6 °F on the thermometer indicates the presence of fever, implying a physical illness. For most physical illnesses, there is clearly marked progression from health to illness. However, the boundary is not so distinct between mental health and mental illness. For example, it may be difficult to appreciate the difference between the emotion of sadness, which is experienced universally and commonly by all, and depression, which is experienced only by about 5% of the population. This delay in the recognition of mental illness contributes to the delay in getting appropriate intervention.

Mental illnesses are one of the leading causes of disability in afflicted persons and contribute significantly to family burden. Sometimes, these can be fatal as well. As per the National Mental Health Survey (NMHS) of India, 2016, 13.7% of the adult population in India suffers from mental morbidity during their lifetime, and is in need of intervention. However, the majority of the persons with mental illness do not receive treatment, though affordable and evidence-based treatments are available for most mental illnesses. It is important to start treatment early since the earlier the treatment is started, the more effective it is.

The key element here is to know how to recognize mental illness. In this chapter, we will focus on the symptoms of mental illness, how to identify and diagnose a mental disorder, types of mental disorders, and, once diagnosed, where and from whom to seek help.

Symptoms of Mental Illness

A person with a mental illness experiences a plethora of symptoms. It is noteworthy that both physical and mental functions are controlled by different areas of the brain. Therefore, a person can experience both physical and mental manifestations of a mental illness. These symptoms are usually accompanied by impairment in functioning.

Mental symptoms: Different mental illnesses can affect different mental functions, like behavior, thinking, mood, perception, cognition and judgment. Thus, symptoms of mental illness can occur in any of these areas and are discussed here.

Behavior: Changes in behavior may indicate mental illness. For example, a person laughing or crying without any reason, talking to self or gesticulating in the air as if talking to someone, disorganized behavior, wandering aimlessly, maintaining odd positions for a long time, etc. S/he may be distractible and may exhibit crying spells, shouting, and abusive or aggressive behaviors. S/he may be ill-kempt or not properly groomed. S/he may also show socially inappropriate behavior.

Thinking: Disturbances in thinking may manifest in various ways. One of the important disturbances in thinking is delusion, which is a false and irrational belief that is held without any evidence, like being suspicious that others are going to harm him/her. Thinking maybe disorganized and may be evident in speech as sentences or words that do not follow an appropriate sequence. A person may have negative thinking; s/he may believe that s/he is worthless, hopeless or helpless. S/he may have ideas of guilt. There may be ideas or attempts at self-harm. Some people may report repeated thoughts even when knowing that these are senseless. Thinking may become slow or fast, which gets reflected in speech as too little or too much talk. Although uncommon, a person may have a vague feeling as if s/he is disconnected from her/himself or from the surroundings and there may be a sense of unreality.

Mood changes: These are frequently seen in individuals with mental illness. A person may be unduly cheerful or sad. S/he may be anxious or restless or fearful without any reason. There may be very rapid shifts in the mood. The person may experience fluctuating mood. There may be a loss of pleasure in previously enjoyable activities or a person may indulge excessively in pleasurable activities.

There may be fear of closed spaces, crowds, heights or social situations.

Perception: Perception is a function of the mind in which a meaning is given to the sensations experienced in response to a stimulus in the realm of hearing, vision, taste, touch and smell. One of the important symptoms of mental illness is a hallucination in which a person may experience sensations in absence of an appropriate external stimulus, like s/he may see a person or hear voices when no one is around or speaking. There may be auditory, visual, tactile, olfactory or gustatory hallucinations.

Cognition: There may be difficulty in paying attention to the task at hand and maintaining concentration. This may manifest as frequent complaints of difficulty in remembering or forgetfulness. In long-standing mental illnesses, there may be problems in understanding complex ideas, and consequently, doing difficult tasks.

Judgment: Due to changes in thinking, mood or perception, a person with mental illness may exhibit impaired reality testing. This means that the person may not correctly understand her/his experiences and the external world, and may also be unaware that her/his behavior is strange. This usually leads to poor judgment, for example, a person who irrationally believes that s/he has become very rich (while in reality, s/he is very poor), may buy three refrigerators of different brands from different shops incurring a significant loan. Sometimes, due to social disinhibition, the person may indulge in embarrassing behaviors. S/he may also not have an insight into her/his illness, which may result in non-recognition of symptoms and consequent refusal of treatment.

Figure 1 summarizes the symptoms of mind in mental illness

Physical symptoms: A person with mental illness may experience difficulty in carrying out biological activities (sleep, appetite, bowel/bladder, sexual, etc.).

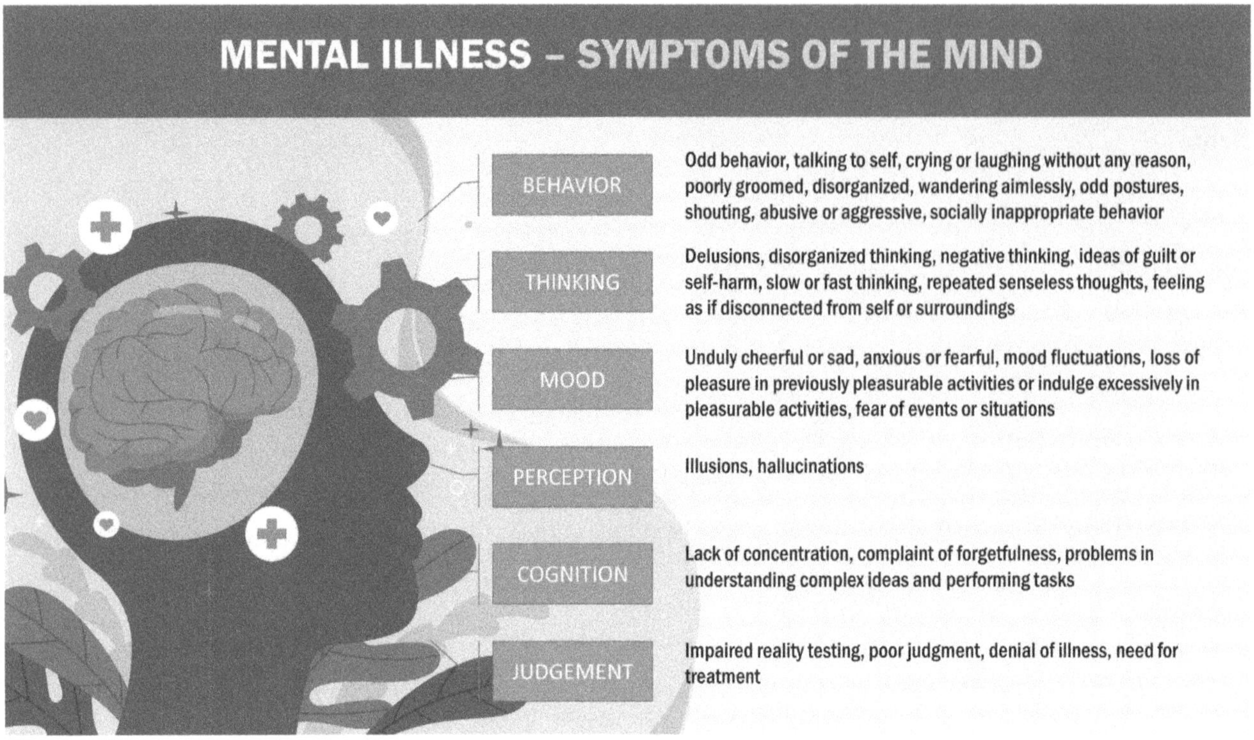

MENTAL ILLNESS – SYMPTOMS OF THE MIND

BEHAVIOR — Odd behavior, talking to self, crying or laughing without any reason, poorly groomed, disorganized, wandering aimlessly, odd postures, shouting, abusive or aggressive, socially inappropriate behavior

THINKING — Delusions, disorganized thinking, negative thinking, ideas of guilt or self-harm, slow or fast thinking, repeated senseless thoughts, feeling as if disconnected from self or surroundings

MOOD — Unduly cheerful or sad, anxious or fearful, mood fluctuations, loss of pleasure in previously pleasurable activities or indulge excessively in pleasurable activities, fear of events or situations

PERCEPTION — Illusions, hallucinations

COGNITION — Lack of concentration, complaint of forgetfulness, problems in understanding complex ideas and performing tasks

JUDGEMENT — Impaired reality testing, poor judgment, denial of illness, need for treatment

Figure 1. *Symptoms of Mind in Mental Illness*

S/he may experience poor sleep, with difficulty in falling asleep or intermittent awakenings or getting up earlier than usual time. S/he may eat poorly and may experience weight loss, which may manifest as the loosening of clothes. Sometimes, a person may sleep excessively or have an increased appetite. S/he may feel fatigued or excessively restless. S/he may have extremely low or high energy levels. S/he may have constipation and repeated urge for urination or defecation. S/he may have reduced or increased libido that may manifest as sexual disinhibition.

An anxious person may experience palpitation, sweating, dizziness or tremors due to increased sympathetic activity. S/he may suffer from headaches, bodyaches and/or heaviness or numbness in the body.

Figure 2 summarizes the symptoms of the body in mental illness.

Functioning: Day-to-day functioning is significantly affected. The domains of functioning in any person's life usually comprise personal activities (bathing, brushing and grooming), social activities (social interactions and relationships with significant others – family, friends, colleagues, etc.), occupational activities (homemaker, student, job, business, etc.) and recreational activities (watching television, reading news, gardening, knitting, etc.). There may be disturbances in these domains in a person with mental illness. A person may neglect personal hygiene, withdraw from social situations, may be unable to perform usual household and occupational tasks or may not engage in recreational activities.

Mental Illness

Some of the symptoms listed above can be present in a person at some point of time in his/her life. But a mere presence of a few symptoms does not mean that s/he has a mental illness.

Mental illness is characterized by the presence of a specific set of symptoms that are present together and have a characteristic course and outcome. This constellation of symptoms should

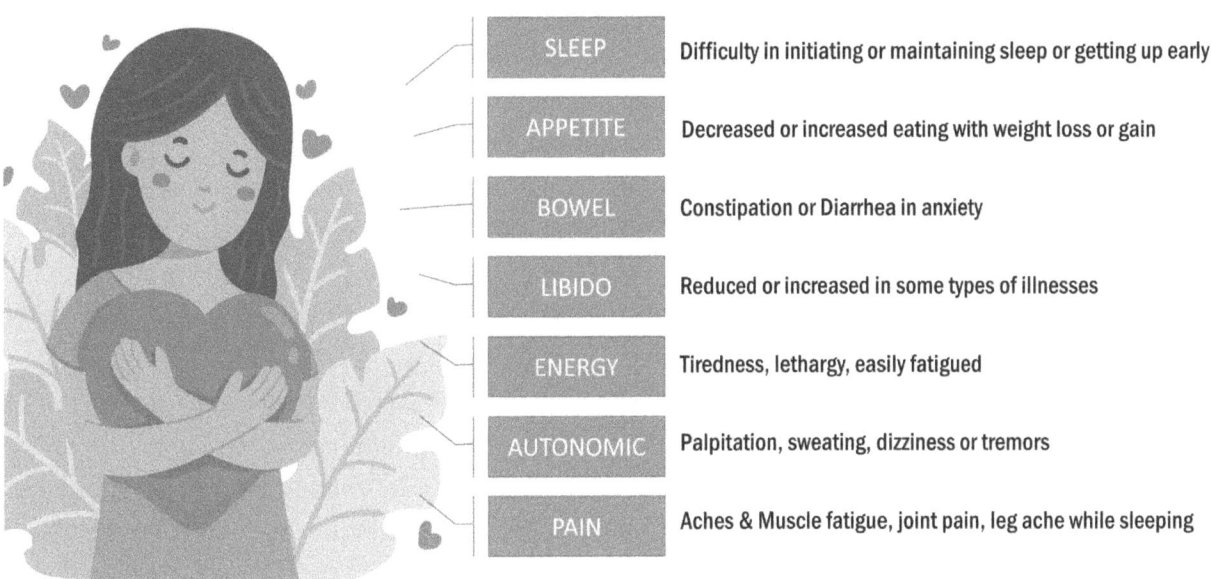

MENTAL ILLNESS – SYMPTOMS OF THE BODY

SLEEP	Difficulty in initiating or maintaining sleep or getting up early
APPETITE	Decreased or increased eating with weight loss or gain
BOWEL	Constipation or Diarrhea in anxiety
LIBIDO	Reduced or increased in some types of illnesses
ENERGY	Tiredness, lethargy, easily fatigued
AUTONOMIC	Palpitation, sweating, dizziness or tremors
PAIN	Aches & Muscle fatigue, joint pain, leg ache while sleeping

Figure 2. *Mental Illness: Symptoms of the Body*

be persistent, which means that these symptoms should last for a significant period of time. These should cause significant distress and disturbance in functioning that should be pervasive across all the domains of functioning (Box 1).

Let's take the example of depression – a common and ubiquitous emotion. We all have felt depressed when we do not get something we want

---

Box 1. Identifying Mental Illness

- Specific set of symptoms, related to thoughts, mood or behavior
- Tend to be persistent
- Cause significant distress
- Lead to pervasive disturbance in functioning
- Symptoms vary from person to person
- Symptoms may devlop gradually over weeks or months or rapidly within hours or days
- May or may not be preceded by stressor

---

desperately or things do not go the way we want or we lose something precious to us. So, does that mean that we have a depressive disorder?

This can be further illustrated by two scenarios.

Mr. A, a 25-year-old young man, while traveling in a metro, lost all his money that he had received as the first payment for his work. He felt very sad and was tearful as this money was needed for important household expenses. He reached home and shared this with his family who reassured him. He felt better and also enjoyed a game of scrabble with his younger brother.

On the other hand, Mr. B, another 25-year-old young man, has experienced depressed mood for last three weeks and has felt tired all day long. He also experiences ideas of helplessness, hopelessness and guilt. Reassurance from his family and friends does not make him feel better. He was fond of reading newspapers and watching movies. He has lost interest in these activies which he previously felt pleasurable. He also feels suicidal. He has stopped taking care of his grooming. He eats and sleeps poorly. He has stopped going to his job.

Mr. A experienced depression in response to the loss of his first paycheck, which is a common feeling experienced by anyone in similar circumstances. The emotional reaction lasted for a very short period of time and did not cause disturbance in his day-to-day functioning. It was not significant clinically and did not warrant medical attention. On the other hand, Mr. B experienced several symptoms of depression - depressed mood, negative thinking, suicidal ideas, loss of pleasure in activities previously considered pleasurable (anhedonia) and tiredness (anergia). These symptoms were present for a long period of time (persistent) and resulted in significant distress (sadness) and problems across different domains of functioning (pervasive). Therefore, this young man appears to have suffered from a mental illness (depressive disorder) and requires medical attention.

An expectable and culturally sanctioned response to a specific situation is not diagnosed as a mental disorder. Also, if an individual holds religious beliefs or political opinions that are not in consonance with the beliefs or opinions held by a larger section of the society, s/he is not considered to have a mental illness.

Symptoms of mental illness vary from person to person. These symptoms may develop gradually over weeks to months or rapidly within a very short span of hours to days. A mental illness may or may not be preceded by stressor/s.

There is always a question in the minds of persons with mental illness and their families that why s/he has a mental illness. There are many reasons which can lead to a person developing mental illness. Similar to chronic medical illnesses, like hypertension or diabetes mellitus, mental illnesses do not occur because of a single factor but occur due to interactions of multiple factors, like biological, environmental and psycho-social factors.

Types of mental illnesses

It is important to take a lifespan approach to mental illness, which can occur in adults, children, elderly, or in pregnant or postnatal women. There are several types of mental illnesses with each having characteristic signs and symptoms, course and outcome. Mental illnesses are broadly classified as severe mental disorders, common mental disorders, addictions, and disorders specific to childhood and adolescence.

Severe mental disorders: These include psychotic disorders, like schizophrenia and bipolar disorder. Nearly 1.9% of the population in India has severe mental disorders.

Psychotic disorders are characterized by disturbances in thinking, perception and behavior. The presence of psychotic disorders is indicated by symptoms, such as remaining lost in oneself, talking to oneself, laughing or crying without reason, being fearful, wandering aimlessly, social withdrawal and poor functioning in various domains. The person may have delusions, hallucinations, disorganized behavior, and impaired reality testing, insight and judgment. Schizophrenia is a type of psychotic disorder.

Bipolar disorder is characterized by episodes of mania (a state of elevated mood) and depression (perssitent and pervasive low mood). Mania is characterized by remaining excessively cheerful without reason, excessive talk, talking big about self, excessive religiosity, over socialization or excessive spending beyond means and poor functioning. Depression is characterized by remaining excessively sad without reason, feeling tired and low energy, negative thinking, reduced talking and social interactions, and poor functioning. Some patients may have episodes of either only mania or of both mania and depression.

Common mental disorders: These include depressive disorders, anxiety disorders and stress-related disorders. These are common mental illnesses and may affect about 10% of the population. Although these cause significant distress and difficulties in functioning, there is no loss of contact with reality or impaired insight. The main symptom of anxiety disorders is excessive anxiety or inner restlessness and lack of concentration that may be present all the time or come in episodes. In phobias, anxiety may be associated with excessive fear of certain objects or situations with a tendency to avoid them. Symptoms of anxiety and depression may be present over the background of acute or ongoing stress.

Addictions: Addictions like alcohol use disorder, moderate to severe use of tobacco and use of other drugs (cannabis – *bhang, charas, ganja,* opioids – *afeem, bhukki, smack,* cough syrups containing opioids, sedatives, etc.) are common and are seen in nearly one-fourth of the adult population in India. Around 21% of the population in India uses tobacco with moderate to high dependence, and 4.6% use alcohol to the extent of dependence or harmful use. Addictions are usually characterized by repetitive and gradually increasing intake of a substance, spending all efforts in procuring and using it, craving, withdrawal symptoms, if unable to take the substance, and continuing the use despite developing complications. Persons with addiction need treatment.

Disorders of children and adolescents: Many different types of mental illnesses are seen in about 14-20% of children and adolescents, like autism, attention deficit hyperactivity disorder, specific learning difficulties, mental retardation and behavioral disturbances, Mental illnesses, that are usually seen in adults, like depression, anxiety, psychotic illnesses, etc., can also occur in children and adolescents.

Early Signs of Mental Illness

Most mental illnesses develop gradually. There may be subtle changes in a person's behavior and routine that may be present for some time before the development of full-blown mental illness. If one is aware of these symptoms, it can help in early recognition of mental illness and timely help-seeking and treatment. Some of early signs of mental illnesses are:

- Change in day-to-day routine for no obvious reason
- Disturbances in mood, lasting for a long period
- Talking too much or too less
- Odd, uncharacteristic or strange behavior
- Making gestures in the air, laughing and talking to oneself
- Ideas of helplessness and hopelessness, poor self-esteem, reduced confidence, thinking oneself to be worthless, death wishes, suicidal ideations or attempt
- Irrational fears, suspiciousness, fearfulness and doubts
- Loss of interest in previously enjoyed activities and hobbies
- Unable to sleep or sleep for a few hours or may get up early
- Loss of appetite
- Poor concentration, memory or illogical thought and speech
- Loss of initiative or desire to participate in any activity
- Keeping to oneself and not interacting with family members, friends or colleagues
- Neglect of personal care
- Reduced functioning in whatever work a person does: studies for a student, household chores for a homemaker or job

The presence of one or two of the symptoms listed above does not indicate a mental illness but may indicate a need for further evaluation.

Whom to approach? Where to go?

If a person is experiencing several symptoms at a time and the symptoms are causing distress and serious problems in her/his ability to function, help should be sought from a mental health professional or physician.

Mental health professionals include psychiatrists (MBBS and MD/DPM/DNB psychiatry), clinical psychologists (MA in psychology and M Phil in clinical psychology), psychiatric social workers (M Phil in psychiatric social work), psychiatric nurses (Diploma or MSc in psychiatric nursing) and occupational therapist (Bachelor of Occupational Therapy). It is important to state here that a family physician or a general physician is often competent to treat common mental health problems and can be the first contact for mental health issues.

Mental health services are available at stand-alone mental hospitals, psychiatry services in general hospitals (that can be a district hospital), medical colleges, multispecialty hospitals, hospitals in major public sector companies and armed forces, and also in office-based practice. These services are available in both public as well as private settings. Private sector psychiatrists practice in their own offices, polyclinics and private general and psychiatric hospitals. Some non-governmental organizations provide mental health services too. Psychiatrists are not available at primary care centers. However, health workers posted in primary health centers are expected to look after patients with mental illness under the supervision of a medical officer (Box 2).

How Diagnosis of Mental Illness is Made?

You must be wondering what will happen when you visit a physician/mental health professional. Usually, evaluation by a mental health professional involves taking a detailed history of the case and doing physical and mental status examinations. Unlike physical illnesses, like tuberculosis or dengue, where specific tests are available for diagnosis, no diagnostic laboratory tests exist for making or confirming a diagnosis of mental illness. Psychometric tests

---

Box 2. Where to Access Mental Health Care?

- Mental health services are available at stand-alone mental hospitals, psychiatry services in general hospitals (that can be a district hospital), medical colleges or hospitals of major public sector companies and armed forces, multispecialty hospitals and office-based practice
- Available in both public as well as private settings
- Private sector psychiatrists practice in their own offices, polyclinics and private general and psychiatric hospitals
- Nongovernmental organizations provide mental health services

---

and psychological tools may help in elucidating information about the mental health of a person but these are not diagnostic of a mental illness.

Mental health professionals collect detailed history with specific emphasis on:

- When did the symptoms start?
- Presence of any stressor
- Duration and severity of symptoms
- Impact of symptoms on functioning
- Use of alcohol or drugs
- History of any physical disease
- Any treatment received and response or side effects related to it
- Past or family history of such symptoms
- Aggressive behavior
- Suicidal ideations/attempt
- Personal history
- Any other significant history

The doctor will do the physical and mental status examinations. The mental status examination is done by detailed interview in which the doctor examines the behavior, thinking, perception, emotions, cognitive functions, judgment and insight of the patient.

It is important to remember that sometimes a mental illness can emerge due to physical (medical/surgical) diseases, including brain-related issues, like dementia, brain tumors and infections; head injury or chronic physical diseases, like diabetes; infections like malaria, tuberculosis, etc.; endocrinological (hormonal) disorders, like hypothyroidism, etc.; or side effects of certain drugs, etc. The list of physical conditions that lead to mental illness is long. It is important to understand that the symptoms of mental illness can emerge due to physical illnesses that need to be ruled out by history, physical examination and relevant investigations. In these cases, the treatment of physical illness is important and leads to improvement in symptoms of mental illness.

Presence of several symptoms that are persistent and pervasive and cause significant distress and difficulties in functioning indicate the presence of mental illness.

The diagnosis of mental illness is made based on history and examination.

Usually, two kinds of treatments are used: pharmacological in form of medications and non-pharmacological in form of psychotherapies (also commonly called 'talking cure'). Hospitalization is indicated if a person is at suicidal risk or has made a suicidal attempt, is not manageable at home, there is a total refusal of food or medications, or there is no improvement with medication given on an outpatient basis. In most patients, short-term hospitalization for 4-6 weeks is indicated. In some cases, electroconvulsive therapy may also be used.

Conclusion

Mental illnesses result in a significant burden for individuals, their families and society. Both physical and mental symptoms are seen in mental illness. Mental illness is characterized by the presence of a specific set of symptoms that are present together and are persistent, pervasive and cause significant distress or dysfunction. There are several types of mental illnesses, such as severe mental disorders, common mental disorders, addictions and childhood and adolescent mental disorders. The presence of one or two symptoms related to mental illnesses does not indicate a mental illness but might suggest a need for evaluation by a mental health professional. Diagnosis of mental illness is based on history and physical and mental status examination. Mental health services are available both in public and private sectors.

KEY POINTS

➢ Unlike physical health and illnesses, the boundary is not distinct between mental health and mental illness. There are no laboratory tests available that confirm mental ill-health.

➢ Mental illnesses result in a significant burden for individuals, their families and society.

➢ Both physical and mental symptoms of several kinds are seen in patients with mental illness.

➢ Mental illness is characterized by the presence of a specific set of symptoms that are present together and are persistent, pervasive and cause significant distress or dysfunction.

➢ There are several types of mental illnesses with each having characteristic signs and symptoms, course and outcome. These are broadly classified as severe mental disorders, common mental disorders, addictions and childhood and adolescent mental disorders.

➤ The presence of one or two symptoms does not indicate a mental illness but may suggest a need for further evaluation.

➤ Diagnosis of mental illness is based on history, physical examination and mental status examination.

➤ Mental health services are available both in public and private sectors.

REFERENCES

1. Chadda RK, Sagar R, Sood M, Ambekar A (2007) Mental Illnesses: Identification and treatment (*Manasik Rog: Pahchan aur Upchaar*) - in Hindi. All India Institute of Medical Sciences: New Delhi.

2. The World Health Report: 2001: Mental Health: New Understanding, New Hope. World Health Organization, Geneva.

CHAPTER 3

Mental Ill-Health and Disease Burden

Rakesh K Chadda

Introduction

Mental ill-health often remains unrecognized and untreated and tends to be chronic. Mental ill-health is often disabling and the affected persons are unable to function with full capacity. Thus, an individual with mental ill health often needs help from others, generally a family member, friends, or social support systems. This need has often been referred to as a burden or a disease burden. Burden, in simple words, refers to additional work or responsibility which is not generally anticipated. In this chapter, we will discuss the disease burden caused by mental ill health, and how to reduce this burden.

Prevalence of Mental Illnesses

Mental illnesses are one of the commonest illnesses afflicting mankind. World Health Organization (WHO) estimates that one in four persons is at risk of developing a mental disorder during their lifetime. In the National Mental Health Survey of India (NMHSI), conducted during 2015-16, the current prevalence of mental disorders amongst the adult population was found to be 10.6% with a lifetime prevalence of 13.7%. In terms of individual disorders, as reported in the survey, the highest annual prevalence was observed for neurotic and stress related disorders (3.5%), followed by depression (2.7%), schizophrenia and related disorders (0.4%) and bipolar disorder (0.3%). In addition, the survey estimated that 22.4% of the adult population in India suffers from substance use disorders (drug addiction), which include tobacco use disorder (20.9%), alcohol use disorder (4.6%) and other substances, such as opioids, cannabis products, etc. These percentages translate to huge numbers considering our population of about 1.4 billion. Thus, about 150 million people in India require mental health care at any time. In the survey, the prevalence of mental disorders in adolescents (aged 13-17 years) was estimated at 7.3%, with depression, agoraphobia, intellectual disability, autism, phobias, and psychosis seen in 2.6%, 2.3%, 1.7%, 1.6%, 1.3% and 1.3% respectively, of the adolescent population. This is important since many of these illnesses might run a continuous or episodic course to the adult life.

Figure 1 summarizes the prevalence of mental and substance use disorders in India.

Disease Burden due to Mental Illnesses

Mental ill-health has been identified as a major contributor to the disease-related disability, measured as disability-adjusted life years (DALYs), contributing to the global burden of the disease. Historically, mental ill-health or mental disorders were never recognized as important from the public health perspective till 1993, when the Global Burden of Disease (GBD) study was published. The study was conducted by the Harvard School of Public Health in collaboration with the World Bank and the WHO. The GBD study used the concept of DALYs to estimate the burden of diseases, besides the conventional mortality and morbidity statistics. (Figure 2)

PREVALENCE OF MENTAL DISORDERS & SUBSTANCE USE IN INDIA

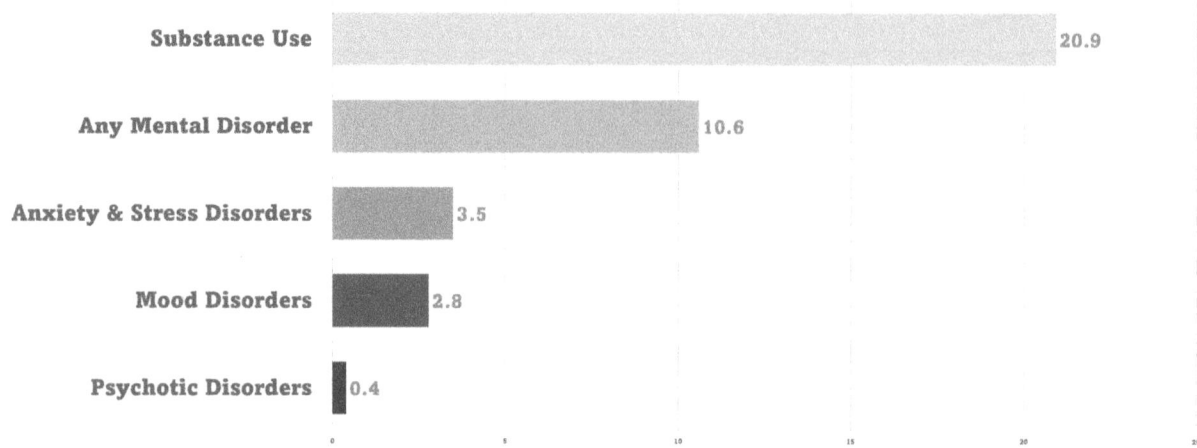

Adapted from the data of the National Mental Health Survey of India (NMHSI), conducted during 2015-16

Figure 1. *Prevalence of Mental and Substance Use Disorders in India*

The GBD study estimated that mental and neurological disorders contributed to 10.5% of the DALYs due to various illnesses. The economic effects of the mental disorders were further illustrated by the World Economic Forum in 2010 with mental disorders estimated to lead to a loss of economic output of around US $16 trillion over a period of 20 years. The GBD study's estimates of 2017 confirmed mental disorders as a consistent contributor to the Years Lived

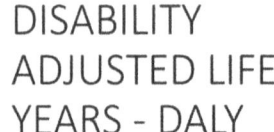

DISABILITY ADJUSTED LIFE YEARS - DALY

- DALY considers both premature death & years lost in disability
- DALY = Total lost years of healthy & productive life
- Mental Disorders = Significant for years lived with disability

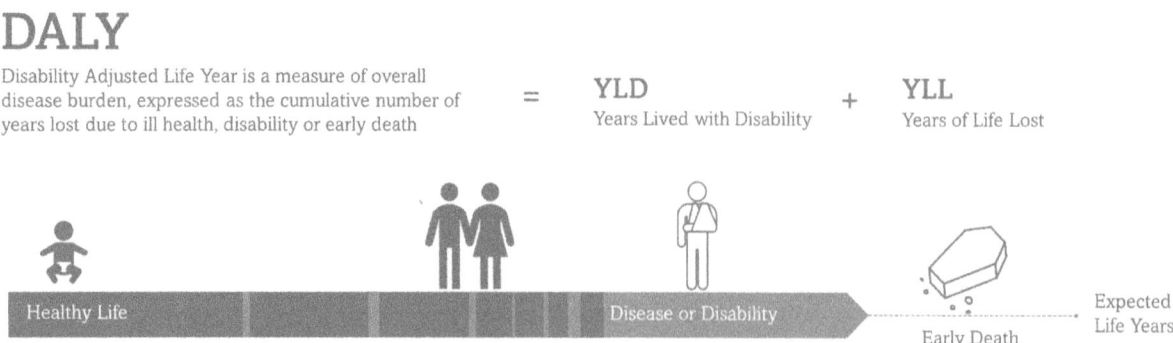

DALY

Disability Adjusted Life Year is a measure of overall disease burden, expressed as the cumulative number of years lost due to ill health, disability or early death

= YLD
Years Lived with Disability

+ YLL
Years of Life Lost

Healthy Life

Disease or Disability

Early Death

Expected Life Years

Figure 2. *Disability and Burden due to Mental Disorders*

with Disability (YLDs) for nearly 3 decades with estimates standing at 14%. This phenomenon has been observed all over the world. Mental disorders predominantly contributing to the global burden include depression, bipolar disorder, schizophrenia and substance use disorders including alcohol. Estimates show that the burden caused by mental disorders is higher than that due to some of the well-recognized serious illnesses, such as HIV/AIDS, tuberculosis, diabetes, urogenital and blood and endocrine diseases. This finding further confirms the need to recognize the public health significance of mental disorders.

In India, one in ten people warrants mental health care at any time. A substantial increase in the contribution of mental disorders to the total DALYs has been reported in India (2.5% in 1990 to 4.7% in 2017). This increase in burden is mainly attributed to mental illnesses, such as depression, anxiety disorders, intellectual disability, schizophrenia and bipolar disorder. (Box 1)

What Leads to Burden in Mental Disorders?

It is well known that mental disorders tend to be chronic and disabling. As we discussed earlier, there is a huge treatment gap due to many patients not

---

Box 1.   Burden Due to Mental Ill Health

- One in seven Indians suffers from mental ill-health during their lifetime
- Nearly 21% of Indian population suffers from different forms of addictions (substance use disorders) to tobacco, alcohol or other drugs
- Mental disorders are a major contributor to the global burden due to various illnesses.

---

seeking treatment for their illness, which further adds to the problem. Estimates show that nearly half of the mental illnesses begin by the age of 14 and around 75% of these illnesses commence by the age of 25. Generally, there is often a delay, ranging from a few months to even years, by the time the mental illness gets recognized and treatment is sought. This happens due to multiple reasons, including lack of awareness, difficulty in differentiating early signs of mental illness from the normal variations during the developmental phase of adolescence and early adult life, and not accessing mental health services due to stigma or non-availability. (Figure 3).

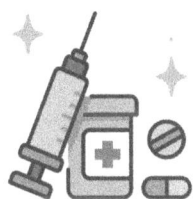

Barriers to Treatment in Mental Disorders

70-91% of the persons with mental disorders in India fail to seek treatment for mental ill health

Stigma and lack of awareness about the problem is an important reason for not seeking treatment

Inequitable and urban centered distribution of mental health services across the country

Figure 3.   *Barriers to Treatment in Mental Disorders in India*

Since most mental illnesses begin at a young age and are experienced during the formative years of life, it affects education, employment and personality growth. Severe illnesses like schizophrenia and bipolar disorder, and even severe depression and obsessive-compulsive disorder can be disabling, and the affected person may have difficulty in sustaining him/herself. The family and caregivers often bear the burden of their member with mental health problems, if s/he is not able to take care of self or earn. The family and caregivers also need to take care of the treatment, taking the patient to a doctor and bearing the costs of treatment. Sometimes, the patients with severe mental illnesses also indulge in odd or aggressive behaviors and the family and caregivers need to take care of this aspect too. Often, the caregivers need to take time off from their jobs to take care of the person with mental ill-health. Persons with mental ill-health are also more prone to physical illnesses due to their inability to communicate or to take proper self-care, a tendency for a sedentary lifestyle and, sometimes, the side effects of the medications. All these factors further increase the burden and disability due to mental illnesses, adding to the global burden.

Treatment Gap

As already stated, one serious problem afflicting mental disorders is the treatment gap, i.e., persons needing treatment not getting adequate services. Estimates from the WHO show that one-third to half of the patients in developed countries and up to 85% of similar patients in the less-developed countries fail to receive treatment even for severe mental illnesses. In India, NMHS of 2015-16 has reported that 70-91% of the persons with mental disorders fail to seek treatment for various reasons, including stigma, discrimination, lack of awareness and lack of adequate mental health services. The treatment gap varies widely with 70.5% for

intellectual disability (mental retardation), 73.6% for severe mental disorders like schizophrenia and related psychotic disorders, 85% for common mental disorders like anxiety disorders and depression and 91.1% for substance use disorders. The maximum treatment gap (91.8%) was found for tobacco-use disorders (smoking, smokeless tobacco, etc.), which is well recognized as a silent killer by being a common cause of cancer of the mouth and lungs.

Barriers to Seeking Help for Mental Illnesses

Several barriers contribute to a large treatment gap for mental illnesses. These include lack of awareness about mental illnesses, mental illness not being considered as requiring treatment, the stigma of accessing mental health services, sociocultural beliefs, and inadequate mental health services. Mental health services are often not easily available and accessible, being concentrated in urban centers or big cities. However, this is not the only reason for not availing help for mental health problems, since the mental health gap has also been found high even in urban sector and also in high-income countries, where all kinds of resources are available. Often, the cost of treatment also acts as an inhibitory factor. This cost includes not only the cost of medications but also the cost of travel since patients need to travel to the treatment facility, which may be located far away. A person with mental illness also needs a family member to accompany him/her to a treatment facility, which further increases the cost. The Government of India and the State Governments in the country have taken several steps to increase the mental health services across the country, especially with wider coverage of the population with the District Mental Health Programme (DMHP). The Government of India and the State Governments also have welfare schemes for persons with mental illness. Such supports include disability pension and reservation of jobs for persons with a benchmark (>40%) disability (Discussed in detail in another chapter).

Possible Solutions to Deal with the Burden of Mental Ill Health

Several strategies can be used to manage and reduce the burden associated with mental ill-health. Most of these involve action at the policy level on part of the local governments, whereas others need initiative at the level of the local community and the persons with mental health issues and their families. Thus, it needs to be a joint effort. The strategies can include policy initiatives, strengthening human resources, ensuring availability of mental health care for all, easy accessibility of services, emphasis on early intervention for mental health problems, raising community awareness about the need for early treatment for mental health problems and targeting stigma related to mental health problems.

India launched its National Mental Health Programme (NMHP) long back in 1982. The program aimed at making minimum mental health care easily available and accessible for everyone, especially the most underprivileged sections; integrating the principles of mental health in general health care; and encouraging community participation in mental health services. Later, districts were identified as the units for implementation of the NMHP with the launch of the DMHP in the 1990s. Currently, DMHP covers most of the districts in the country. The Government of India launched the Mental Health Policy on 10th October 2014. Thus, the Government has undertaken several initiatives that are at various stages of implementation. However, there is still a gross deficiency of manpower in India to meet the huge requirements of our country with the population reaching nearly 1.4 billion. This is also true for most of the low- and middle-income (LAMI) countries across the world.

It is noteworthy that mental health resources are not uniformly available across the country. Rural areas, Northeastern states and states like Uttar Pradesh, Bihar and Chhattisgarh in general, have poor access to mental health services. Unfortunately, countries with higher levels of socioeconomic deprivation, like those in Africa, South America or South Asia, have much lower mental health resources compared to the western countries. In fact, the number of psychiatrists of Indian origin working in western countries is more than twice the number of psychiatrists available in India. This is also true for many LAMI countries.

In recent years, the Government of India has also taken initiatives to expand human resource capacity that would help in reducing the treatment gap, leading to early detection and treatment of mental ill-health and help in reducing the burden due to mental disorders. The Government has upgraded the mental health services across various state-run medical colleges and psychiatric hospitals and increased the training facilities in mental health, including those for psychiatry, clinical psychology, psychiatric social work and psychiatric nursing.

It needs to be emphasized here that all persons with mental disorders don't need to be seen and treated by psychiatrists. Most of the common mental illnesses, like depression and anxiety disorders, can be treated by the family physician or primary health care doctor. In this context, the focus in DMHP has been on strengthening the mental health services in primary care settings. Under DMHP, training programs on mental health have been regularly conducted for the doctors working in primary care, and also for nurses and paramedical workers to strengthen their skills in identifying and managing common mental health issues in the population visiting primary care settings. For a simple comparison, mild mental health problems, such as anxiety, stress or mild depression, are just like common cold or fever, and don't need to be treated by a psychiatrist. The family doctor or a doctor working in a government dispensary or a primary health center is fully competent to treat such problems.

Need for Priority to Mental Health at Multiple Levels

It goes without saying that mental health needs to be prioritized at all levels with services needing strengthening at all levels, including primary, secondary and tertiary care. The steps need to be taken at the level of policy-making by the Governments. This book is also an attempt at spreading the message of prioritizing mental health care. Media, including print media, virtual media and audio-visual channels, all play an important role in spreading awareness about the need for adequate mental health care and not avoiding but availing the mental health services, whenever needed. Mental health is an integral component of health and needs to be taken care of. Certain simple methods as discussed in Chapter 1, if

followed properly, can help reduce the burden related to mental disorders.

Conclusion

Mental ill-health is highly disabling and is responsible for burden across multiple spheres to the family members, the society and the nation. Most mental disorders have an onset in the early phase of life and tend to be chronic. A delay in identification and treatment further adds to the related burden. In addition, a substantial proportion of patients with mental illness don't seek treatment for various reasons, such as lack of awareness, stigma and lack of adequate and easily accessible mental health care services. Many steps have been taken at the national level to deal with the problem, like expanding and strengthening the mental health services in the community at multiple levels, manpower development and initiating community awareness programs on mental health.

KEY POINTS

➢ Mental ill-health contributes substantially to disability and burden.

➢ Burden results from multiple factors, such as treatment-related costs, a person's inability to work or function and time to be taken off work by the family members to care for the person with the illness.

➢ If the ailment is identified early and the treatment is started in time, the disability and burden associated with mental ill-health can be reduced.

➢ All persons with mental ill-health need not be seen by psychiatrists. Common mental illnesses can be easily managed by the family physician or primary care doctor.

➢ Governments need to take policy initiatives and steps to strengthen mental health services to reduce the burden associated with mental disorders.

REFERENCES

1.   GBD 2017 Disease and Injury Incidence and Prevalence Collaborators. Global, regional, and national incidence, prevalence, and years lived with disability for 354 diseases and injuries for 195 countries and territories, 1990–2017: A systematic analysis for the global burden of disease study 2017. Lancet. 2018;392(10159):1789-1858. https://doi.org/10.1016/S0140-6736(18)32279-7.

2.   Gururaj G, Varghese M, Benegal V, Rao GN, Pathak K, Singh LK, et al. Bengaluru: National Institute of Mental Health and Neuro Sciences; 2016. National mental health survey of India, 2015-16: Prevalence, patterns and outcomes. NIMHANS Publication No. 129.

3.   New Pathways New Hope: National Mental Health Policy of India, 2014. New Delhi. Ministry of Health and Family Welfare, Government of India.

CHAPTER 4

Myths and Misconceptions About Mental Health

U C Garg and Kashypi Garg

Introduction

Cambridge Dictionary defines 'Myth' as "an ancient story or set of stories, especially explaining the early history of a group of people or about natural events and facts". It includes traditional beliefs based on past experiences or events, or the local religious and cultural values and norms. Myths may provide a model of behavior to emulate effective rituals with a specific purpose and establish cult sanctity.

A misconception is a mistaken belief or wrong idea, defined as a common viewpoint or factoid that arises from conventional wisdom, stereotypes and a misunderstanding of science, and becomes accepted in the current times as truth.

Mental health has been defined by the WHO as an individual's state of well-being, realizing one's abilities, being capable of coping with normal stresses of life, being productive and fruitful and making contributions to the community. It is an individual's capacity to feel, think and act. Mental health has gained significant attention in the 21st century, yet it is still prejudiced by the old, disturbing, discriminating myths and misconceptions about mental illnesses. Myths and misconceptions are prevalent in the population, whether uneducated or educated and the young or the old.

Myths about Mental Illnesses

India has a diverse population with widely varied ethnocultural and linguistic backgrounds associated with their own belief systems. This is further complicated by an additional layer of inequitable distribution of education and economic mobility, often in a complex interaction with prevailing cultural and societal norms. Some of the commonly encountered myths and misconceptions in India related to mental health are discussed below:

Mental health problems are uncommon or rare. It is an established fact that mental disorders are common. According to the WHO, worldwide, one in four persons is likely to suffer from a mental disorder during their lifetime. The National Mental Health Survey of India has estimated the lifetime prevalence of mental disorders at 13.7%.

People with mental disorders cannot work. Contrary to the stereotype, most people with psychiatric disorders have jobs, have families and make it through their daily life quite easily. Although some psychiatric disorders can be crippling for people, most of the persons with mental illnesses are productive in society.

Mental health problems are signs of weakness. Having a mental illness does not make a person weak or lacking in 'resilience'. One does not choose to have a mental illness; anyone can develop a mental health problem. It takes a lot of strength and courage to recognize the need to seek help for a mental illness.

Mental illness is permanent/Once you get a mental illness, it is for a lifetime. It is a known fact that a large proportion of people with mental illnesses get better and make a complete recovery. Recovery in health refers to the ability to live, learn and actively participate in society. To help people towards these goals, a range of treatments and community support services are available.

Mental illness is 'Uppari chakkar', that is, it is a result of possession by ghosts or outside influences. India has a large number of cases with possession, trance, fugue states and hysterical fits. Many patients attribute their symptoms to unknown supernatural causes. Indian ideology proposes that the suffering in mental illness arises from the *Karma* (deeds) of the past life. A cultural belief and myth in reincarnation and polytheism is a well-recognized reason for possession phenomena, further popularized by many Indian movies. Mental illnesses occur due to interplay of multiple factors including biological, psychological and sociological ones.

Children don't suffer from mental illness. Research has established that up to half of mental illnesses develop by the age of 14. Mental illness affects almost 1 in 5 children and adolescents around the world. Nearly 50 million Indian children and adolescents are estimated to be living with mental disorders. Suicide is a common cause of death in adolescents and young adults and most suicides have been attributed to mental illnesses.

Marriage can 'cure' a person with mental illness. Any disturbance in mental health needs to be treated by a mental health professional, Marriage, by putting the person in a new, unfamiliar environment with new responsibiities may create more adjustment problems. Thus, marriage is not at all an answer for curing mental illness.

Seeking help is a sign of weakness. The idea of seeking professional help can sometimes seem daunting for the patients due to the stigma associated with mental illness. However, it represents a strength rather than a weakness. Actively seeking psychological help has many immediate and long-term benefits and helps build better relationships. Steps taken towards promoting well-being and improving mental health can benefit everyone.

Mental illness is a family problem. Certain adverse events or circumstances like poverty, unemployment, violence, etc. may affect the mental well-being of a person, members of the family and the relationships among them. It is not uncommon for patients' families to be blamed for mental illness if any member(s) of the family develops a mental illness. It is a known fact that some mental illnesses have a genetic basis, but that does not mean that the family is responsible for the genesis of the illness.

People who need psychiatric care are locked away in 'institutions' and 'given electric shocks'. Just as hospitalization is not necessary for all physical illnesses, it is not mandatory for all mental illnesses as well. Most people with mental illnesses are treated as out-patients. Similarly, electro-convulsive therapy, which has been established to be of immense value for a small subset of patients, is practiced in line with modern medical science, at par with minor surgery, under general anesthesia.

Psychiatric medications are addictive. Most psychiatric medications do not have addictive potential. Only a limited number of medicines used in psychiatry have dependence potential, and these are used only for a limited duration.

Figure 1 summarizes myths about mental illnesses.

Misconceptions About Mental Illnesses

Mental illness is not a real illness, 'It's all in the head'. It is now well established that mental illnesses are a result of disturbances in the function of the brain, a result of neurochemical imbalances. Unfortunately, since mental illnesses don't always have visible physical manifestations

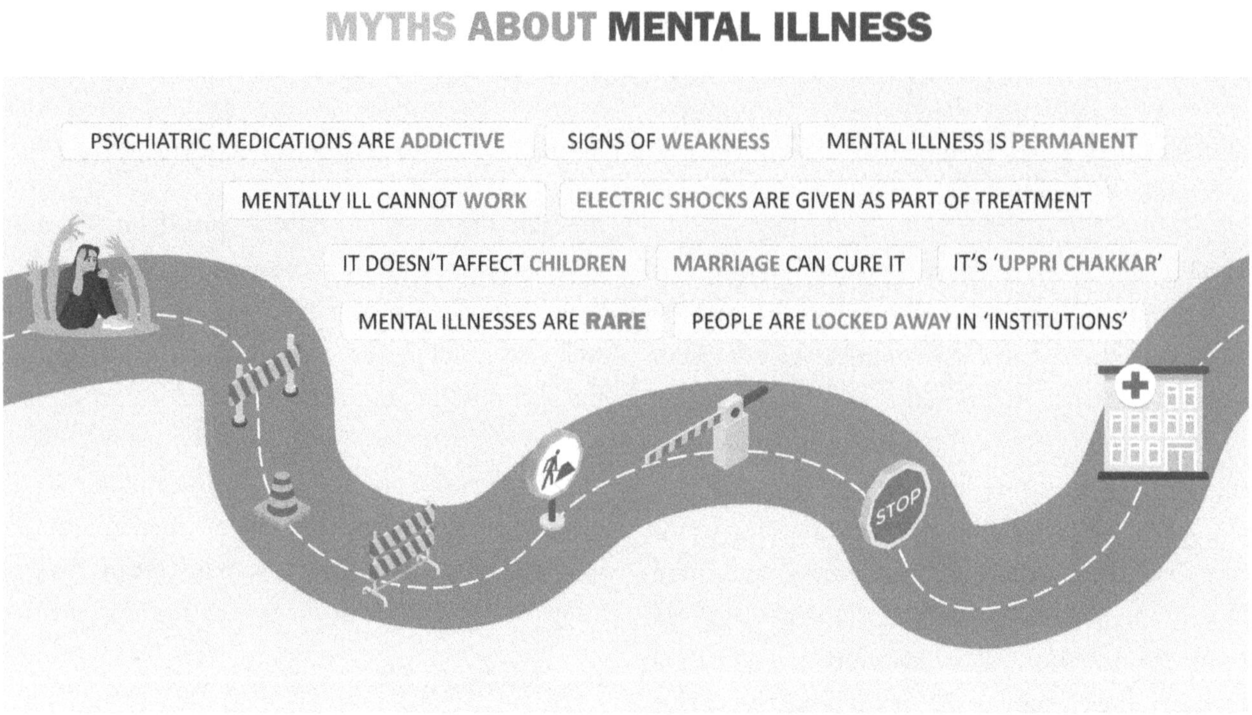

MYTHS ABOUT MENTAL ILLNESS

PSYCHIATRIC MEDICATIONS ARE ADDICTIVE · SIGNS OF WEAKNESS · MENTAL ILLNESS IS PERMANENT

MENTALLY ILL CANNOT WORK · ELECTRIC SHOCKS ARE GIVEN AS PART OF TREATMENT

IT DOESN'T AFFECT CHILDREN · MARRIAGE CAN CURE IT · IT'S 'UPPRI CHAKKAR'

MENTAL ILLNESSES ARE RARE · PEOPLE ARE LOCKED AWAY IN 'INSTITUTIONS'

Figure 1. *Myths about Mental Illnesses*

or demonstrable pathological markers, it is not uncommon for a sudden change in a person's behavior to be dismissed as a flaw in his/her personality. Along with this, many culture-bound syndromes occur throughout the world, some of which tend to be psychiatric disorders but are named differently in different parts of the world (Table 1 lists some culture-bound syndromes commonly seen in India).

People with psychiatric illnesses are 'crazy'. Hurtful words like 'crazy', 'cuckoo and 'insane', and their local vernacular versions actively feed into traditional stereotypes about mental illnesses, and that affected people are 'wild', 'uncontrollable', and 'always severe'. In reality, mental health and illness are part of a wide spectrum, and any odd behavior does not mean that a person has a mental illness.

Mental illness is God's way of 'punishing us for our past sins'. Many people believe that the symptoms of mental illness are some kind of 'divine punishment', and subsequently, may refuse to go for treatment thinking they do not deserve to be relieved from their suffering and only be 'cured by prayers'. In addition to being obstructive to treatment, these beliefs can also subject patients to harmful and exploitative practices by faith healers. In India, people attribute their ideas of guilt or reference in depression and persecutory delusion in psychosis to deeds of past lives or Karma.

Only severely depressed people die by or attempt suicide. The notion is possibly risky, because friends, families and sometimes even health professionals may presume, mistakenly, that people without severe depressive symptoms are 'safe' and do not need any psychological attention. Among those who attempt suicide, up to a sixth of them do not meet the criteria of major depression and 10% suffer from schizophrenia or substance use disorders. In addition to these, many other disorders (personality disorders, obsessive-compulsive disorder, etc.) are associated with an increased risk of suicide.

Table 1. *Culture-bound syndromes in India*

Nomenclature	Description
Culture-Bound Suicide	Sati: A widow immolates herself on her husband's pyre; the custom used to be followed by Brahmins and Kshatriyas. Santhara/Sallekhana: It is voluntary fasting unto death over a long time for religious purposes to attain God/Moksha. It is commonly observed in the Jain community.
Mass Hysteria	Also called collective hysteria or collective obsessional behavior, where large groups of people start believing and behaving in a manner, that is not their usual pattern
Dhat Syndrome	A state of distress that occurs most frequently in young males caused by anxiety over the loss of dhatu (semen).
Jhin Jhini	It is a feeling of bizarre involuntary contractions and spasms with no underlying pathology.
Ascetic Syndrome	This syndrome mostly affects adolescents and young adults characterized by social withdrawal, serious sexual abstinence, practicing religious austerities, disregard for self-care and considerable weight loss.
Possession Syndrome or *"Devi Mata"*; being possessed by the Mother Goddess	The trance and possession syndrome is characterized as a 'spirit' controlling a person's personality; during such episodes, the person is aware of the existence of the possessor.
Bhanmati Sorcery	It is the belief that magical spells produce evil spirits, thus causing symptoms of mental illness such as conversion, somatization, anxiety, dysthymia, psychosis, etc.
Gilhari Syndrome	The affected person feels a small swelling on the body changing its place from time to time as if a *gilhari* (squirrel) is running inside the body.
Koro	There is fear of genital retraction into the abdomen and ultimately death. It is reported in both sexes. Some people may even apply external retractors, such as chains, clamps, etc., to stop the genitalia from retracting.
Suudu	It is described as pain while urinating and pelvic 'heat', attributed as rising in 'inner heat' of the body often due to dehydration. Reported in both sexes.

Self-harm or suicidal attempt is an attention-seeking behavior. The negative implication of the term is that an individual's self-harm attempt is 'just to get attention'; however, it is rarely, if ever, the main motivation. It is important to understand that the reason behind self-harm can be the manifestation of a mental disorder. As stated earlier, suicide is also a major cause of death among people in the age group of 15-29 years. All suicide attempts must be treated as though the person has the intent to die and should not be dismissed as being an attention-gaining device. This is an important suicide prevention strategy, further discussed in the chapter on Suicide Prevention.

Mental illness makes people violent. Multiple studies have shown that people with mental illnesses are far more likely to be victims of violence rather than perpetrators. Most people with mental disorders are no more likely to be violent than anybody else.

Patients with mental disorders should not have similar rights as normal people. Less than half of the countries across the world have plans and policies for mental health according to the human rights accords. This then manifests as some or other form of restriction, exclusion or disenfranchisement of the person, resulting in a vicious cycle of stress and negative emotional impact. The Mental Health Care Act (2017) of India is a welcome progressive step towards aligning the rights of people with mental illnesses with the bare minimum human rights enshrined in the law.

Using psychiatric 'labels' for persons with mental illnesses. Psychiatric labels like schizophrenia and mania can be stigmatizing. It needs to be clarified here that for many people, having an explanation for their distressing experiences can, in fact, be a process with therapeutic implications. While it cannot be dismissed that psychiatric diagnosis is sometimes used as a derogatory term, it is up to the practitioners and policymakers to change that perception with wider education and awareness.

Schizophrenia means having 'multiple personalities'. This misconception is surprisingly very common and continues to be propagated by popular mainstream media and cinema, thus now has cemented its place in popular culture. In reality, persons diagnosed with schizophrenia, or any other mental disorder do not possess more than one personality. Schizophrenia is a severe psychotic disorder marked by disturbances in the perception of reality, ability to think coherently and having distressing thought and perceptual disturbances (delusions and hallucinations). Multiple personality disorder is a completely different disorder that falls under the domain of dissociative disorders.

Scholars and people with a lot of friends have nothing to be depressed about; they do not have any mental health problems. Depression is a complex disorder arising from multiple social, psychological and biological factors. Depression can affect any person, young or old, rich or poor, rural or urban, illiterate or educated. For example, adolescents and young adults may feel pressurized to perform well in school or college, leading to stress and anxiety; some may face difficulties at home and some may show signs and symptoms of depression for no particular reason.

Challenges

Herein, we have made a precursor attempt to enumerate and discuss some of the most common myths and misconceptions regarding mental health in India as well as South Asia. The issues discussed here are, by no means, exhaustive or exclusive but can serve as a starting point for discussion and acknowledgment of beliefs that form a barrier in the identification and management of mental disorders. These discussions then also need to be bolstered by the identification of challenges that propagate and provide resistance against attempts at addressing these myths.

- **Word of mouth**: Some such beliefs have spread across multiple generations by verbal communication and prevalent societal and cultural narratives.
- **Desire for 'early answers' and 'quick fixes'**: It is human nature to prefer explanations that offer fool-proof promises and painless behavior changes, or appeal to emotions rather than reason. This forms a major reason that drives attendance at faith healers' places (also contributed to by lack of awareness) for a quick and easy fix to their problems.
- **Inferring causation from the association**: It is often, and incorrectly, inferred that if two events co-occur statistically frequently, then they must be causally related to each other. Co-occurrence doesn't imply causation.
- **Misleading cinema and popular media portrayals**: Mental health issues in cinema are often portrayed as an 'explanation' for violence, crime or psychopathy. This occurs due to the lack of proper research and not consulting a psychiatrist with priority on commercial profits and over-dramatization. This feeds into stereotypes of mental illness. Bollywood movies like Damini, Khamoshi, Jewel Thief, etc. have shown methods like brain stimulation

to cause more problems and memory loss and no improvement in mental health.

- **Knowledge and awareness gaps**: There is a lack of knowledge and awareness about mental health problems and treatment among the illiterate as well as the literate. Sometimes, even health professionals don't give due consideration to mental health issues while dealing with physical illness.
- **Reaching out**: Stigma of mental illness puts a barrier between the patient and the treatment needed. This also puts a negative impact on health-seeking behavior among the people needing help.
- **Social interaction**: Poor interaction and support create more distance between a patient with mental illness and society.
- **Financial burden**: Mental illnesses lead to great financial burden to the affected persons and their families.

Need to change

There has been a gradual expansion of the mental health care services all over the world, though a large section of low- and middle-income countries still have a huge treatment gap for mental disorders. Ignorance about mental health, including the prevalent myths and misconceptions about mental illnesses, is one of the main reasons for this problem.

Thus, it is of utmost and imminent importance to combat stigma, myths and misconceptions about mental illnesses, enhance prevention, ensure early recognition of mental illness, encourage active interventions and promote community participation as a means of increasing awareness about mental health.

The ability to access, understand and use the information to promote and maintain good health has been labeled as mental health literacy, which needs to be prioritized. The National Mental Health Programme and National Mental Health Policy of India have also emphasized on this aspect.

We need to facilitate the dissemination of the correct knowledge about how to seek all mental health-related information, the right attitude that facilitates recognition and help-seeking in mental illness, and identification of the signs of mental health distress.

Some Strategies to Correct Myths and Misconceptions

Some of the strategies that can be used to combat the myths and misconceptions related to mental illness include:

Education: The persons who are well informed about mental illnesses are less likely to endorse stigma and discrimination. In other words, awareness runs the power to replace the myths about mental illness with correct concepts. Implementation of a mental health-related curriculum is highly advisable in school and college education and can help towards de-stigmatization and early detection, promoting relevant discussions (e.g., the relationship between mental illness and violence, depression and self-harm, etc.). Wide-reaching public awareness drives are also helpful. India has a long and successful history of employing such strategies and utilizing grassroots infrastructure for many illnesses, such as polio, malaria and tuberculosis, and population control. Audio-visual, virtual and print media can be used to spread awareness about mental health problems.

Facilitating meaningful contact: Direct interaction with patients with mental illness can help challenge misconceptions. Social media, in its various forms, is demonstrating an ever penetrating and increasing reach amongst the younger population. A carefully curated message or narrative can truly transform the delivery of effective mental health strategies with targeted amplification. Media has been pivotal in connecting people to mental health literacy. Celebrities endorsing mental health and sharing of experiences (e.g., as recently done by Bollywood actress Deepika Padukone when she shared her episodes of depression), along with succinct advertising slogans and rich narratives and documentaries are some key pointers towards constructive use of media.

Protesting harmful narratives: In addition to promoting accurate and helpful narratives, it is equally important to challenge the harmful ones. It is crucial to declare the idea of prejudice against patients with psychiatric disorders as morally untenable, by drawing parallels from other untenable positions toward vulnerable people. These programs can be seen being reflected in street plays organized by various NGOs, government-run health missions, accredited social health activist (ASHA) workers and educational institutions.

Conclusion

A large section of the population continues to subscribe to myths and misconceptions about the treatment and etiology of mental disorders. This creates a treatment gap and a challenge while implementing mental health care services. The patients and their caregivers do not believe in the interventions offered and are rather driven to faith healers or unqualified health practitioners, running the risk of further worsening the ailment and exploitation. Thus, it is of utmost importance to increase mental health literacy to reduce the stigma and distress faced by patients with mental illnesses and to assist in the prevention and early intervention.

KEY POINTS

➤ Mental illness is very much real and is very common.

➤ Most of the persons with mental health-related problems can be helped.

➤ Myths and misconceptions related to mental illness need to be systematically challenged and corrected.

➤ Media platforms can be a helpful tool in spreading mental health awareness and correcting the myths and misconceptions related to mental illness.

REFERENCES

1. Mental health - WHO | World Health Organization https://www.who.int/mental-health accessed on 10th January 2022.

2. Pakaslahti, A. (2014). Family-centered treatment of mental health problems at the Balaji temple in Rajasthan. Studia Orientalia Electronica, 84, 129–166. Retrieved from https://journal.fi/store/article/view/45132

3. Gonsalves PP, Hodgson ES, Michelson D, et al. What are young Indians saying about mental health? A content analysis of blogs on the It's Ok to Talk website. BMJ Open 2019;9:e028244.

4. Pathak A, Biswal R. Mental illness in Indian Hindi cinema: Production, representation, and reception before and after media convergence. Indian J Psychol Med. 2021;43(1):74–80

CHAPTER 5

Dealing with Common Mental Illnesses

Siddharth Sarkar

Introduction

Mental illnesses are a common occurrence in any society. Some mental illnesses can be of limited duration (few days to weeks), while others can be of a longer duration (many months). Mental illnesses can present with a variety of symptoms, which may include anxiety, depression, disordered substance consumption, hallucinations, delusions, impairment in mental capacity, obsessions, etc. A cluster of psychiatric symptoms forming a well-defined pattern is categorized as a mental illness or disorder. Often, mental illnesses result in difficulties either for the patients themselves (like inability to perform day-to-day activities) or for others (like violence). Fortunately, most mental illnesses can be addressed through therapeutic interventions, either using medicines or psychotherapy or both. This chapter briefly discusses common mental illnesses and how to deal with them.

What are Common Mental Illnesses?

Simply put, common mental illnesses are those that are very common in the general population. Common mental illnesses and their typical presentation are described as below:

Depression: Depression is one of the most common mental illnesses encountered in the community. It is a mood disorder, characterized by sadness that is persistent and pervasive. Such sadness persists for at least several weeks. There are negative thoughts, and the person may feel that there is nothing to look forward to in the future. The person may have suicidal thoughts and may even attempt to kill self. He/she may also suffer from insomnia and low appetite. He/she may feel guilty and is generally unable to concentrate well. Depression often occurs in the form of episodes lasting 3-6 months, and the episodes have a natural course of remission over a period of a few months, even without treatment. Episodes of depression can occur spontaneously or may be precipitated by a life event.

It is important to treat depression since it is very distressing and disabling and the person runs the risk of committing suicide.

A case vignette of a person suffering from depression is presented below:

A 23-year-old college student started to experience sadness after failing his exams. He feels low all through the day and does not even enjoy binge-watching, which he previously used to enjoy. He feels tired when getting out of bed and does not have any good sleep either. He does not feel like eating food and says that he has lost taste. He feels that life is not worth living anymore due to failure and thinks that his career has been severely affected now. He does not go out to meet others and has reduced his self-care.

Generalized anxiety disorder: Generalized anxiety disorder is a condition associated with continuous and free-floating anxiety, which is difficult to control. Such anxiety is present on trivial issues and occurs most of the day. Individuals with generalized anxiety disorder have difficulty concentrating and may have difficulty falling asleep due to anxiety. They may also present with forgetfulness due to difficulty in concentration, palpitations, excessive sweating and tremors of the hands. Sometimes, due to increased muscle tension, the person starts experiencing aches and pains in different body areas, like headache, chest pain, backache or pain in the extremities.

Panic disorder: Panic disorder is characterized by recurrent episodes of panic attacks that occur spontaneously without any provocation. A panic attack is an episode of intense anxiety where the person feels that he/she is going to die or lose control. An attack may be associated with palpitations (feeling the heart beating), difficulty in breathing, tremulousness, sweating or urgency of going to the toilet. Patients may feel that they are having a heart attack and may need to go to the emergency services, where on physical examination and investigations, no evidence of any heart problem is found. A patient with panic disorder may avoid going out alone due to the fear of the next attack.

Phobias or phobic disorder: Patients with phobic disorders have an irrational fear of objects or situations that are not feared generally. This can include fear of closed spaces, fear of spiders, fear of social situations, etc. Avoidance behavior is associated with fear, for example, people with a phobia of closed spaces may avoid lifts, and hence, take the stairs. Individuals with phobic disorders realize that their fear is excessive and irrational, but they are not able to control their fear.

Alcohol dependence: Patients with alcohol dependence exhibit gradually increasing use of alcohol over many years, followed by difficulty in controlling its intake. Alcohol takes greater precedence for the person, and other things that

Table 1. *Clinical Presentation of Common Mental Illnesses*

Illness	Typical presentation
Depression	Sadness, continuing throughout the day and pervasive; lack of interest in previously pleasurable activities; feeling fatigued; ideas of hopelessness, helplessness and worthlessness; wish to die, suicidal thoughts; negative views of self; feelings of guilt; lack of sleep; decreased appetite; and poor attention
Generalized anxiety disorder	'Free floating' anxiety (i.e., anxiety occurring all the time, worries about minor things) and difficulties in controlling the worries. Anxiety is present for months together and is not limited to specific things or issues. May cause difficulty in sleep, inability to concentrate and headache.
Panic disorder	Recurrent panic attacks occur all of a sudden and often not triggered by specific situations. During a panic attack, the person feels extremely anxious and may feel that he/she is going to die or may lose control. Symptoms like racing heartbeat, sweating, dryness of mouth, tremors, etc. may be present. Due to several such unanticipated attacks, the person may avoid going out alone.
Phobic disorder	Fear of a specific situation (like fear of heights or closed spaces) or an object (like fear of spiders or blood). Due to fear, the person avoids facing the situation or the object. Exposure to the situation or the object can lead to a panic attack.
Alcohol dependence	Alcohol becomes an important part of a patient's life to the extent that other activities are given less importance. The person is unable to cut down on use, has an intense desire for alcohol use, has withdrawals if does not consume alcohol, needs more amounts of alcohol to get the previous effects and continues drinking despite adverse consequences.

had a greater value previously, are relegated to the background. The person continues to drink despite negative health consequences and may experience an intense craving to consume alcohol and withdrawals in the form of lack of sleep or tremors when he/she does not get alcohol.

Burden of Common Mental Illnesses

Globally, it is estimated that one in every three persons worldwide has a lifetime history of a common mental illness and one in five individuals has experienced a common mental illness in the past 12 months. There are geographical variations in the prevalence of common mental disorders. Incidence of common mental disorders also shows a considerable variation with gender. Anxiety and depressive disorders are more common in women, while substance use disorders are more common in men.

Indian data suggests that one in ten individuals (excluding tobacco and other substance use disorders) suffers from mental illness. Among the common mental illnesses, depression and alcohol dependence are the more common ones (with a lifetime prevalence of about 5% each in

the population). Depression and anxiety disorders are twice more common in women as compared to men. Alcohol use disorders are much more common in men as compared to women.

A worrying fact is that in India, only one in six persons with common mental disorders receives treatment. Even in Western countries, a large majority of persons with common mental illnesses remain untreated. This large untreated population, also referred to as 'treatment gap', is worrisome as this leads to the perpetuation of the problems of the patients, leading to the experience of distress and impaired functioning. From an individual and societal point of view, the 'treatment gap' leads to the inability of the person to function to his/her usual level. Additionally, some psychiatric disorders may become more difficult to treat as time progresses. So, early intervention can be helpful in improving the outcomes of patients with common mental illnesses.

There are several reasons for this huge treatment gap. Some of the reasons for this treatment gap are summarized in Figure 1. Different sets of reasons may be applicable in different situations. Often, more than one of these reasons may be applicable in a given scenario. Steps are being taken to

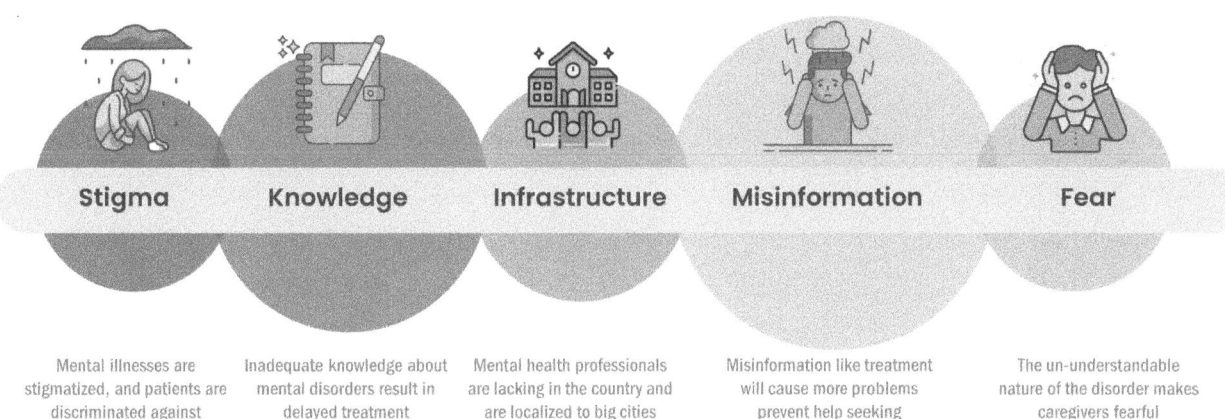

Figure 1.   *Reasons for Treatment Gaps for Common Mental Disorders*

systematically address the issues leading to a high treatment gap.

Identification of Common Mental Illnesses

The features of different common mental illnesses are summarised in Table 1. Essentially, the common mental disorders (like depression, generalized anxiety disorder, panic disorder, phobic disorder and alcohol dependence) can be identified by the specific constellation of symptoms, and the impact they have on day to day functioning of the individuals. The constellation of symptoms forms a defined set and can be differentiated from the other sets of symptoms.

Recapitulating briefly, depression presents with sadness, which is prolonged (more than a couple of weeks) and affects most domains of a person's life. There are negative thoughts, which may include thoughts of suicide or self-harm. Generalized anxiety disorder presents as a worried behavior, which is difficult to control and the worry jumps from one trivial issue to another.

There may be associated muscle tension and headache due to the worries, and difficulties in falling asleep. Panic disorder refers to a condition where a person experiences multiple attacks of intense anxiety when there is no reason for such anxiety (panic attacks). Such attacks typically last for a few minutes, but the person may feel that he/she is going to die or will lose control. Phobic disorders are those that manifest with fear of a specific object or situation, leading to avoidance of such objects and situations (like closed spaces, social events, heights, etc.). Alcohol dependence is a maladaptive pattern of alcohol consumption that manifests as difficulty in controlling its use, intense urge for consumption and other aspects of life gradually becoming secondary to alcohol use.

Myths and Misconceptions About Common Mental Illnesses

Some of the myths and facts about common mental illnesses are listed in Table 2.

Table 2. *Myths and facts about common mental illnesses*

Myth	Fact
A common mental illness is forever.	Many of the common mental illnesses undergo resolution on their own. Most of the common mental illnesses can be treated effectively with medications.
Patients with common mental illnesses cannot perform marital/family responsibilities.	Most patients with common mental illnesses are able to perform their marital and family responsibilities.
Patients with common mental illnesses cannot hold an employment.	Most patients with common mental illnesses can hold employment and perform their duties appropriately.
Common mental illnesses afflict only those who are 'weak'.	Common mental illnesses can develop in anyone and can be addressed by suitable treatment.
Common mental illnesses can be simply remedied by proper discipline.	Often, common mental illnesses require treatment for improvement. Treatment can be in the form of medications or psychotherapy.
Medications for treatment have to be taken lifelong.	In many situations, a person with a common mental illness can be safely withdrawn from medications.
Treatment for common mental illnesses largely comprises sleeping pills.	Most of the anxiety and depressive disorders are treated with antianxiety drugs or antidepressants that are not sleeping pills. Sleeping pills are generally prescribed for a short period of time as an add-on medication.

Whom to Approach?

When a common mental illness is suspected, it might be a good idea to approach a mental health professional or a primary care physician who is adept at treating these illnesses. Mental health professionals include psychiatrists, clinical psychologists, psychiatric nurses and psychiatric social workers, who have been formally trained in the identification of psychiatric disorders and their treatment. Among them, psychiatrists are able to prescribe medications for a range of common mental illnesses. Many general physicians also have good training in the treatment of common mental illnesses and are capable to provide good psychiatric care to patients.

Treatment for these conditions is available in several settings. Both general hospitals and dedicated psychiatric hospitals provide treatment for common mental illnesses. Apart from them, treatment can be provided in primary care settings. Many clinicians have their own clinics or practice and these conditions can be treated in the outpatient setting as well. Figure 2 summarizes the places where treatment for common mental illnesses is provided.

Available Treatments

Common mental illnesses are primarily treated by two approaches. One of them comprises medications (pharmacotherapy) and another comprises structured counseling sessions conducted in a systematic manner and following specific theoretical principles (psychotherapy).

Pharmacotherapy: Medications form one of the important components of the treatment of common mental illnesses. Usually, antidepressants are prescribed for the treatment of depression,

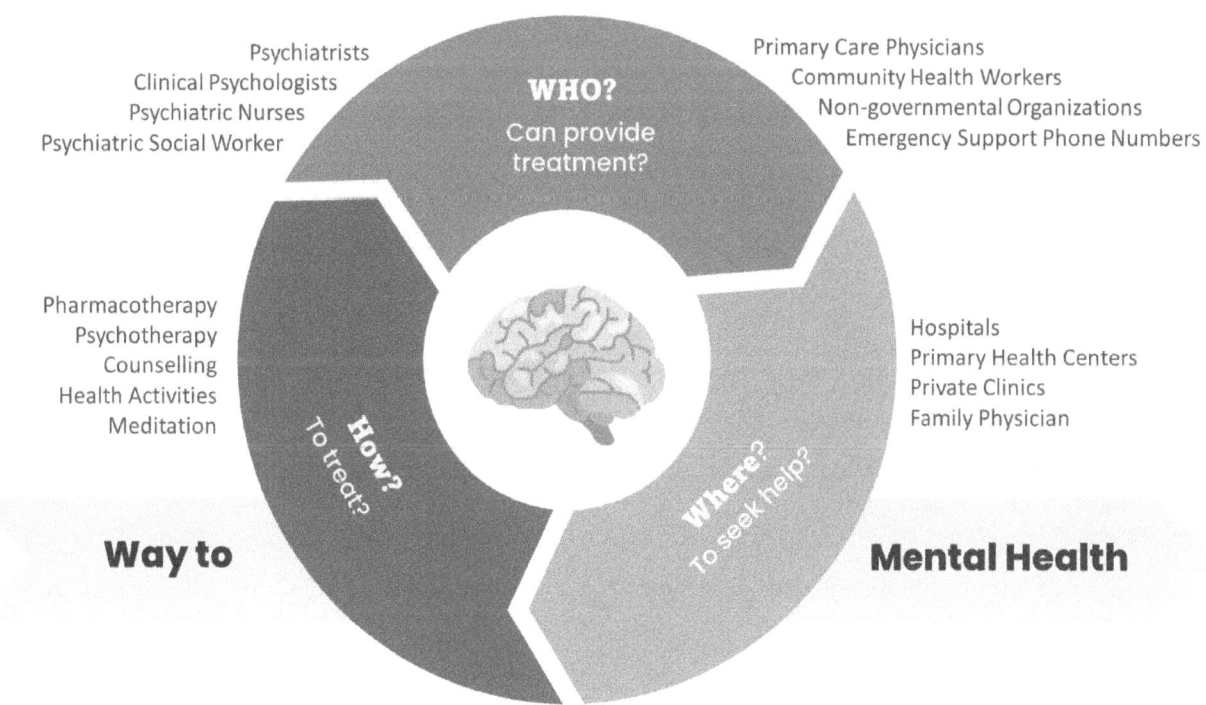

Figure 2. *Treatment Approaches*

generalized anxiety disorder, panic disorder and phobic disorders. Selective serotonin reuptake inhibitors (SSRIs), such as escitalopram, fluoxetine, sertraline and paroxetine, are the most widely used group of antidepressants used nowadays. One of the reasons for their popularity is a good safety profile and fewer adverse effects. Apart from SSRIs, another class of antidepressants, known as tricyclic antidepressants (TCAs), like imipramine or amitriptyline, mirtazapine, trazodone and others, are also used widely. Generally, all antidepressants have similar levels of efficacy (they seem to work for about two-thirds of the cases). Major deciding factors, hence, are the safety profile of the drug and the preferences of the patient/treatment provider. Most of the patients can tolerate the medications well for prolonged periods of time. Apart from antidepressants, other medications can be used on a case-to-case basis. For example, benzodiazepines, such as lorazepam or clonazepam, can be given for insomnia or to address an episode of a panic attack. These drugs are generally prescribed for a shorter period of time (typically less than 4 weeks), so as to prevent dependence.

Psychotherapy: Psychotherapy or psychological treatment sessions are conducted by mental health professionals trained in a particular technique. Various approaches can be used, though cognitive behavior therapy (CBT) is probably the most commonly used approach for the treatment of common mental disorders. CBT is a collaborative and systematic approach that aims at targeting thoughts and behaviors to modify emotions. In some patients, psychotherapy can be combined with medications for better effect.

Treatment of alcohol dependence: It generally comprises two steps – detoxification (i.e. safely quitting alcohol) and maintenance (prolonging abstinence). Detoxification is done using benzodiazepines, such as chlordiazepoxide or diazepam, given in high doses, but tapered within 7 to 10 days. In the maintenance phase, medications like disulfiram are used, which cause an unpleasant and potentially fatal reaction when alcohol is consumed and hence given after telling the patient all details and taking a consent. During this phase, medications like naltrexone (to reduce the desire for alcohol) or acamprosate (to reduce craving) are also used. Psychotherapy and group therapy are also used. The topic is discussed in detail in another chapter (Chapter 9).

Initiating and Continuing Treatment

Before initiating treatment, diagnosis is made on the basis of the cluster of symptoms present. The treating clinician needs to rule out other causes that may masquerade as symptoms of common mental disorders. For example, individuals suffering from hypothyroidism may exhibit some of the symptoms of depression like fatigue. Hence, the treating doctor may like to get some tests done to rule out other potential ailments. Also, some investigations may be suggested based on the type of treatment being planned (for example, an ECG may be considered for an elderly patient who is to be started on imipramine).

Any medication is initiated after the discussion with the patient and/or their family members about the need for medicines, tentative duration and common side effects. Often, antidepressant medicines are started at lower doses and escalated to target doses. Achieving the target dose is easier and quicker for SSRIs, and the target dose may be the initial dose for some patients (for example, escitalopram is started at 5-10 mg and the same dose is used throughout treatment). Common side-effects of SSRIs include gastrointestinal complaints (dyspepsia or 'acidity', diarrhea or constipation) or a mild headache, which usually resolve spontaneously. With correct doses of medicines, the desired effect may begin in 10-15 days and optimum benefits can be observed within 4 to 6 weeks.

Psychotherapy is initiated by explaining the procedure of psychotherapy and the expected frequency, setting up the time and day of the sessions, discussing the payment formalities, etc. *(this topic is discussed in detail in Chapter 22)*.

Continuing treatment is important especially when the patient exhibits some improvement with treatment. Discontinuation of treatment does not immediately lead to the re-emergence of symptoms; it takes a few weeks for symptom re-emergence. If the patient faces any discomforting side effects, these should be addressed by the treating professional. A change in medication or treatment approach can also be tried. In certain cases, like sudden worsening of symptoms, admission may need to be planned. However, for common mental illnesses such situations are rare. Once the patient's symptoms have been under control for a fairly long period (may vary from 6-12 months), and he/she is well functional in different domains of life, the treating professional may decide that treatment is not currently necessary and the medications can be gradually withdrawn over a few months under guidance. However, the patient and their family members should preferably be not in a haste to stop the treatment.

Case vignette (contd...)

The student was, as described above, taken to a psychiatrist in a hospital. A diagnosis of depression was made. He was started on escitalopram (antidepressant) given 5 mg per day that was increased to 10 mg per day after a week. He started to show improvement in mood within the first two weeks and his depression remitted within four weeks. He was also given clonazepam (sleeping pill) 0.5 mg at night for the initial 10 days only to help him sleep. He was able to resume his studies after 6-7 weeks. Traetment was continued for about 9 months and then gradually stopped over the next 3 months.

Conclusion

Mental illnesses are common in the community. About one in ten Indians is likely to suffer from common mental illnesses. Depression, generalized anxiety disorder, phobic disorders, panic disorder, and alcohol dependence are some of the common mental illnesses. Fortunately, effective treatment options are available for these disorders. Most patients with these conditions improve with treatment and become functional enough to perform their responsibilities.

KEY POINTS

➢ A considerable proportion of the general population is affected by common mental disorders.

➢ Common mental disorders generally include depression, general anxiety disorder, panic disorder, phobic disorder and alcohol dependence.

➢ Effective treatment options are available for the treatment of common mental disorders in the form of medicines (pharmacotherapy) and structured counseling (psychotherapy).

➢ Improvement is not immediate and often takes a few weeks for anxiety and depressive disorders.

➢ The treatment should be discontinued only after due consultation with a trained professional.

REFERENCES

1. Gautham MS, Gururaj G, Varghese M, Benegal V, Rao GN, Kokane A, et al. The National Mental Health Survey of India (2016): Prevalence, socio-demographic correlates and treatment gap of mental morbidity. Int J Soc Psychiatry 2020;66(4):361–72.

2. National Collaborating Centre for Mental Health (UK). Common Mental Health Disorders [Internet]. British Psychological Society (UK); 2011 [cited 2022 Jan 10]. Available from: https://www.ncbi.nlm. nih.gov/books/NBK92254/

3. Steel Z, Marnane C, Iranpour C, Chey T, Jackson JW, Patel V, et al. The global prevalence of common mental disorders: a systematic review and meta-analysis 1980–2013. Int J Epidemiol 2014;43(2):476–93.

4. Verhaak PF, Prins MA, Spreeuwenberg P, Draisma S, van Balkom TJ, Bensing JM, et al. Receiving treatment for common mental disorders. General Hospital Psychiatry. 2009;31(1):46-55.

CHAPTER 6

Dealing with Severe Mental Illnesses

Mamta Sood

Introduction

Schizophrenia and related psychotic disorders, and bipolar disorders are grouped under severe mental illnesses (SMIs). These are so called as these cause significant disability and burden for the individuals, families and the society due to an inherent tendency to be chronic, inadequate recovery in many patients and suboptimal functioning. SMIs impact all domains of functioning, including personal care, work and social and family life.

Schizophrenia and related psychotic disorders, also known as non-affective psychotic disorders, are characterized by disturbance in thinking, perception and behavior. Bipolar disorder is a mood disorder, characterized by a predominant disturbance in emotions accompanied by a range of other symptoms.

According to the National Mental Health Survey (2016) of India, 1.9% of the population in India suffers from a SMI at some point in their life (lifetime prevalence) and 0.8% currently have a SMI (current prevalence). SMIs often begin at an early age (late childhood and adolescence) and are 2-3 times more common in urban areas as compared to rural areas.

Early treatment can result in early symptom resolution and improved functioning. Although there have been efforts for improving access to treatment, there remains a huge treatment gap, and about three-fourths of persons with SMIs – bipolar disorder (70%), and schizophrenia and related disorders (75%) – do not receive any treatment.

Persons with SMIs suffer from the stigma that results in delay in treatment-seeking, which, in turn, increases the time spent being ill and increases the disability and burden. Stigma also limits the opportunities for education, finding work and meaningful relationships – marriage and friends. Most of the persons with SMIs in India stay with their families at home. The families help in identification, help-seeking and ensuring treatment for the illness. Family members not only experience significant stigma but also have to miss their work to take care of the affected individual, especially during the acute or florid phase. Families also need to spend a significant amount of money on the treatment of their ward with a mental illness.

This chapter discusses various aspects of SMIs: symptoms and identification, related myths, and available options for treatment.

What are Severe Mental Illnesses?

It is important to know what these conditions are. In the description below, technical terms used by mental health professionals to describe these conditions are explained.

Schizophrenia and related psychotic disorders are a group of mental illnesses generally referred to as psychosis. Schizophrenia is the most known condition in this group. Others include delusional disorder, acute and transient psychotic disorders and schizoaffective disorder.

Psychosis refers to a broad group of illnesses presenting with delusions, hallucinations or disorganized behavior, with impairment of reality testing and judgment. It includes schizophrenia and related disorders and mania.

Hallucinations are false perceptions occurring in absence of an adequate external stimulus. Thus, a person perceives something that does not exist. Hallucinations can occur in any sensory system, like hearing, vision, smell, touch or taste, and are thus called auditory, visual, olfactory, tactile and gustatory hallucinations, respectively.

Delusions are false and unshakable beliefs that are not based in reality, which are held on inadequate grounds and cannot be corrected by any amount of reasoning or evidence to the contrary. These beliefs cannot be explained by the sociocultural background of the person. Delusions can have persecutory, grandiose or other themes.

Disorganized behavior may occur in the form of extreme excitement or slowing of motor activities. A person may smile or laugh without any reason, may become aggressive or violent, adopt odd postures, wander aimlessly, etc. A person may become mute or become completely immobile or become excited and grimace or show unusual mannerisms or maintain awkward postures. Symptoms related to over and under activity come under the group of **catatonic symptoms**.

Thinking may also get disorganized and this is evident in form of irrelevant and disorganized speech, also called formal **thought disorder**.

A person with psychosis is often unaware that these experiences may be imaginary or her/his behavior is strange, and therefore, may be reluctant to seek medical help. There may be gradual withdrawal from the events/activities and the person stops socializing and isolates him/herself. This constitutes a parallel reality for the person with psychosis. This may result in difficulty for the person to tease out 'real' from 'not real', thereby resulting in **impaired reality and judgment**.

Delusions, hallucinations, disorganized behavior and thinking are also called **positive symptoms**.

Negative symptoms are so called, as there is a loss or decrease in certain areas of mental functioning, like emotions and behavioral abilities. Unlike positive symptoms that are obvious to even a layman, these symptoms are difficult to identify. Negative symptoms include anhedonia, apathy, alogia, avolition and asociality. Family members may mistake these symptoms for laziness. **Anhedonia** refers to a loss of interest in previously pleasurable activities. **Apathy** refers to loss of emotions and can be reflected as gross indifference to day-to-day events. **Alogia** refers to no or minimal speech output. **Avolition** refers to a reduced ability to initiate or carry out daily activities. **Asociality** refers to stopping of socializiation,

Cognitive symptoms are the third set of symptoms that are most difficult to appreciate as these are very subtle and impact the ability of the affected person in day-to-day functioning.

A person with psychosis may experience difficulties in concentrating on any task at hand. S/he may have forgetfulness because of poor concentration and there may be difficulty in registering new information. Difficulty in decision-making and problem-solving tasks manifests in daily life as an inability to understand and carry out complex tasks.

Schizophrenia is a type of psychotic disorder characterized by positive, negative and cognitive symptoms, along with functional impairment. The symptoms should be present for a minimum duration of at least one month for making a diagnosis.

Delusional disorder is a type of psychotic disorder in which the predominant symptom is the presence of delusions that are well systematized. Functioning is relatively better preserved than in schizophrenia.

Both schizophrenia and delusional disorder often tend to be long-standing or chronic illnesses.

Acute and transient psychotic disorder is characterized by the presence of psychotic symptoms that devlop rapidly. Usually, it resolves in 2-3 months.

Schizoaffective disorder is characterized by the presence of both schizophrenic and mood symptoms in the same episode. A person may have either depressive (schizodepressive) or manic (schizomanic) symptoms during the same episode.

Bipolar disorder and depressive disorder are two major types of mood disorders. Depressive disorder has been discussed in the chapter 'Dealing with Common Mental Illnesses'.

Bipolar disorder was earlier called **manic-depressive psychosis** or **MDP**. It is an episodic and recurrent mental illness and is characterized by episodes of mania/hypomania and depression. A person may have only episodes of mania/hypomania or both mania/hypomania and depression.

The core feature of a **manic episode** is **elevated mood**, which may be on a spectrum from cheerfulness to excitement and ecstasy. Some persons may have irritable mood. **Lability of mood** may also be seen, which refers to a rapid change of mood from sudden cheerfulness to crying or vice versa. The person may feel very **energetic** and may have a **reduced need for sleep**, which means that the person may not feel tired even after minimal sleep.

Increased psychomotor activity is another important symptom of mania. The patient may be physically over-active and may start/carry out multiple activities without finishing any. S/he may be mentally overactive, which manifests in excessive and loud speech, talking nonstop on any topic/object/event that catches her/his attention. Sometimes, the person talks so much and so fast that it is difficult to interrupt them - **pressure of speech**. S/he may report getting too many thoughts and multiple ideas - **racing of thoughts**. Her/his speech may be full of superfluities, like songs, rhymes, puns, jokes, etc., and may jump from topic to topic, termed as a **flight of ideas**. He/she may have **ideas of grandiosity** in form of having special abilities, powers or worth. The symptoms should be present for a minimum of one week for a diagnosis of mania to be made.

Hypomania is a milder form of mania and generally does not need any treatment.

The core feature of a **depressive episode** is depressed mood. The depressed mood has a distinct quality, which is different from the normal emotion of sadness and is very distressing. There may be a slowing of both physical and mental activities. Speech may be of low volume, slow and monotonous. This slowing is called **reduced psychomotor activity**. **Anhedonia** refers to a loss of interest in previously pleasurable activities. **Anergia** refers to a feeling of having reduced energy or fatigue. A person with depression may have **depressive cognitions** – ideas of hopelessness, helplessness and worthlessness. S/he may have ideas of guilt and may falsely hold oneself responsible for past or present misfortunes. The symptoms are associated with disturbances in all domains of functioning.

The symptoms should be present for a minimum of two weeks for a diagnosis of depression to be made.

The episode of mania or depression may vary in severity from mild and moderate to severe, depending on the number of symptoms and functional impairment. In severe cases, a person may exhibit psychotic symptoms, like delusions and hallucinations, and may also develop catatonic symptoms.

How do Severe Mental Illnesses Present?

The initial symptoms in persons with SMIs may not be noticeable. Usually, a change of behavior in patients is picked up by people in close contact, like family members, colleagues at work, friends or teachers. This is in contrast to common mental illnesses like anxiety or depression, where persons suffering from illness identify themselves that something is wrong and may initiate help-seeking.

The symptoms may develop rapidly over days to weeks or may develop slowly over weeks to months.

Symptoms vary from person to person. All the symptoms of schizophrenia and related psychotic disorders or bipolar disorder may not be present in one person.

Schizophrenia and related psychotic disorders

As the illness advances, all the symptoms may become severe. Symptoms may progress as follows:

- Sleep disturbance is one of the earliest symptoms – sleeping late or intermittent awakenings or getting up early
- Remaining preoccupied with certain thoughts or meaningless work
- Appear anxious or bewildered or fearful or irritable
- Express beliefs not based on reality and continue to have these beliefs even when explained about the falsity of the beliefs, like expressing suspicion or ideas that others are talking about her/him
- Report hearing voices or seeing things that do not exist in reality
- Smile, laugh or cry, or mutter or talk to self, or shout loudly without any apparent reason
- Make gestures in the air as if talking to someone
- Poor appetite
- Decreased interaction with family, friends or colleagues or may avoid company altogether

- Remaining ill-kempt and ignoring hygiene - May need coaxing to take care of themselves
- Neglect work
- Appear restless
- Sudden or unexpected changes in behavior or clumsy, uncoordinated movements or maintaining awkward postures
- Emotional indifference, lack of interest in pleasurable activities, like watching TV, reading newspaper, going to market, etc.
- May become abusive and aggressive
- May refuse to take food

Figure 1 summarizes the clinical features of schizophrenia and related disorders.

Bipolar disorder

Manic/hypomanic episode

- Get up early in the morning, feel fresh and energetic even after reduced sleep
- Appear happy and cheerful
- Talk excessively, shifting from one topic to another
- Easily distractible
- Express ideas of self-importance: enhanced abilities, powers, being on a special mission
- New and exciting ideas and plans
- Restless, move around more often and always on run, easily distractible
- Overconfident
- Wearing new and bright clothes and eating fancy foods; meeting people, even strangers, and talking too much on phone (a change from the previous routine)
- May spend money unnecessarily
- May indulge in risky or exciting ventures/ schemes/business enterprises
- Increased use of alcohol or illicit drugs
- May make inappropriate advances towards the opposite sex
- May become irritable, angry and abusive
- Neglect of work

Psychosis

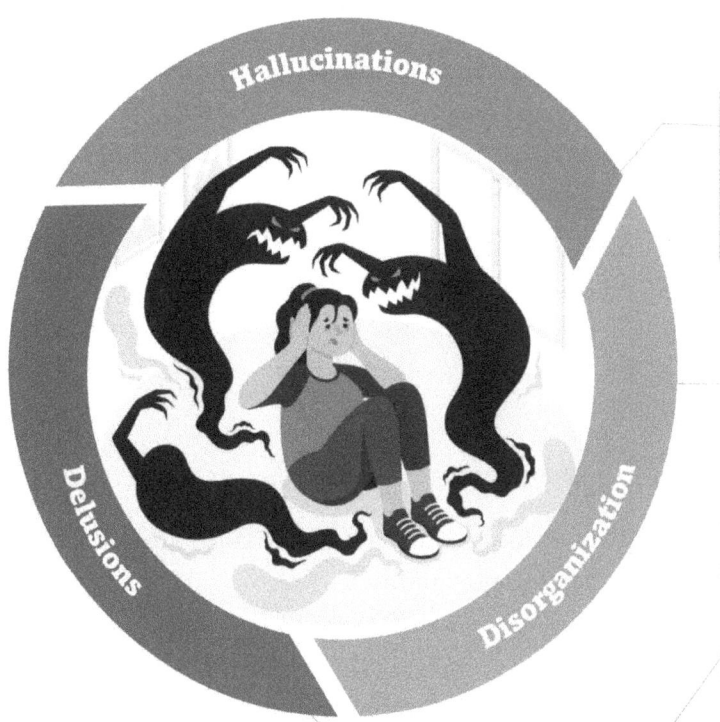

Hallucinations
Delusions
Disorganization
False perceptions occurring in absence of an adequate external stimulus:
• Seeing people around
• Hearing voices
• Feeling insects crawling under skin
Smiling or laughing without any reason, may become aggressive or violent, adopt odd postures, wander aimlessly. Thinking also gets disorganized and this is evident in form of irrelevant and loosening of speech
False and unshakable beliefs that are not based in reality, which are held on inadequate grounds and cannot be corrected by any amount of reasoning or evidence to the contrary

Figure 1. *Presenting Features of Psychotic Disorders*

Bipolar Disorder

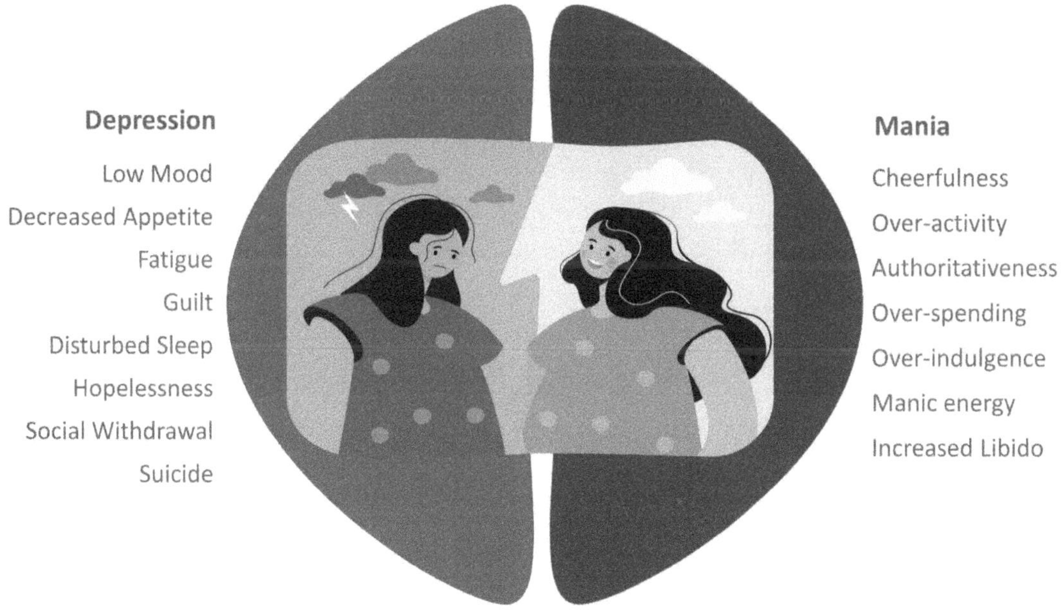

Depression
Low Mood
Decreased Appetite
Fatigue
Guilt
Disturbed Sleep
Hopelessness
Social Withdrawal
Suicide
Mania
Cheerfulness
Over-activity
Authoritativeness
Over-spending
Over-indulgence
Manic energy
Increased Libido

Figure 2. *Presenting Features of Bipolar Disorder*

As the illness becomes severe, all aspects of functioning become severely impaired. The person may become aggressive and assaultive and express beliefs not based on reality, especially related to special abilities. Figure 2 summarizes the clinical features of bipolar disorder.

Depressive episode

In a manic episode, the symptoms are not difficult to identify due to rapid development and drastic changes in behavior. In contrast, in a depressive episode, it takes longer to recognize that something is amiss. A person in depressive episode presents with:

- Not feeling fresh after getting up from sleep
- Feeling sad; sadness does not get better in response to changes in circumstances and is worse in the morning
- Lack of energy to complete day to day tasks and tiredness
- Neglect of personal grooming; preferring to stay alone
- Loss of interest in day-to-day activities
- Inability to enjoy activities that one used to feel pleasurable
- Neglect of work/job
- Forgetfulness with an inability to concentrate and think clearly
- Slowing of speech, walking speed and other actions
- Gloomy and negative thoughts - negative view of self, future and the world, blaming self for any mishappening in the family
- Decrease in self-confidence
- Recurrent thoughts of death and suicidal ideas
- May have physical symptoms - body aches, headache, nausea, dizziness, constipation
- Sleep disturbances - getting up early or difficulty in falling asleep

- Lack of appetite and weight
- Loss of interest in sexual activities

As the illness becomes severe, all aspects of functioning become severely impaired; the affected person may remain confined to bed; have frequent suicidal ideas and sometimes make a suicidal attempt; express beliefs not based on reality, especially related to negative thinking; self-blame, poverty, and report seeing or hearing things that do not exist. Sometimes, s/he may become completely mute or not move at all.

Diagnosis

Diagnosis of SMIs is made based on detailed history and examination. There is no laboratory test that can diagnose these conditions. However, detailed physical examination and lab investigations help to rule out physical diseases that may lead to symptoms similar to those of schizophrenia and related disorders and bipolar disorders. This has been discussed in detail in the chapter 'Recognizing Mental Illness'.

Management

Both pharmacological and non-pharmacological treatments are available for the management of SMIs. Both kinds of treatments go hand in hand to achieve the goals of treatment, which are to:

- Reduce symptoms and time spent in the disease state
- Improve functioning and return to a pre-illness level of functioning
- Prevent relapse and recurrence of future episodes

The overall goal of management is 'recovery'. Traditionally, the goal of management has been only in terms of the cessation of symptoms and

---

Box 1.   Treatment for Severe Mental Illnesses

- Evidence-based affordable pharmacological and non-pharmacological treatments are available.
- Early identification of illness and early initiation of medications in an adequate dosage and adequate duration of treatment helps in recovery.
- Psychoeducation is a non-pharmacological strategy and is an essential component of treatment.
- Most patients can be treated in an outpatient setting.
- Improvement in symptoms takes place slowly over weeks. Treating doctors should not be changed frequently in the hope of quick recovery.
- Physical health needs to be looked after by eating nutritious and balanced food, regular physical exercise and physical health check-ups.
- Family members play an important role by supervising medications, ensuring follow-up, providing support and encouragement, remaining vigilant for early symptoms of relapse and not being critical, hostile or overinvolved.
- Relapse can be prevented by taking medications as prescribed, sleeping for about 8 hours at night and avoiding addictive substances.

---

no further hospitalization. However, in the last few decades, the concept of recovery has redefined the scope of the outcome for persons with SMIs. Recovery means that a person with SMI can recover even when the illness is not cured and that the process of recovery can proceed in the presence of continuing symptoms and disabilities.

After making assessments and diagnoses, the first decision that needs to be taken is whether the person needs hospitalization for management. Most patients can be managed on an outpatient basis while staying at home with family. Hospitalization is needed if a person with SMI shows grossly disorganized or inappropriate behavior or has history of suicidal ideations/attempts or is violent or unmanageable like complete refusal of food or there is a need for clarifying the diagnosis. Usually, a short hospitalization of 4-6 weeks is required. In some cases, electroconvulsive therapy may be needed, especially in persons having catatonic symptoms, high suicidal risk and complete refusal of food.

Box 1 summarizes the treatment for severe mental illnesses.

Pharmacological (medication) treatment

Pharmacological treatment is essential for both types of SMIs. It is important to start treatment at the earliest as delay in treatment prolongs the duration of illness and may also contribute to poor response to treatment.

A variety of medications are used in the treatment. There are some **common principles** about medication use that need to be remembered:

- Only a qualified physician can prescribe. Within medication groups (antipsychotics, mood stabilizers and antidepressants), no one medication is superior to others. A specific drug is chosen depending on the side effect profile and history of previous response to it in the person or a family member.
- Medicines are given at a low dose initially and gradually increased to a dose on which improvement is seen; different persons may need different dosages
- Improvement in symptoms takes place slowly over weeks. This is an important fact to

remember. At the start of treatment, many patients and their family members change the treating psychiatrist frequently in the hope of quick recovery which is counterproductive.

- Medication needs to be taken for a minimum duration of 4-6 weeks in adequate dosage to assess its effectiveness.
- Medication needs to be continued beyond the point of improvement and should not be stopped without consultation with the treating doctor

Prevailing **myths** about medications used for treatment are: these are 'sleeping pills' and would result in 'dependence/addiction' or turn the person into a 'zombie/sleeping all the time' or side effects would be very disabling.

It is true that these medications cause sedation as a side effect. However, the main therapeutic effect is on the core symptoms of SMIs, like delusions, hallucinations, mood symptoms, etc. These medications do not produce any high/kick or joy like an addicting substance but improve the abnormal behavior by restoring the normal functioning of the brain. Side effects are usually mild and are regularly monitored.

Schizophrenia and related psychotic disorders –

The mainstay of treatment is antipsychotic drugs. A variety of antipsychotic drugs are available as tablets and solutions. Antipsychotic drugs are also available in the form of injections for acute control of agitation or in case of medication refusal. Depot injections are available for use in persons who may not take oral medications and can be given at 2-4 weeks intervals.

With treatment, sleep, appetite and agitation improve first. Psychotic symptoms improve after that. Negative and cognitive symptoms improve last of all.

Bipolar disorders - Mood stabilizers are the mainstay of treatment. These are used for the treatment of the episode and also for the prevention of further episodes (prophylaxis). For acute control of manic episodes, antipsychotics are used. Antidepressants are used for the treatment of depressive episodes.

After treatment, sleep, appetite and psychomotor symptoms improve first, followed by improvement in mood and thinking. In depression, there is often a lag period of about 2 weeks, before the medicines begin their specific beneficial effect.

Maintaining Adherence with Treatment: Adherence to treatment is an important issue that plays a significant role in recovery from SMIs. It refers to the extent to which a person with illness follows the recommended treatment plan. Non-adhherence to treatment is common in nearly half of the patients with SMIs.

Some of the reasons for poor drug adherence are as follows:

- Negative view about medications, side effects of medications
- Co-occurring psychoactive substance misuse
- Persons with SMI may not consider themselves ill
- Inadequate explanation by prescribing doctor about dosage and timing of medications
- Patients and their families may not have understood the instructions for medications
- Lack of availability of medications

Adherence to treatment can be improved by some of the following strategies:

- Know the name, correct dose and timing of medications by asking your doctor. You can also request her/him to write this in the language you understand

- Ask about likely side effects of the medications; how serious these are and what to do, if side effects develop
- Most of these medications can be given at night as a single dose; the schedule of medications can be in sync with the workday or with routine activities like meals
- Use of tablet/pill boxes
- Procure medications in advance and have adequate stock of medications
- In case of development of a side effect, discuss with the treating doctor
- In case of non-availability of a medication, discuss it with your doctor. S/he may prescribe another medication
- Depot injections are given once in 2-4 weeks

Physical health of persons with SMIs is often neglected. Due to a sedentary lifestyle, unhealthy eating habits and smoking, there is an increased risk for lifestyle diseases, like obesity, diabetes mellitus, hypertension and cardiovascular diseases. Also, the medications used in treatment lead to an increase in appetite that may result in weight gain. Therefore, it is important to eat healthy nutritious and balanced food. It is also important to regularly do physical exercise like brisk walking. It is important to get a regular physical health check-up.

Non-pharmacological treatment

Psychoeducation is the most important and essential non-pharmacological treatment for both illnesses. Persons with SMIs and their family members are educated about the symptoms, available treatment options, benefits and side effects of medications, the importance of treatment compliance and the course of illness. They are also explained about how to identify early symptoms of relapse and seek help.

The following steps by the family members of persons with SMIs can be useful in the management of persons with SMI:

- Supervise medications and bring the patient for regular follow-up
- Provide encouragement and support
- Start the process of encouraging the person with SMI to get back to pre-illness normal role/activities early along with the treatment. However, this does not have to be rushed and has to be slow and gradual.
- Involve in household matters and decision-making. Start with assigning small tasks and responsibilities
- Avoid over-involvement/overprotection, critical remarks and hostility, since these hamper recovery
- Remain vigilant for early symptoms of relapse/recurrence

It is important to acknowledge that family members of persons with SMIs experience significant stress and burden. Therefore, they should also take care of their mental and physical health by finding time for recreation, socialization and physical activities.

For preventing relapse or recurrence, **four simple actions** can help:

- Take medications regularly. Do not miss medications.
- Sleep for eight hours at night. Shift duties are known to cause relapse, especially in bipolar disorder.
- Avoid the use of addicting substances, like alcohol, tobacco, cannabis, etc., as this may lead to relapse.
- Know symptoms of illness so that if relapse occurs, it can be identified early and treatment can be started early.

How Long to Continue Medications?

For persons with schizophrenia and related psychotic disorders, after improvement, the medications should not be stopped. In persons with the first episode, the medications should be continued for a period of 1-2 years after improvement. If there is no recurrence, the dosages can be decreased over a few months and then stopped. The affected person and her/his family members should know the symptoms of the illness so that if it recurs, medications would be restarted. In persons with multiple episodes and incomplete improvement, the medications may be continued indefinitely. Continuing antipsychotic medications reduces the risk of future psychotic episodes. In some cases, relapses occur despite taking regular medications. If a relapse occurs while on medications, the patient experiences illness with a shorter duration and lesser severity.

For persons with bipolar disorder too, after improvement, medications should not be stopped. In a person with the first episode, the medications need to be continued for a minimum period of 6-9 months after the symptoms have subsided. Chances of recurrence are very high in bipolar disorder. After the second episode, prophylactic treatment needs to be given, which may need to be continued till the person is free of episodes for a period of 3-5 years.

Course of Illness

Among schizophrenia and related psychotic disorders, acute and transient psychotic disorders have good chances of recovery. About 45% of patients with schizophrenia recover after one or more episodes, 20% of patients show unremitting symptoms and increasing disability and around 35% of patients show a mixed pattern with varying degrees of improvement and relapses. Factors related to better chances of recovery are late age of onset, good social and work history prior to the onset of illness, support from family, being married, presence of positive symptoms, acute onset and presence of stressors at the time of onset. With regular treatment and family support, most patients are able to lead a reasonably satisfactory life and also meet their social and family responsibilities.

Bipolar disorder is a recurring disorder and usually starts with depression in 60-75% of cases. Most patients experience both depressive and manic episodes, though 10-20% experience only manic episodes. About 40-50% of persons may experience a second manic episode within 2 years of the first episode and 5-15% become rapid cyclers (having four episodes within a year). As the disorder progresses, the time between episodes often decreases and the duration of episodes increases. A person may experience 2-30 (average - 9) episodes during his/her lifetime, if not treated. Factors related to a good prognosis are short duration of illness, late age of onset, few suicidal thoughts and few coexisting psychiatric or medical problems.

Conclusion

Schizophrenia and related psychotic disorders and bipolar disorder are SMIs with substantial burden and large treatment gap. Evidence-based and affordable treatment for SMIs is available. Early treatment results in early symptom resolution and improved functioning. Diagnosis is made based on detailed history and examination. Antipsychotic and mood stabilizer drugs are used for treatment. Psychoeducation is an essential component of treatment. Supervision of medications and encouragement and support from family members is essential for recovery. Most of the persons with SMIs can recover and lead productive lives with available pharmacological and non-pharmacological treatments.

KEY POINTS

➤ Schizophrenia and related psychotic disorders and bipolar disorders are severe mental illnesses (SMIs).

➤ Schizophrenia and related psychotic disorders are a group of mental illnesses that are characterized by disturbance in thinking, perception and behavior.

➤ Bipolar disorder is a mood disorder and a recurrent, episodic illness characterized by predominant disturbance in emotions as episodes of hypomania/mania (excessive and sustained mood of elation) and depression (excessive and sustained low mood).

➤ Both pharmacological and non-pharmacological treatments are available for the management of SMIs.

➤ Early identification of illness and early initiation of medications in an adequate dosage and for adequate duration helps in recovery.

➤ Most patients can be managed on an outpatient basis while staying at home with family.

➤ For schizophrenia and related psychotic disorders, antipsychotics, and for bipolar disorders, mood stabilizers are the mainstay of treatment.

➤ Improvement in symptoms takes place slowly over weeks.

➤ Psychoeducation is a non-pharmacological treatment and involves educating persons with SMIs and their family members about symptoms, available treatment options, benefits and side effects of medications, and need for adherence to treatment.

➤ The physical health of persons with SMIs is often neglected. It is important to eat healthy, nutritious and balanced food, do regular physical exercise and undergo physical health check-ups.

REFERENCES

1. Chadda RK, Sagar R, Sood M, Ambekar A (2007) Mental Illnesses: Identification and treatment (*Manasik Rog: Pahchan aur Upchaar*) - in Hindi. All Indian Institute of Medical Sciences: New Delhi.

2. Bipolar disorder. https://www.rcpsych.ac.uk/mental-health/problems-disorders/bipolar-disorder

3. Bipolar disorder: for parents, carers and anyone working with young people. https://www.rcpsych.ac.uk/mental-health/parents-and-young-people/information-for-parents-and-carers/bipolar-affective-disorder-for-parents-carers-and-anyone-who-works-with-young-people

4. Gururaj G, Varghese M, Benegal V, Rao GN, Pathak K, Singh LK, et al. Bengaluru: National Institute of Mental Health and Neuro Sciences; 2016. National Mental Health Survey of India, 2015-16: Prevalence, patterns and outcomes. NIMHANS Publication No. 129.

5. Schizophrenia. https://www.rcpsych.ac.uk/mental-health/problems-disorders/schizophrenia

6. Schizophrenia for parents and carers. https://www.rcpsych.ac.uk/mental-health/parents-and-young-people/information-for-parents-and-carers/schizophrenia-for-parents-and-carers

CHAPTER 7

Obsessive Compulsive Disorder

Abhijit R. Rozatkar, Geetesh Kumar Singh and Raveena Saroye

Introduction

Obsessive compulsive disorder (OCD) is a highly distressing psychiatric condition where patients are troubled by frequent intrusive and unwanted thoughts, commonly known as obsessions. These obsessions generally cause severe anxiety, forcing the sufferer to carry out repetitive behaviors or rituals to decrease the worry. Such behaviors are clinically called 'compulsions'. Although completing the compulsive behavior provides a short-lived respite to the patient, obsessions invariably come back within hours or even minutes, resulting in a never-ending cycle of suffering. Over time, patients with OCD start avoiding persons, places or objects that trigger obsessive thoughts, become severely home-bound and require repeated reassurance for every mundane activity.

What are Obsessions?

Obsessions are repetitive, irrelevant, intrusive and uncontrollable thoughts. The thoughts may refer to worries, persistent images, impulses, fear, doubts or a combination of these. Obsessions are always recognised as undesirable, disturbing and intrusive, thereby affecting patients' ability to function effectively on an everyday basis.

Persons with OCD generally know that their obsessive thoughts are unreasonable, and are excessive and unwarranted. They have no difficulty in appreciating that these thoughts are their own, but feel a loss of control over them, as the thoughts continue despite patients' effort to 'let them go'.

Over time, patients succumb to compulsions as the only way to relieve their distress.

Obsessive thoughts can be grouped based on their content and nature. The thought of contamination, where patients find everything around them to be dirty, is the commonest form seen by doctors. Other forms, which include doubts and fears, are summarised in **Figure 1**, along with the associated behavioral compulsions.

What are Compulsions?

Compulsions are repetitive physical or mental actions that a person is forced to do as a consequence of one's obsessive thoughts. The natural initial response of any person with OCD is to fight with one's intrusive and distress-provoking thoughts. Over time, however, the person resorts to carefully chosen, ritualistically performed behaviors, to help him/her decrease the anxiety associated with obsessive thoughts. For example, persons obsessed with dirt and contamination may initially resist the thought by self-assurance - 'it is OK'. However, over time, as resolve fails, they go on to develop a pattern of repeated handwashing to help them cope with the same thoughts. Thus, repeated washing becomes a compulsion. As a counterpoint, a 'normal' person will also wash one's hands when they are dirty and 'see' that they are dirty. However, individuals with an obsessive focus on contamination would keep washing their hands until they are completely assured of absolute cleanliness, often taking hours.

In addition, their OCD convinces them to rewash their hands immediately after completion of one set of washing, repeating the whole process as the thoughts recur. Thus, a vicious cycle ensues, forcing patients to go through 20-30 handwash cycles per day, where each handwash cycle must be done in a proper way, with 20-30 times of soap rinse, taking 10-15 minutes, with any mistake resulting in repetition of the whole process.

The primary purpose of all compulsive behaviors is to relieve the anxiety triggered by the obsession. This leads to compulsions generally following the obsessive demands, a phenomenon called 'yielding'. Sometimes though, persons with OCD may resort to 'neutralizing' compulsions to avert harm resulting from the obsessions. For example, some patients with OCD might suffer from blasphemous or 'dirty thoughts' whenever they see a deity or visit a religious place. These patients might then resort to compulsive praying to counteract the harmful thoughts. Compulsions are mostly 'observable', such as washing hands frequently, checking the door to ascertain if it is locked, etc. Less frequently, compulsions might be 'covert,' such as repeating a specific phrase in the mind or mental counting, without any associated behavior. Generally, obsessions and compulsions go together, although rare cases of obsessions without compulsions and isolated compulsions without obsessions are also seen clinically.

Types of OCD

There are numerous types of obsessive thoughts and compulsive behaviors, but a person's OCD can be categorized into the following five categories, with some degree of overlapping of symptoms:

Contamination and Washing: The fear of being or getting dirty is an obsessive worry and the individual is anxious that the contamination with dirt or germs will hurt himself/herself or his/her loved ones. Common compulsions are to wash or clean hands and avoid physical contact with people or objects. This may include avoiding hospitals and public places and may extend to hamper marital life by avoiding intimacy and sexual acts.

Doubting and Checking: The obsession is that of self-doubt, characterized by repeated thoughts of 'have I heard it correctly?' or 'have I understood it correctly?' or 'have I done it correctly?'. Such doubts are associated with anxiety to prevent damage or harm to self or others due to any form of accident or neglect. Commonly associated compulsions include double-checking locks, switches, gas burners, etc. In addition, people with OCD may frequently check their pockets/bags/purses for items like keys, cash, cards, phones or documents. Checking is often repeated multiple times, sometimes for hours, resulting in being late for work, school, social engagements or other significant events.

Symmetry and Orderliness. A person having an obsessive thought that everything should be neat, clean and in order leads to the compulsive act of aligning the objects to prevent the perceived harm or to feel 'just right'. Sometimes, compulsion is associated with the feeling of having everything not just right, and the person may spend a significant amount of time doing so.

Ruminations. Rumination is a form of OCD characterized by only obsessions without compulsions. Ruminations refer to constant preoccupation with a single thought, generally referring to trivial objects or events. Ruminations are not unpleasant like other obsessions and patients often like to ruminate than to resist. For example, an individual may ruminate about what would happen after death. However, most ruminations never lead to a solution or satisfactory conclusion. The thoughts are irrelevant and repetitive and lead to distress, not because of the content but because of the time consumed and intrusiveness.

Hoarding. Hoarding is a form of OCD with only compulsions without identifiable obsession. Hoarding is characterized by an inability to remove unnecessary or useless belongings or physical objects. A person with hoarding compulsion can collect a range of items with no use or economic value. Containers like jars, plastic boxes or bags, clothes, newspapers, books, magazines, letters, emails and other household items are the most hoarded objects. Hoarding is different from collecting, where the collector seeks out specific objects of value (e.g., postage stamps, coins, etc.). Hoarding is associated with ambivalence and anxiety of letting things go in apprehension that they may be required later. Compulsive hoarding is also different from household prudence, where families often hold on to old objects of occasional use or due to sentimental value. Persons suffering from hoarding disorder often have homes overflowing with wrappers and packets to the extent that liveable space becomes insufficient.

Figure 1 shows a graphic representation of common obsessions and compulsions.

What Causes OCD?

Researchers believe that an imbalance of neurotransmitters and faulty connections within the brain lead to OCD. Often children with OCD have a past history of throat infection and tics, suggesting the involvement of basal ganglia, an area of the brain associated with control of planned behavior. Stress and environmental factors can also trigger or exaggerate obsessive and compulsive symptoms. In many patients, a family history of OCD or related disorders is present and genetic markers associated with the serotonin neurotransmitter have been implicated in the causation of the OCD.

Figure 2 depicts the cycle of obsessions and compulsions.

Prevalence of OCD

The National Mental Health Survey of India (NMHS) (2015-16) estimated that around 0.8% of the adult population in India suffers from OCD. Nearly 85% of perons with OCD fail to seek help for various reasons including lack of awareness about it being an illness.

Consequence if Untreated

If untreated, OCD can be severe enough to significantly impact all areas of a person's life, including studies, employment, relationships with family and friends, and even self-care. As the severity of OCD differs among patients, some individuals may be able to hide their distress from their friends and family. Nevertheless, the disorder does negatively impact their social relationships, leading to familial and marital discord or dissatisfaction, separation or divorce. Understanding OCD, identifying it early and accepting the need for treatment can significantly improve the outcome and the quality of life in these patients.

Comorbidity with OCD

Due to the chronic and distressing nature of the illness, more than two third of patients with OCD suffer from some other associated psychiatric disorders. Patients with OCD have a higher rate of comorbid depression, anxiety disorders and tics. Neurodevelopmental comorbidities, like tics, are common in young children, while in the elderly, neurodegenerative disorders, like Parkinson's disease, are frequent. Adults can have associated anxiety or mood disorders.

Obsessions in Other Mental Illnesses

OCD needs to be differentiated from normal health and from several other mental illnesses. Phenomena similar to obsessional thoughts and compulsive behaviors are found in a range of other mental illnesses. However, a close inspection generally separates them from true OCD.

Common Types of Obsessions & Compulsions

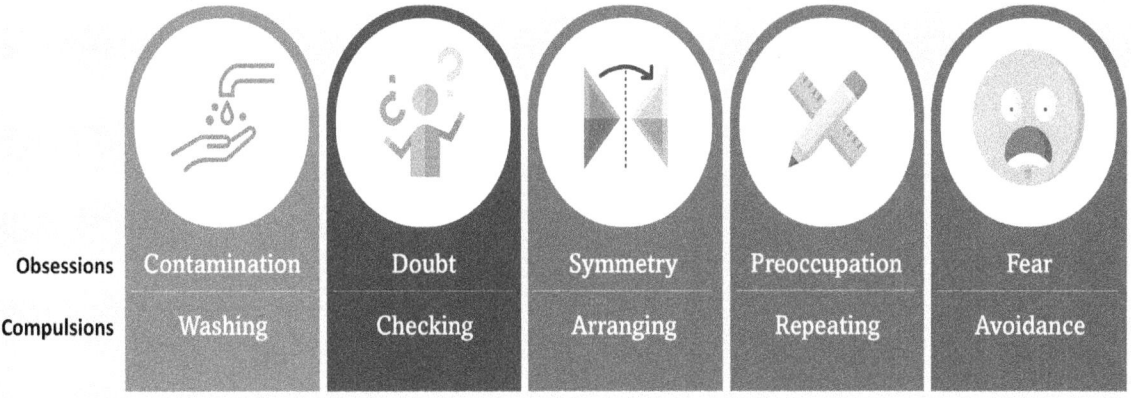

	Contamination	Doubt	Symmetry	Preoccupation	Fear
Obsessions	Contamination	Doubt	Symmetry	Preoccupation	Fear
Compulsions	Washing	Checking	Arranging	Repeating	Avoidance

Figure 1. *Common Types of Obsessions and Compulsions*

The OCD Cycle

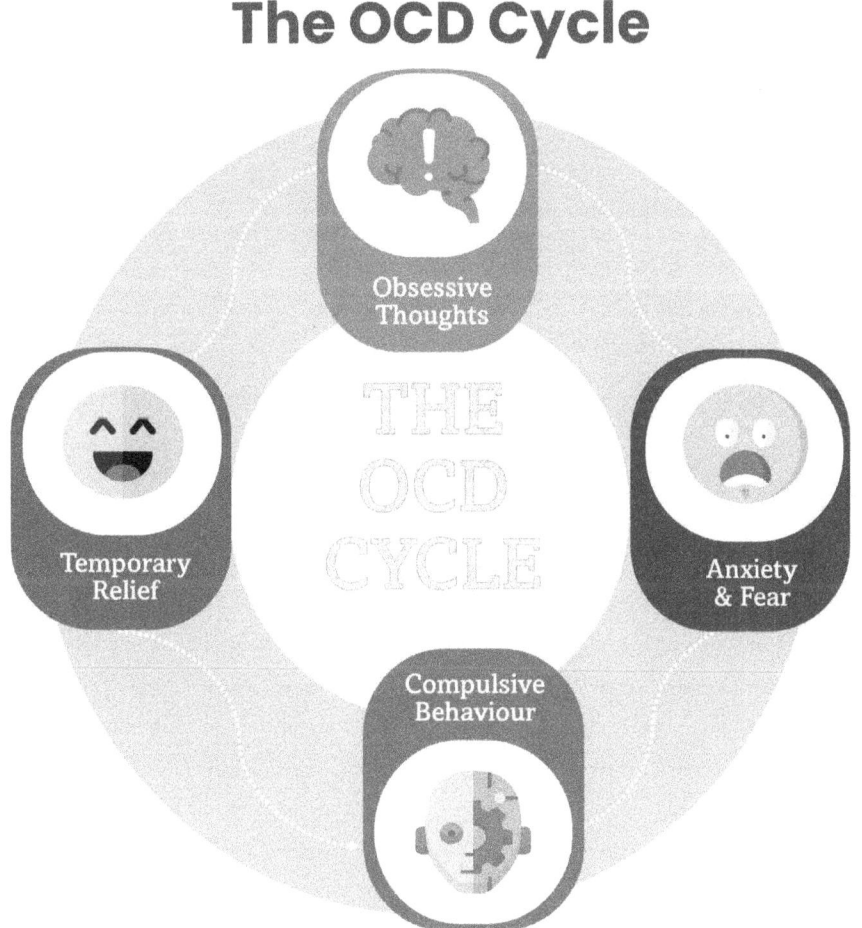

Figure 2. *OCD Cycle*

Table 1. *Myths associated with obsessive compulsive disorder*

Myth	Fact
We all have a little bit of OCD at some times.	OCD is different from normal doubts about cleanliness or orderliness. It is a real illness with evidence of malfunctions in the brain.
OCD is no big deal. Such people should relax and stop worrying.	People who have OCD face significant, often unbearable anxiety over their 'obsessions'. Symptoms can be overwhelming and cause disruptions in their quality of life.
OCD is about handwashing, checking, cleaning and being neat.	Persons with OCD can also have obsessions related to various other things, like losing control over self and circumstances, hurting others accidentally or intentionally, unwanted sexual thoughts, blasphemous thoughts, etc.

- **Depression** - Depression may have depressive ruminations, which are primary repetitive thoughts about self-criticism, failure, regret or guilt. However, the depressed patient believes them to be true and does not consider such thoughts irrational.

- **Anxiety** - Patients with generalized anxiety disorder can have similar repeated worries about real concerns and future events. However, they too consider them as valid worries and not irrelevant thoughts.

- **Trichotillomania (characterized by repeated pulling of hair) and other impulse control disorders** - This group of illnesses may look like OCD. However, here the person feels the urge to do the action. In addition, the act of doing it is pleasurable and satisfying, unlike in compulsion, where the act is neither pleasurable nor satisfying, but the patient is driven to perform it out of distress.

- **Obsessive-compulsive personality disorder (OCPD)** - OCPD is a disorder of personality where the patient has an excessive preoccupation regarding perfection in all tasks, orderliness and neatness of things. However, unlike OCD, the preoccupation is not related to a specific theme but is a character trait.

Myths and Facts About OCD

There are many myths associated with OCD, which are listed in Table 1.

Whom to and Where to Approach for OCD?

Perons with OCD need to be evaluated by a psychiatrist. Treatment includes psychotropic medication and psychological therapies involving problem assessment, crisis intervention, individual and group therapies, supportive counseling, etc. Any psychiatrist, clinical psychologist or even a general medical practitioner can be the first contact to evaluate and guide appropriate therapy for individual patients.

Treatment

A range of medications, like fluoxetine, fluvoxamine, clomipramine, and others, are currently available for the treatment of OCD. Fluoxetine is often used as a first-line drug. It is quite cheap and also effective. Fluoxetine is included in the essential medicines list of the Government of India and hence is available free of cost at most government institutions. A range of non-pharmacological methods, like behavioral therapy, cognitive behavior therapy (CBT) and exposure and response prevention (ERP), have been found to be effective in the treatment of OCD. The treatment outcome is considered best when using both medicines and behavioral therapy. However, due to the nature of the illness, medicines need to be continued for a period of 1-2 years and medicine discontinuation should only be done after consultation with the treating psychiatrist. Clinical research shows that early discontinuation of medication can increase the chances of relapse. The decision to discontinue medications or behavioral therapy would be made by the clinician based on various factors, such as the number of symptoms, the severity of symptoms, total duration of illness, history of recurrence of symptoms on discontinuation, residual symptoms while on treatment, comorbid psychological or neurological disorders, etc.

In psychotherapy, ERP encourages patients to identify their problems and be aware of the inaccurate thinking, emotions and beliefs associated with them. ERP teaches the patient to experience obsessions and concomitant anxiety without resorting to compulsive behavior.

During CBT, patients are expected to be open and honest, stick to the treatment plan and do their homework. Any difficulty arising in the process should be discussed with the therapist and most importantly, clients should not expect instant results. Guidelines recommend continuing therapy and medication for at least 1-2 years even after attaining remission to prevent the re-emergence of symptoms.

Conclusion

People with OCD often experience recurring intrusive and unpleasant obsessional thoughts. These thoughts are very distressing and compel the person to carry out repetitive behaviors as dictated by their obsessions. However, effective treatment options are now available for OCD. In addition to effective medications, a variety of psychotherapy options have been found to be of proven value in treating OCD. Making family members aware of the condition and including them as partners in therapy often leads to gratifying results.

KEY POINTS

➤ According to the National Mental Health Survey of India, 0.8% of India population suffers from OCD.

➤ Obsessive symptoms can occur in many other illnesses, like depression and anxiety disorders.

➤ OCD is a highly distressing and disabling illness and can be treated.

➤ Treatment for OCD includes medications and behavioral therapy.

REFERENCES

1. Obsessive-compulsive disorder (OCD). https://www.rcpsych.ac.uk/mental-health/problems-disorders/obsessive-compulsive-disorder accessed on 26th February 2022

2. Obsessive-compulsive disorder in children and young people: information for parents and carers. https://www.rcpsych.ac.uk/mental-health/parents-and-young-people/information-for-parents-and-carers/obsessive-compulsive-disorder-in-children-and-young-people-information-for-parents-and-carers accessed on 26th February 2022

3. OCD: for young people. https://www.rcpsych.ac.uk/mental-health/parents-and-young-people/young-people/ocd-young-people accessed on 26th February 2022

CHAPTER 8

Personality Disorders

Pratap Sharan and Nileswar Das

Introduction

Personality disorders are a group of mental illnesses characterized by long-term patterns of thoughts and behaviors that are unhealthy and inflexible. These behaviors can lead to significant problems in relationships and work performance. People with personality disorders find it difficult to deal with everyday stresses and problems.

What is Personality and Personality Disorders?

Personality is defined as a deeply ingrained pattern of behavior, which includes the way one relates to, perceives, and thinks about the environment and oneself.

Personality disorders are diagnosed when personality traits lead to inflexible and maladaptive ways of dealing with inner and external issues to the extent that it significantly interferes with how a person functions in society or causes the person a lot of emotional distress.

Personality disorders are characterized by an enduring pattern of inner experiences and behaviors that:

- is markedly different from the variations expected in the individual's culture
- is pervasive (seen in most contexts) and inflexible
- has an onset in adolescence or early adulthood, and
- leads to distress or impairment in various areas (e.g., educational/occupational and/or family/social) of life

Personality disorders are usually not diagnosed until adulthood, because personality traits often change till then. Personality development is influenced by heredity, temperament, experiential learning and social interactions.

Epidemiology

Personality disorders are relatively common, occurring in 6-13% of the general population. They occur with greater frequency in clinical groups, e.g., the frequency of personality disorders is 30-50% in mental health outpatient settings. This means that about half of those with a primary diagnosis of another mental illness also have a coexisting personality disorder that significantly complicates the treatment of the primary mental disorders.

Personality disorders are associated with significant distress to self as well as to those living or interacting with the affected person, especially the family members and co-workers. This group of illnesses often remains under-recognized and under-treated.

Clients with personality disorders have a higher death rate, especially because of suicide; they also have higher rates of suicide attempts, accidents and emergency department visits and increased rates of separation, divorce and involvement in legal proceedings regarding child custody.

Personality disorders are highly correlated with criminal behavior (70% to 85% of incarcerated individuals have personality disorders), alcohol dependence (>50% of those with alcohol dependence have personality disorders) and drug abuse (>50% of those who abuse drugs have personality disorders).

What Causes Personality Disorders?

The exact cause of personality disorders is unknown. However, genetic, familial and environmental factors, as well as early life experiences play an important role in the development of personality disorders.

Types of Personality Disorders

Personality disorders are broadly grouped under three clusters:

Cluster A Personality Disorders

Includes people whose behavior appears odd or eccentric and comprise paranoid, schizotypal and schizoid personality disorders

- *Paranoid personality disorder:* Characterized by mistrust and suspiciousness; clients with this disorder interpret others' actions as potentially harmful
- *Schizoid personality disorder:* Characterized by a social detachment and a restricted range of emotional expression in interpersonal settings.
- *Schizotypal personality disorder:* Characterized by social and interpersonal deficits marked by discomfort with and reduced capacity for close relationships; and by idiosyncrasies related to thought (e.g., persecutory ideas), perception (e.g., illusions) and behaviors (e.g., eccentricities).

Cluster B Personality Disorders

Includes people who appear dramatic, emotional or erratic and comprise antisocial, borderline, histrionic and narcissistic personality disorders

- *Antisocial personality disorder:* Characterized by disregard for and violation of the rights of others, deceit and manipulation
- *Borderline personality disorder* (most common personality disorder found in clinical settings): Characterized by unstable interpersonal relationships, self-image and mood, as well as marked impulsivity
- *Histrionic personality disorder:* Characterized by excessive emotionality and attention-seeking
- *Narcissistic personality disorder:* Characterized by grandiosity (in fantasy or behavior), need for admiration and lack of empathy

Cluster C Personality Disorders

Includes people who appear anxious or fearful and comprise avoidant, dependent and obsessive-compulsive personality disorders

- *Avoidant personality disorder:* Characterized by social discomfort and reticence, low self-esteem and hypersensitivity to negative evaluation
- *Dependent personality disorder:* Characterized by excessive need to be taken care of, which leads to submissive and clinging behavior and fears of separation; these behaviors are designed to elicit caretaking from others
- *Obsessive-compulsive personality disorder:* Characterized by preoccupation with perfectionism, mental and interpersonal control and orderliness at the expense of flexibility, openness and efficiency

Whom and Where to Approach for Help?

Management of personality disorders generally needs a multidisciplinary team consisting of psychiatrists, clinical psychologists and social workers.

Detailed psychiatric assessment is needed to diagnose personality disorder. In many cases, persons with personality disorders may also suffer from other mental health conditions, like depression, and may harbour suicidal thoughts and impulses. Treatment includes psychotherapy and medications.

A psychiatrist may help by prescribing medications and/or giving psychotherapy. Clinical psychologist conducts psychological assessment to further understand the problem and can administer specialized psychological treatments, e.g., cognitive behavioral therapy, dialectical behavior therapy, etc. Multiple sessions of psychotherapy (at least 12-16 sessions but often more) are needed to reduce the distress and dysfunction associated with personality disorders.

School- and college-going students and their parents can approach counselors in schools and colleges, if they feel that the student has personality related issues. The counselor will be able to provide further guidance about the need to go for psychiatric assessment.

In cases of self-harm attempts and injuries, it is better to approach the emergency services.

Assessment of Personality Disorders

People with personality disorders may have trouble realizing that they have a problem. To them, their thoughts are normal and they often blame others for their problems. When they do seek help, it is usually because of their problems with relationships or work.

Diagnosis of personality disorders is based on clinical assessment and psychological testing.

Assessment of the patient includes particular attention to:

Mood: Usually, the mood is dysphoric, involving unhappiness, loneliness, boredom, frustration and feeling "empty".

Thought: Thinking about self and others is often polarized and extreme, which is sometimes referred to as splitting. Patients tend to adore and idealize other people even after a brief acquaintance but then quickly devalue them if they do not meet their expectations in some way.

Ineffective coping: Affected person is unable to learn or change behavior based on past experience or punishment.

Social interactions: There are unsatisfactory interpersonal relationships even with family, friends and co-workers.

History of abuse and neglect: Many individuals may have disturbed early relationships with their parents; about 50% may have experienced childhood physical or sexual abuse; even more may have experienced verbal and emotional abuse and neglect. Many patients have a family history of alcohol dependence.

Intellectual processes: Individual's intellectual capacities are generally intact and the person is fully oriented to reality.

Risk assessment is an important component of the assessment. Persons with personality disorders may have:

- Risk for suicide related to low frustration tolerance
- Risk for self-harm related to impulsive behavior
- Risk for other directed violence related to lack of feelings of remorse

Some investigations may occasionally be needed in persons with personality disorders:

- *Toxicology screen:* Substance abuse is common in subjects with personality disorders.

- *Screening for HIV and other sexually transmitted diseases:* Persons with personality disorders often exhibit abnormal impulse control and may act without regard to risk; such behavior can lead to infection with a sexually transmitted disease.
- *Radiological assessment:* Radiological assessment is needed for injuries from fighting, motor vehicle accidents or self-mutilation.

Management

Management for persons with personality disorders includes the following:

Vigilance related to risk behaviors:

- Person's safety and care if injured
- Safety of others (and property)
- Control of impulsive behavior

Plans are also needed for the following:

- Person's progress toward self-reliance
- Improving problem-solving skills
- Improving the ability to verbalize needs and distress to enable the person to progress towards greater satisfaction with relationships

The main forms of treatment for personality disorders are psychotherapy and medications.

A. *Psychotherapy:* Psychotherapy is the mainstay of care for personality disorders. Since personality disorders produce symptoms due to poor or limited coping skills, psychotherapy aims to improve perceptions of and responses to social and environmental stressors.

Psychotherapy aims to:
o **Promote client's safety:** Therapists should seriously consider suicidal ideation and plans, access to means for enacting the suicidal plans and self-harm behaviors, and institute appropriate interventions.

o **Promote therapeutic relationship and establish boundaries:** The therapist must provide both empathy and structure - the latter may involve setting limits, e.g., seeing the patient for scheduled appointments of a predetermined length rather than whenever the patient comes and demands attention.

o **Teaching effective communication skills:** It is important to teach basic communication skills, such as eye contact, active listening, taking turns while talking, validating the meaning of other person's communication and using "I" statements.

o **Helping patients to cope with and to control emotions:** The therapist can help the patients identify their feelings and learn to tolerate them without exaggerated responses, such as destruction of property or self-harm. Keeping a record or a diary often helps patients gain awareness of feelings.

o **Reshaping thinking patterns:** Cognitive restructuring is used to change patterns of thinking by helping the patients recognize negative thoughts and feelings and replace them with positive patterns of thinking.

o **Structuring the client's daily activities:** Minimizing unstructured time by planning activities can help clients manage time alone. Clients can make a written schedule that includes appointments, shopping, reading the paper, going for a walk, etc.

Psychotherapy helps an individual gain an understanding of the disorder and figure out what is contributing to symptoms. Psychotherapy also helps people understand the effects of their behaviors on others.

Gradually, they learn to cope with symptoms and manage behaviors causing problems with work functioning and relationships.

The type of treatment depends on the specific personality disorder, how severe it is, and the individual's circumstances.

B. *Pharmacologic Management*

There are no specific medications for treating personality disorders. However, medications, such as antidepressants, anxiolytics or mood stabilizers may help in partially treating some features of personality disorders and other comorbid mental illnesses. They also act as an adjunct to psychotherapy and help the client productively engage in psychotherapy.

o **Antidepressants:** Selective serotonin reuptake inhibitors (SSRIs) and newer antidepressants are safe and may be effective in lifting depression at least partially. However, because the depression of most individuals with personality disorders stems from their limited range of coping capacities, antidepressants are usually less effective in those with personality disorders than in individuals with uncomplicated major depression.

o **Anticonvulsants**: Anticonvulsants demonstrate some efficacy in suppressing impulsive and particularly aggressive behavior in patients with personality disorder. However, these agents are somewhat less effective in stabilizing the extremes of mood in personality disorders as compared to their effectiveness in bipolar disorders.

o **Antipsychotics:** Response to antipsychotics in individuals with a personality disorder is less dramatic than it is in psychotic disorders, but symptoms such as fearfulness, anxiety, hostility and sensitivity to rejection may be reduced.

Occasionally, clients may need to be admitted to general hospitals, usually to take care of self-harm or injuries. Sometimes, they may need psychiatric inpatient care for comorbid conditions, like depression, or for assessment and intensive treatment of personality disorders. The length of stay should usually be kept to a minimum to avoid dependency that may hinder recovery from the circumstances, prompting hospitalization.

Role of Family

Family members can work with the treatment team on the most effective ways to help and support a person with a personality disorder.

Conversely, having a family member with a personality disorder can be very stressful. Family members need support and may benefit from talking with a mental health provider who can help them cope with such difficulties.

In addition to actively participating in a treatment plan, some self-care and coping strategies can be helpful for people with personality disorders. These include:

o **Learning about the condition:** Knowledge and understanding empowers and motivates (towards change) the individuals.

o **Physical activity and exercise:** These can help manage symptoms like depression and anxiety.

o **Avoiding alcohol and drugs:** Alcohol and drugs can worsen symptoms or interact with medications.

o **Routine medical care**: Physical check-ups/ vaccinations should be done as indicated and/ or care for injuries.

o **Diary** may be kept to express one's emotions.

o **Relaxation and stress management techniques** like Yoga and meditation are helpful.

o **Staying connected** with family and friends is of great help.

Myths About Personality Disorders

MYTH: Individuals with personality disorders are weak.

Difficulties in self-esteem and self-image and social stigma make the lives of individuals with personality disorders difficult. However, despite their struggles, many of them achieve success; suggesting that they are anything but weak.

MYTH: Individuals with personality disorders fake sadness.

Contrary to popular belief, individuals with personality disorders are more prone to depression and other common mental illnesses. Because of poor interpersonal relationships, they are often lonely. There is a need to manage the co-occurring conditions like depression and stress reactions as these may increase the risk of self-harm.

MYTH: Suicide attempts in personality disorders are attention-seeking behaviors.

Repeated self-harm is commonly associated with personality disorders (especially with a borderline personality disorder). Many of these occur in reaction to acute stress and are misinterpreted as manipulative. However, these should be taken as an expression of distress ("cry for help") rather than as attention-seeking strategies. The risk of enduring damage and death due to such acts is high as seen in morbidity/mortality statistics. An understanding of the person's perceived difficulties may guide the clinician and the caregivers to make appropriate arrangements that could help decrease the need to self-harm.

Conclusion

- Personality disorders are a common group of mental health conditions, which often remain unrecognized
- There are three groups of personality disorders: odd and eccentric, dramatic and emotional, and anxious and fearful
- Persons with personality disorders can be helped with appropriate treatment

KEY POINTS

➢ Personality disorders are associated with high mortality and morbidity.

➢ Various treatments for personality disorders significantly improve quality of life.

➢ Psychological interventions are first-line treatment options for personality disorders.

➢ Pharmacotherapy can be used along with psychotherapy to address specific issues related to personality disorders (e.g., aggression, mood swings, etc.) as well as other co-occurring mental illnesses.

➢ Self-help is an important aspect of management and caregivers need support too.

REFERENCES

1. Bateman, A. W., & Tyrer, P. Psychological treatment for personality disorders. *Advances in Psychiatric Treatment 2004; 10(5)*, 378–388.

2. Kessler, R. C., Aguilar-Gaxiola, S., Alonso, J., Chatterji, S., Lee, S., & Ustün, T. B. (2009). The WHO World Mental Health (WMH) Surveys. *Psychiatrie (Stuttgart, Germany), 6(1)*, 5–9.

3. Personality Disorders. https://www.rcpsych.ac.uk/mental-health/problems-disorders/personality-disorder accessed on 12th March 2022.

4. Sharan, P. An overview of Indian research in personality disorders. *Indian Journal of Psychiatry 2015, 52*(Suppl 1), S250-254. https://doi.org/10.4103/0019-5545.69241

5. Tyrer, P., Reed, G. M., & Crawford, M. J. Classification, assessment, prevalence, and effect of personality disorder. *Lancet 2015, 385*(9969), 717–726. https://doi.org/10.1016/S0140-6736(14)61995-4

CHAPTER 9

Dealing with Drug Addiction

Atul Ambekar and Shalini Singh

Introduction

A drug or a substance is any chemical that alters the state of mind to a feeling of pleasure, 'euphoria' or relaxation. These chemicals are also called '**psychoactive**' substances. In common parlance, people who use drugs are often called '**drug addicts**' and substance use disorder is called '**drug addiction**'. However, the term 'addict' is considered pejorative, which adds to the stigma of substance use. The preferred and technically correct terms are '**substance use disorder (SUD)**' and '**substance user**' for the condition and the user. While the phenomenon may still be regarded as addiction, the affected individual is best referred to as a person with substance use disorder.

Which Drugs are Used?

The following classes of psychoactive substances have been identified to be leading to addiction (substance use disorder), as also recognized by the World Health Organization.

- Alcohol
- Opioids
- Cannabis and synthetic cannabinoids
- Sedatives and hypnotics
- Cocaine
- Other stimulants, including caffeine (coffee)
- Synthetic cathinones
- Hallucinogens and dissociative drugs
- Nicotine (tobacco)
- Volatile inhalants

Humans have been using one or the other psychoactive substances for thousands of years. Indeed, the use of a chemical substance to achieve an altered mental state has been a prevalent practice in all civilizations and in all periods of time. In recent years, however, we have witnessed many such substances being produced and used across the world, including in India.

A brief description of common psychoactive (addictive) substances is discussed as below:

Alcohol

Alcoholic beverages contain ethyl alcohol as an 'active' ingredient. Different kinds of alcoholic beverages contain varying percentages of ethyl alcohol. 'Distilled spirits', also known as 'Indian Made Foreign Liquor' in India, include whisky, brandy, rum, vodka and gin. Their ethyl alcohol content ranges between 35-50% (usually about 42% in India). Some other kinds of beverages contain a comparatively lesser concentration of ethyl alcohol: beers contain around 4-8% and wines contain around 12%. The effect of drinking depends on the blood alcohol concentration, which, in turn, depends upon the amount consumed and the speed of consumption.

Alcohol is a general brain depressant. At lower blood levels, it leads to a reduction in anxiety, disinhibition and incoordination. At higher levels, loss of consciousness and even coma and death may occur. Besides the risk of accidents and violence under the influence of alcohol, long-term use of alcohol is associated with a wide variety of health risks.

Cannabis

Cannabis products are derived from the cannabis or hemp plant, which is commonly found in India. The type of cannabis preparation depends on which part of the plant is used to make it, each containing a varying concentration of active molecules. Bhang, the least potent preparation, is derived from dried leaves, while Ganja is the dried flowering stem of the plant. Charas, hashish or hash oil – the most potent preparations – are extracted from the plant's resin. Interestingly, while Bhang – used orally – is legally available in many states of India, other cannabis preparations (Ganja, Charas, etc., which are smoked) are illegal.

Cannabis consumption evokes a feeling of well-being and an altered state of reality. Other effects include delayed reflexes and impaired hand-eye coordination. As a result, certain actions, such as driving and operating heavy machinery, under its influence can have dangerous consequences. A user may experience a 'bad trip' characterized by a state of paranoia and heightened anxiety. Such symptoms and full-blown psychosis can be precipitated with the use of high-dose and high-potency preparations.

Opioids

Opioids are drugs that act on opioid receptors in the human body. Opium is a naturally occurring opioid that is extracted from the poppy plant. This plant is legally cultivated in India to manufacture medicines. Other opioids include natural products of the poppy plant (such as *doda* or *phukki* i.e. poppy husk) as well as chemicals extracted from the plant (such as morphine and codeine). There are some synthetically developed chemicals (not derived from the poppy plant), which act like

opioids too. The use of opioids leads to intense euphoria, pain relief and a dream-like state characterized by decreased responsiveness to the environment.

Heroin is the commonly used opioid in India. It is also called 'smack', 'brown sugar' or 'chitta'. The routes of its intake are smoking, chasing (inhaling the vapors obtained by heating heroin on an aluminum foil) and injecting. Opioids are very useful as medicines (as pain killers and cough suppressants), however, people may use prescription opioids for recreational use and may develop an addiction to them.

Nicotine

All tobacco products contain nicotine as their active ingredient. Being a stimulant, nicotine generally causes an increased sense of alertness. Regular users report irritability, restlessness, poor concentration and insomnia, especially while trying to quit. Smoking and chewing are common routes of use, but tobacco can also be applied to gums, sucked and gargled to derive desired effects. Consumption of tobacco products represents a significant public health risk factor globally.

Sedative/hypnotics

These medications are prescribed as sleeping pills and anxiolytics. They are also addictive if used without adequate medical supervision. Certain medications like diazepam, nitrazepam, alprazolam and pheniramine are widely used. These may be used either in tablet preparation, as injections or as cough syrups.

Cocaine

Cocaine is a common psychoactive substance used in western countries. It is extracted from the leaves of *Erythroxylon Coca*, a plant that grows in

Latin American countries. As of now, it is largely available only in some big cities in India, since it is very expensive. Cocaine is generally snorted in its white powdery form but can also be smoked. As a stimulant drug, cocaine causes a brief, intense and highly pleasurable feeling, which induces a strong urge to use it again.

Stimulants

Stimulants work by activating excitatory neurochemicals in the brain, leading to a state of high energy, alertness, intense joy and increased activity. Therefore, they are also used as performance-enhancing drugs. The prototype drug of this group is amphetamine, hence the name for the category 'Amphetamine Type Stimulants' (ATSs). They are also not commonly used in India but are gradually making inroads.

Hallucinogens

Hallucinogens are a group of drugs that alter reality and cause vivid sensory distortions and hallucinations. Due to these effects, they are called psychedelics. Examples include LSD (Lysergic Acid Diethyamide), PCP (Phencyclidine) and ecstasy. Their use is rather uncommon in India.

Inhalants

Inhalants are substances that evaporate at room temperature. Vapors are inhaled through mouth (huffing), nose (sniffing) and re-breathing from a bag (bagging). The calming sensation upon inhaling leads to repeated and continuous use. Glues, paint-thinners and petroleum products are essentially chemicals that are not designed to be ingested by humans. Long-term and heavy use of these products is harmful, leading to multi-organ damage. Nerve damage is also common. In India, these products are often used more by children and adolescents as opposed to adults and are a kind of entry drug to the development of addiction.

Is the Use of any Drug an Addiction?

It is important to recognize that while all the substances that we talked about are psychoactive or addictive, use of each of these will not necessarily lead to addiction. Many people are able to use some psychoactive substances without experiencing any negative effects. Some people may develop serious problems even with occasional use. It is necessary to differentiate between drug use and addiction (or drug use disorder).

- **Use:** Use is simply the ingestion of a psychoactive substance without experiencing any negative consequences. It may be social use (in parties), recreational use, experimentation and group activity by the youth, dietary practice or a part of religious or cultural ritual.
- **Harmful use:** If use becomes frequent, it can turn into 'harmful use', which can be a single episode or a pattern of use that causes damage to physical or mental health or results in behavior leading to harm to the health of others. Harm to the health of the individual may result from intoxication, toxic effects on body organs and systems or a harmful route of administration. Harm to the health of others includes physical harm or mental harm.
- **Dependence:** This is the final stage of the pattern of consumption of a psychoactive substance. Dependence is understood as a 'cluster of physiological, behavioral and cognitive phenomena in which use of a substance takes on a much higher priority than other behaviors that once had a greater value'. So, essentially, dependence is a pattern of use where the individual finds it difficult to stay away from the substance. Earlier, the term 'addiction' was used for dependence.

Together, the categories of harmful use and dependence constitute SUDs. SUDs are considered chronic non-communicable, relapsing health conditions, like diabetes, hypertension or depression, and need to be treated accordingly.

How common is substance use in India?

A substantial number of people use psychoactive substances in India, and substance use exists in all the population groups. Tobacco is the most commonly used psychoactive substance. About 29% of Indians (aged 15 years or more) consume tobacco, with smokeless tobacco (chewing) being a more common form compared to smoking. For other substances, the statistics on substance use in the 10-75-year-old population are provided in Table 1. After tobacco, alcohol is the commonest substance used in India. Among illegal or illicit drugs, the category of opioids (especially heroin) is the drug of most concern in India. Data also shows that there are wide variations in terms of statistics on drug use across various states in India. In general, substance use is higher among adult men, as compared to children and women.

Table 1. *Substance Use in India (general population, aged 10-75 years) ***

Substances	Prevalence of current use (in %)	Prevalence of harmful and dependent use (in %)
Alcohol	14.60	5.20
Opioid	2.06	0.70
Cannabis	2.83	0.66
Sedatives	1.08	0.20
Inhalants	0.70	0.21
Cocaine	0.10	0.02
Amphetamine type stimulants	0.18	0.02
Hallucinogens	0.12	0.03

*National Survey on Extent and Pattern of Substance Use in India (2019)

Box 1. Etiology of Addiction

Addiction has a complex etiology. It develops due to biological, psychological and environmental factors, which interact with each other and make a person susceptible to substance use and substance use disorders.

It is also important to note that India's figures for the prevalence of substance use are much lower than the global average in the case of most of the other substances. However, our opioid use prevalence (about 2.1%) is much higher than the global average (about 0.7%).

What are the Causes of Addiction? (BOX 1)

Genetic and biological causes

Substance use disorders have some genetic component, i.e. a person may be predisposed since birth to develop substance use problems. Such data is most widely available for alcohol as compared to other drugs.

Certain areas of the brain are responsible for generating a feeling of pleasure – 'the reward pathway'. These brain areas get activated after indulging in any activity, which is perceived as pleasurable or enjoyable (and hence, such activities are repeated!). In simpler terms, psychoactive substances act on the same mechanism of the brain, which is responsible for giving us pleasure. Over time, with repeated use, this pleasure area of the brain gets taken over by the psychoactive substances with the user experiencing various features of addiction.

Environmental causes

The ease of availability and social acceptability of a drug determines its popularity and pattern of use within a community. The cost plays a big role for legal or licit drugs, such as alcohol and tobacco. In the case of illicit drugs, such as heroin, scarcity of the drug causes many smokers to shift to injecting route of drug use as a way to make its use more economical. Another key environmental factor is the route of administration. Smoking and injecting result in instant drug delivery. This makes it more addictive than oral intake.

There are many social, cultural and legal factors that influence drug use and addiction. An individual's connectedness with his/her community plays a big part in his/her likelihood of using drugs. Certain parts of the world are considered 'dry regions' because alcohol use is prohibited due to various reasons, for example, Iran, Saudi Arabia, etc. Peer pressure is an important contributing factor to drug use initiation. Permissiveness at home towards a particular drug and family dysfunction are other contributing factors. Family conflict due to substance use by a family member can make the user feel targeted and can nudge him/her further towards the drug-using peer group. Incarceration

of drug users often leads them to learn to use harder drugs in jail, and thus punishment rarely works, as a deterrent for drug use.

Psychological causes

Self-medicating to relieve psychological pain is a common reason why people use drugs. For example, alcohol is commonly considered a social lubricant, and on the same spectrum, it is used to curb panic and social anxiety. The continued use of a drug for these reasons can lead to a harsh rebound of symptoms upon discontinuation and precipitation of psychiatric illness.

Each of the biological, environmental and psychological factors predispose to drug use directly or by aggravating other risk factors for addiction. A detailed inquiry into how addiction developed reveals a complex interplay of all these factors. The simple illustration below (Figure 1) shows how various factors contribute to the phenomenon of substance use.

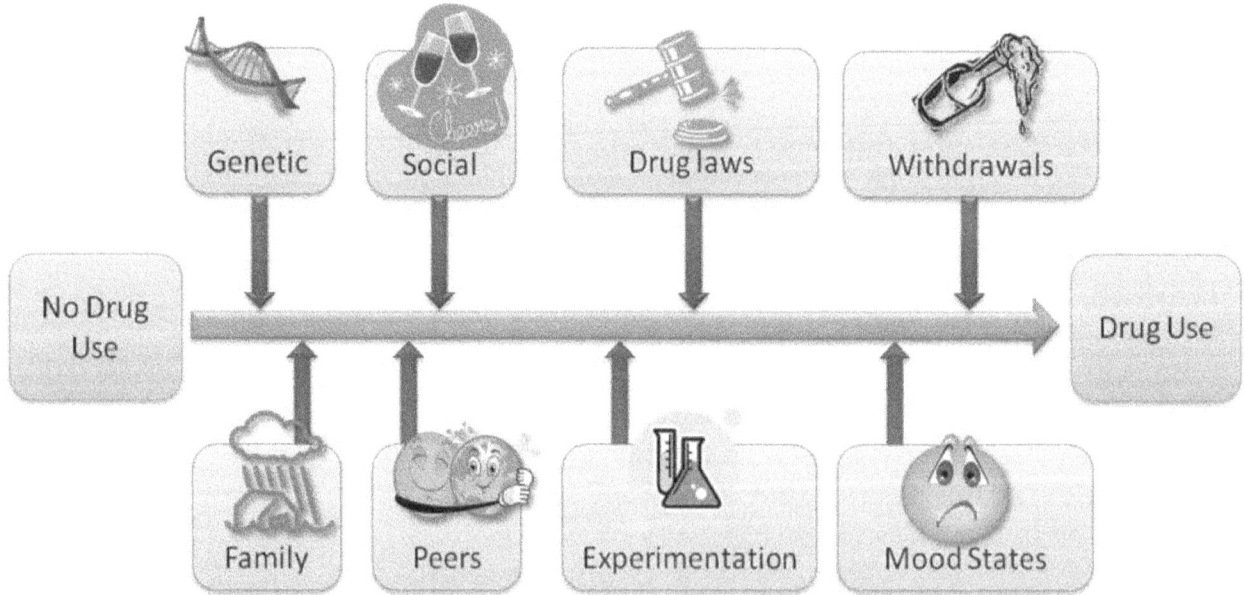

Figure 1. *Illustration Depicting Various Factors That Lead to Substance Use*

Source: Ambekar and Sinha-Deb (2011) *Problems of Substance Abuse (Block 1), MCFTE-003, Substance Abuse Counselling and Therapy*, New Delhi: Indira Gandhi National Open University

What are the Consequences of Substance Use?

Physical health consequences: Firstly, intoxication and overdose can have harmful consequences for physical health. For example, bingeing on alcohol can cause accidents, unconsciousness, severe vomiting, bleeding in the stomach and sedation, progressing to coma and ultimately death. Opioids, particularly when injected, are known to enhance the risk of overdose and death. Long-term drug use pervades all organ systems. Jaundice and liver diseases (alcohol), dementia (alcohol), cardiac problems (alcohol), cancer (tobacco and alcohol), asthma (tobacco), viral hepatitis and HIV infection (among those who inject drugs) represent only a tiny fraction of the list. Even sudden stoppage of drugs by a dependent user can cause severe physical symptoms in the withdrawal state, which sometimes may be fatal.

Mental health consequences: Many mental health conditions have a bi-directional relationship with substance use. Psychological problems and symptoms may be a factor underlying the use of psychoactive substances and vice-versa. Alcohol use is associated with the onset of depression and anxiety. Cannabis use is strongly linked to the onset of acute psychotic episodes and schizophrenia. Chronic opioid and amphetamine use can lead to depression and psychotic illness. Chronic drug use tends to worsen the course and prognosis of an underlying mental illness.

Social/familial/economic consequences: Drug use has a far-reaching impact on the entire community. The effect is all the more damaging because the demographic typically affected is the young adult male. Besides the direct cost of drug use, financial loss is compounded by reduced productivity at work, frequent absenteeism and job loss. Afflicted users drop out of school and college, which diminishes their future earning capacity. The health burden of drug use translates into a high economic burden due to hospitalization costs and disability due to physical complications. Stigma plays a major hurdle in recovery as it leads to reduced chances of employment and prevents re-assimilation into the community.

Substance use causes serious strain on family functioning. Family conflicts increase, financial difficulties worsen and no family member is able to escape the stigma related to drug use by one of their own. The entire community suffers due to increased crime rates, an unsafe environment within the community and an overall loss of productivity among its members.

Legal consequences: Substance users often suffer legal complications. If using illegal or banned drugs, they are often incarcerated and a life revolving in and out of jail follows, thereby severely hampering any gainful employment.

Is it Possible to Quit Taking Drugs?

As explained earlier, SUDs are chronic, relapsing health conditions. This implies that it is not easy for someone to quit taking drugs once they develop an addiction. However, this does not mean that people who are suffering from addiction do not want to quit taking drugs. Indeed, the inability to reduce or quit drug use despite making attempts to do so is a hallmark of addictions. So why do people find it difficult to quit?

Long-term use of psychoactive substances results in changes in the physiological functioning of many body organs, including the brain. Once a user develops a dependence on a drug, any attempt to reduce or quit results in the emergence of specific withdrawal symptoms. These withdrawal symptoms are highly distressing and painful (sometimes dangerous and potentially fatal), and hence force the user to continue taking drugs. Another common characteristic of SUDs is the presence of craving - the intense desire to use drugs. Withdrawal symptoms and cravings make it very difficult for the person to quit drug use without any external professional help, despite strong motivation to quit.

As we discussed earlier, SUDs are bio-psycho-social conditions, hence the treatment approaches also typically involve a combination of psychological, biological (i.e. medicines) and social strategies. Box 2 lists some of the important functions of medicines used for the treatment of SUDs. This treatment is best offered by trained mental health professionals. While all psychiatrists are qualified to provide treatment for addictions, some non-specialist doctors – after receiving appropriate training – can provide treatment to non-complicated cases too.

It is also important to note that treatment of addictions does not necessarily require hospitalization or admission to a 'de-addiction center'. In fact, a large majority of patients can be provided treatment at the outpatient level, involving consultation with a doctor and counselor, taking medications as advised by the doctor, making lifestyle changes and maintaining contact with the treatment providers.

Relapse (restarting drug use after quitting) is yet another distinctive feature of SUDs. Indeed, if not given appropriate long-term treatment, more than 80% of patients of SUDs may relapse within one year of quitting. This relapse does not indicate failure of treatment or poor motivation of the patient but is a part and parcel of the recovery process. Many patients, despite treatment, may go through multiple cycles of treatment-abstinence-relapse-treatment before achieving sustained recovery. As in all chronic conditions, the patient, family members and the treating team need to display patience and understanding in face of setbacks during the treatment process.

How can the Family Help?

Family members can play a very important role in preventing drug use and successfully quitting once someone develops an addiction. In general, a positive, supportive, loving and nurturing family environment acts as a protective factor against substance use. Once someone in the family develops substance use problems, it is important not to chide or punish the user but to provide support and care to help him/her quit. Indeed, stigma and discrimination are among the biggest hurdles for many patients who seek to come out of the clutches of addiction. Helping the patient access proper professional help and supporting him/her throughout the process of recovery is crucial. It is vital that all treatment and help is provided with explicit consent and knowledge of the patient. Forcing someone to undergo treatment or providing treatment without their knowledge (like slipping some pills in their food) is ineffective, dangerous, unethical and illegal. Box 3 summarizes various myths and facts related to drugs.

Conclusion

A substantial number of people across population groups use psychoactive substances and develop an addiction to them in India. Different psychoactive substances lead to varied mental and physical consequences. The treatment of addiction requires

---

Box 2. Role of Medicines in the Treatment of Substance Use Disorders (SUDs)

- Reversal of acute effects (intoxication and overdose)
- Relief from withdrawal symptoms
- Decline of craving
- Prevention of relapse
- Restoration of normal physiological functions

Box 3.   Substance Use: Myths and Facts

Myth	Fact
Drug users are people with bad character.	Substance use and addiction have multifactorial causation. Anyone can be affected by substance use disorders.
A small amount of alcohol is good for the health/heart.	Alcohol is toxic to the human body in any amount. No amount of alcohol use can be recommended as a health promotion strategy.
Illegal drugs are more harmful to health as compared to legal substances like alcohol and tobacco.	The legal status of a substance is a poor indicator of its health effects. Alcohol and tobacco are toxic to human health and have been ranked among the top harmful drugs.
People with addiction should be left alone and should not be mingled with.	Lack of interaction with non-substance using peers results in further isolation/enhanced influence of drug-using peers. A supportive social environment is helpful.
Putting people who use drugs in jail is a deterrent against using drugs.	Criminalizing substance use is not just ineffective but has been shown to be harmful to society.
Anyone can stop taking drugs anytime provided they have strong will-power.	While a strong motivation helps, withdrawal symptoms and many other factors make it difficult to quit without professional help for most of the patients. 'Will power' or motivation is a dynamic phenomenon; it keeps waxing and waning.
Treatment essentially involves admission to a de-addiction or rehabilitation center for a very long period.	Out-patient management can suffice for most patients; however, treatment needs to be continued over a long period.
Relapse indicates failure of treatment and/or poor motivation to quit.	Relapse is the part and parcel of the recovery process. Each instance of relapse brings the patient closer to sustained recovery.

long-term efforts as it is a chronic relapsing illness. Both pharmacological and psychosocial strategies are important, but the treatment must be provided by expert professionals with full consent and participation of the patients. With proper treatment and social support, a healthy and productive life free of addictions is indeed possible for all the affected patients.

KEY POINTS

➢ Drug use is very common and has been a part of society since ancient times.

➢ There are a number of myths and misconceptions associated with the use of drugs.

➢ Drug use has multiple harmful psychosocial and health effects.

➢ Persons who use drugs can be helped with treatment.

➢ Relapse of drug use following treatment is not to be feared upon since relapses can occur in any illness and can be treated.

REFERENCES

1. Alcohol and Depression. https://www.rcpsych.ac.uk/mental-health/problems-disorders/alcohol-and-depression

2. Ambekar A, Agrawal A, Rao R, Mishra AK, Khandelwal SK, Chadda RK on behalf of the group of investigators for the National Survey on Extent and Pattern of Substance Use in India (2019). Magnitude of Substance Use in India. New Delhi: Ministry of Social Justice and Empowerment, Government of India.

3. Cannabis and mental health: for young people. https://www.rcpsych.ac.uk/mental-health/parents-and-young-people/young-people/cannabis-and-mental-health-information-for-young-people

4. NIDA. 'Drugs, Brains, and Behavior: The Science of Addiction.' *National Institute on Drug Abuse*, 3 Aug. 2021, https://nida.nih.gov/publications/drugs-brains-behavior-science-addiction/preface Accessed 14 Feb. 2022.

5. United Nations Office on Drugs and Crime (UNODC) and World Health Organisation (WHO) (2008). Principles of Drug Dependence Treatment. Retrieved from https://www.who.int/publications/i/item/principles-of-drug-dependence-treatment

CHAPTER 10

Behavioral Addictions

Pawan Sharma and Yatan Pal Singh Balhara

Introduction

Traditionally, addictions have been associated with the use of alcohol, tobacco and other drugs (collectively called psychoactive substances). The term 'addiction' is used to represent a pattern of use of substances that can alter one or more functions of the mind, characterized by loss of control after the use of these substances. Moreover, this pattern often continues despite harmful consequences. It has been observed that besides the consumption of psychoactive substances, there are certain behaviors that offer a rewarding experience. Consequently, one repeatedly engages in these behaviors despite awareness and experience of adverse consequences. 'Behavioral addictions' is the term used to represent such patterns. Behavioral addictions are similar to addictions to alcohol, tobacco and other drugs. A major difference between the two is that while addiction to psychoactive substances involves the use of alcohol, tobacco or another drug, behavioral addictions, as indicated in the name, have a prominent behavioral focus.

Definition

Behavioral addictions have clinical features somewhat similar to that seen in cases with addiction to alcohol, tobacco and other drugs (psychoactive substances), but with a behavioral focus rather than consumption of a psychoactive substance. Behavioral addictions are also known as non-substance addictions. While behavioral addictions do not involve the use of alcohol, tobacco

and other drugs (psychoactive substances), some core indicators of behavioral addiction are similar to those of psychoactive substance addiction.

Types of Behavioral Addictions

There is no widely accepted formal classification of behavioral addictions. Different types of behavioral addictions have been described in the literature. The most commonly reported behaviors that have been described to have a potential to cause addiction are excessive internet use, gambling, video gaming, excessive use of mobile phones or social media, excessive sexual behavior, excessive buying and shopping, or excessive eating and food consumption. Some reports have suggested the possibility of the addictive nature of excessive exercise and excessive work. The commonly reported and widely studied behavioral addictions include gambling disorder, gaming disorder and internet addiction (also called problematic internet use). In recent years, there is an increase in reporting of mobile addiction, social media addiction, pornography addiction, shopping addiction and food addiction. Box 1 lists some of the common behavioral addictions.

Burden, Prevalence, Treatment Gap and Its Reasons and Consequences If Untreated

Behavioral addictions have been identified as an emerging public health problem globally. There is variability in the reported incidence rates of

Box 1. Commonly Reported Behavioral Addictions

- Gambling disorder
- Gaming disorder (including internet gaming disorder)
- Internet addiction
- Mobile addiction
- Social media addiction
- Shopping addiction
- Sex addiction
- Food addiction

Table 1. *Commonly reported co-occurring psychiatric disorders and substance use disorders with behavioral addictions*

Anxiety disorders	Panic disorder with or without agoraphobia
	Generalized anxiety disorder
	Social anxiety disorder
	Specific phobia
Mood disorders	Depressive disorder
	Dysthymia
	Bipolar disorder
Substance use disorders	Nicotine dependence
	Alcohol use disorders
	Other substance use disorders
Personality disorders	Antisocial personality disorder
Childhood externalizing disorders	Attention deficit hyperactivity disorder (ADHD)
	Conduct disorder
Sleep disorders	Insomnia
	Sleep-wake cycle disturbances

behavioral addiction from different parts of the world. The prevalence of generalized internet addiction is documented to be about 7%. The worldwide prevalence of gaming disorder is around 3%. The pooled prevalence of internet gaming disorder among adolescents is estimated to be around 4.6%. The prevalence of gambling disorder is as high as 11% among older adults and up to 12 % among adolescents.

Additionally, behavioral addictions are commonly associated with a range of psychiatric disorders and substance use disorders. The most frequently reported co-occurring psychiatric and substance use disorders among persons with behavioral addictions include anxiety disorders, mood disorders, personality disorders, sleep disturbance and childhood externalizing disorders (Table 1). These co-occurring psychiatric and substance use disorders may play a contributory role in the emergence of certain behavioral addictions. Conversely, co-occurring psychiatric and substance use disorders may also be the consequence of behavioral addiction. Also, these can coexist without any causal association.

Despite an increasing focus on behavioral addictions in the past decade, the proportion of patients seeking help for these disorders remains low. There are many factors that contribute to the

treatment gap for behavioral addictions. First, there is limited awareness about behavioral addictions in the general population. Many behavioral addictions involve behaviors that constitute normal behavior in day-to-day living. These include gaming, shopping and eating, among others. Consequently, such behaviors, even when excessive and associated with adverse consequences, do not lead to consideration of the possibility of an underlying mental health problem. Second, the motivation of those experiencing behavioral addictions for help-seeking can be poor due to the inherent pleasurable and gratifying nature of such behaviors. Third, the clinical services for the management of behavioral addictions remain limited.

Behavioral addictions, if left untreated, have been associated with many adverse consequences. These adverse consequences can be observed in different domains, including physical health, mental health, or familial, social, academic, occupational,

Table 2. *Adverse consequences associated with behavioral addictions*

Physical health	Mental health	Familial	Social	Academic/ Occupational	Financial	Legal
- Obesity - Visual problems - Musculoskeletal problems - Headache - Seizures	- Sleep disturbances - Increased aggressiveness - Enuresis - Encopresis - Depressive and/or anxiety features and disorders	- Interpersonal discord - Familial altercations	- Stigma	- Absenteeism - Poor academic performance - Poor work performance	- Loss of savings - Debt	- Certain behaviors are illegal (e.g. gambling in many parts of the country)

financial and even legal spheres. Some of the adverse consequences associated with behavioral addictions are listed in Table 2.

Identification

Characteristic features of behavioral addictions include repeated engaging in the behavior, remaining preoccupied with the addictive behavior, short-lasting satiation, impaired control, preoccupation with the behavior, experiencing negative consequences and continued engagement in behavior despite adverse consequences.

Behavioral addictions have six major components, namely salience, mood modification, tolerance, withdrawal, conflict and relapse, which are briefly elaborated below (Figure 1):

- **Salience** means that the behavior is the single most important activity in one's life and dominates one's thought process, emotions and actions.
- **Mood modification** refers to the experiences that one reports because of engaging in the activity.
- **Tolerance** is the process where increasing indulgence in the behavior is needed to experience the mood-modifying effects.

- **Withdrawal symptoms** are the unpleasant emotional and/or physical states that are experienced when one is not able to engage in the desired behavior.

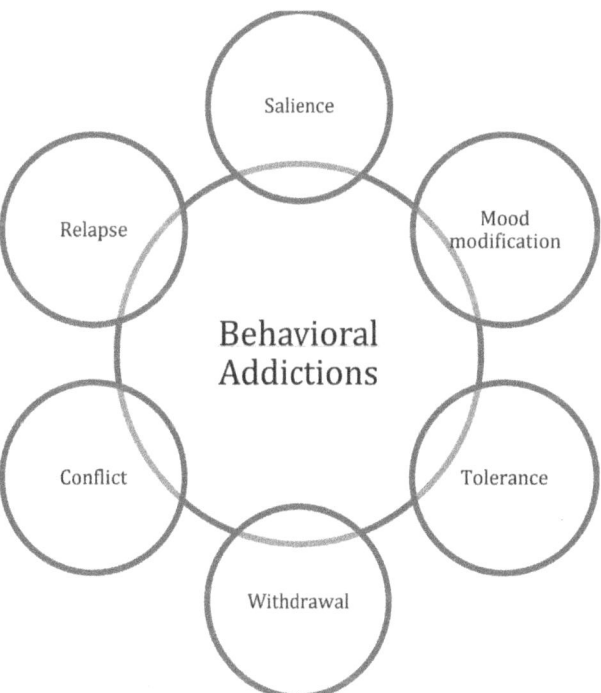

Figure 1. *Components of Behavioral Addictions*

- **Conflict** can reflect in different contexts. First, it can be between the person and those around. Second, it can be with other activities, like job, social life, leisure time activities and interests. Third, it can be from within, also called intrapsychic conflict, leading to a feeling of loss of control.

- **Relapse** means repeatedly reverting back to previous patterns of excessive behavior.

It is important to differentiate behavioral addiction from common behaviors that humans engage in. Certain pointers may help with the early identification of behavioral addictions, which are listed below:

- The behavior tends to be excessive and is engaged in despite potential adverse consequences or neglect of alternate responsibilities and/or interests
- Efforts to hide the behavior
- It is difficult to resist the desire to engage in the behavior
- Engaging in the behavior with an aim to handle stress or challenging emotions
- Becoming defensive when confronted about the behavior
- Feeling an excessive amount of guilt after engaging in the behavior
- Promising to reduce or stop the behavior but not being able to do so
- Getting irritated or upset when not able to engage in the behavior

The presence of one or more of these features in the context of excessive engagement in a particular behavior is a pointer toward the possibility of behavioral addiction.

Myths

While the concept of behavioral addiction is relatively new, there are many myths around behavioral addictions.

- **While addiction to tobacco, alcohol and other substances has been associated with withdrawals, the occurrence of withdrawals in the context of behavioral addictions remains debatable.** While those with behavioral addictions might not experience physical discomfort when they are not able to engage in the specific behavior, they may experience agitation, irritability, unhappiness, low mood, etc. as a part of withdrawal.

- **Behavioral addictions are restricted to teenagers and are not observed among people from other age groups.** While certain behavioral addictions are more common among adolescents (e.g., gaming disorder), behavioral addictions are not restricted to a particular age group and can be experienced across diverse age ranges.

- **There is often a blurring of the boundaries between normal or normative behaviors and behavioral addictions.** The fact that many of the behaviors that are associated with behavioral addictions are engaged in by a large section of the population as a normal behavior does not necessarily preclude the possibility that some of those who engage in these behaviors might end up developing addictions.

There is a common misunderstanding and lack of awareness about the role of therapeutic interventions in the management of behavioral addictions. An increasing body of research has explored the interventions that can be offered to help those with behavioral addictions. Hence, it is important to seek professional consultation at the earliest when indicated.

Self-help interventions for behavioral addictions

Self-help strategies can be used to prevent the development of behavioral addictions (Box 2). Also, self-help interventions are used to manage these disorders. One needs to be aware of the addictive potential of certain behaviors. There

---

Box 2.   Self-Help Strategies for Behavioral Addictions

- Be aware of potential adverse consequences associated with behavioral addictions
- Engage with technology (mobile phones, internet, social media) in an age- and context-appropriate manner
- Have a balanced lifestyle
- Engage in gaming, internet use and social media use at specified times (avoid use at night)
- Learn and practice emotion regulation techniques
- Do not use social media as a substitute for in-person interactions
- Do not engage in the use of the internet, mobile phones and social media in contexts and situations where it may be hazardous and interfere with other responsibilities
- Seek help from family, friends and mental health professionals in case a problem emerges
- Parents should be aware of the extent and pattern of use of the internet and mobile devices by their children

is a need to be cognizant of the reasons behind engaging in such behaviors, the amount of time spent and the level of control one has over such behaviors. One should try to strike a balance between different responsibilities and leisure activities and should ensure that engagement in a particular behavior does not become detrimental to other activities.

Family members and caregivers also play a crucial role here. They can help identify the problematic behavior early by noticing the daily routines, moods, preferences and changes in interests. They can play a crucial role in identifying the mental health professional to seek professional help as well as support the therapeutic adherence by reminding about the medications and appointments. The family members and caregivers can also help with the homework assignments that are offered as part of the treatment process. The family members and caregivers are also crucial in offering the much-needed support. For those who have developed a behavioral addiction, such as a gambling disorder, self-help groups such as Gamblers Anonymous (GA) have been established that offer intervention based on a 12-step program model. In addition, individual and self-directed options, such as

bibliotherapy (e.g., workbooks), internet-based interventions, telephone-based interventions or in-person therapy, have also been developed to manage certain behavioral addictions. For the cases of internet gaming disorder and internet addiction, some approaches like interactive web-based self-help using principles of motivational interviewing are available.

Whom to/Where to Approach?

It is recommended to seek help as early as possible if you are experiencing a behavioral addiction. A delay in help-seeking is likely to add to the distress and dysfunction and is not advisable. Help-seeking can be initiated by the person with behavioral addiction or by their family members and caregivers. Excessive engagement in one or more behavior that is associated with loss of control, preoccupation and adverse consequences warrants a consultation with a health professional (Figure 2). Several screening tools are available for the purpose of identification of those who are likely to have a behavioral addiction. However, the final diagnosis of behavioral addiction is made only after a detailed clinical evaluation.

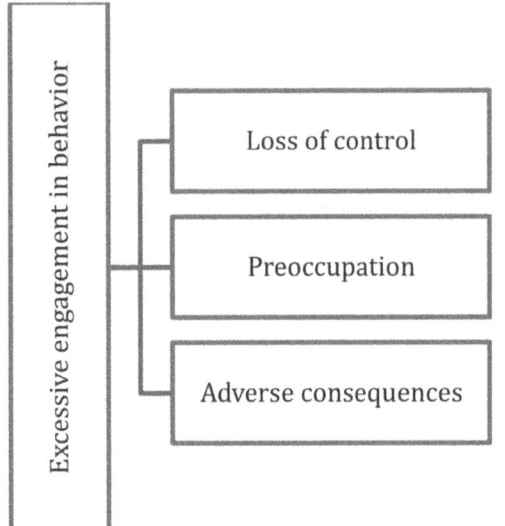

Figure 2. *Indicators for Seeking Professional Help*

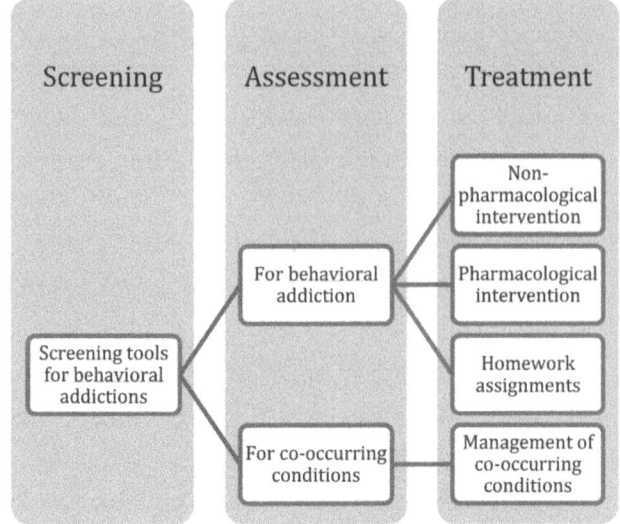

Figure 3. *Scheme of Management of Behavioral Addictions*

Available Treatment

Management of behavioral addictions begins with a detailed evaluation. Such assessment helps in confirming the diagnosis of behavioral addiction. The assessment involves gathering information from different sources, including the patient, family members, friends, other caregivers and teachers' reports. Previous medical records, if any, are also reviewed. Besides the identification of the behavioral addiction, the assessment is also aimed at identifying any associated mental and substance use disorder. The adverse consequences experienced due to the behavioral addiction are also documented. Further investigations and evaluation are guided by the presence of indicators of adverse health consequences during history taking and clinical examination.

Once the diagnosis of behavioral addiction is established, the treatment begins (Figure 3). An integrated approach with a mix of non-pharmacological and pharmacological interventions is recommended. Various non-pharmacological interventions have been studied for their effectiveness in the management of behavioral addictions. These interventions are based on principles of motivational therapy, cognitive behavioral therapy, relapse prevention and contingency management, time management, coping skills training and identification of alternate interests. Certain medications have also been studied for this purpose. The treatment is extended over at least a few sessions. The required number of sessions is determined by the underlying diagnosis, severity of the ailment, presence of co-occurring disorders, choice of treatment modality and rate of response. The therapy is usually supplemented with homework exercises. Treatment is also initiated for the co-occurring mental and substance use disorders, if any. Retention in treatment and adherence are important predictors of the outcome of the treatment. For those who are not well motivated to enter the treatment, there are specific interventions targeted at building the motivation.

Treatment for behavioral addictions can be sought from mental health professionals. Some specialized clinics catering to the needs of persons with behavioral addictions (Behavioral Addictions Clinic) have also been set up all over the country, although the number of such clinics is low.

Conclusion

Behavioral addictions are a growing public health problem. Various types of behavioral addictions have been identified. It is important to demarcate behavioral addictions from normal behaviors. Behavior addictions are associated with adverse effects in various domains, including physical and mental health, and in family, social, academic, occupational, financial and legal areas. Certain myths around behavioral addictions, coupled with limited awareness, lead to a delay in help-seeking for these problems. Family members and other caregivers play a crucial role in early detection and help-seeking. Treatment for behavioral addictions can be sought from mental health professionals.

KEY POINTS

➢ Behavioral addictions, while a relatively new concept, are a growing public health problem.

➢ Behavioral addictions, if left untreated, can lead to significant distress and dysfunction in multiple domains.

➢ There is limited awareness about behavioral addictions that contributes to delayed help-seeking.

➢ Early and effective intervention can help in reducing the dysfunction.

➢ Treatment for behavioral addictions can be sought from mental health professionals and specialized behavioral addiction clinics.

REFERENCES

1. Grant JE, Potenza MN, Weinstein A, Gorelick DA. Introduction to Behavioral Addictions. Am J Drug Alcohol Abuse. 2010;36(5):233–41.

2. Mudry ET, C. Hodgins D, el-Guebaly N, Cameron Wild T, Colman I, B Patten S, et al. Conceptualizing Excessive Behaviour Syndromes: A Systematic Review. Current Psychiatry Reviews. 2011 1;7(2):138–51.

3. Griffiths MD. Classification and treatment of behavioural addictions. Nursing in Practice. 2015; (82):44–6.

4. Balhara YPS, Bhargava R, Chadda RK. Service Development for Behavioural Addictions: AIIMS Experience. Ann Natl Acad Med Sci. 2017;53(3):131–9.

CHAPTER 11

Suicide Prevention

Roy Abraham Kallivayalil and Bettina Sara Mathew

'But in the end, one needs more courage to live than to kill himself.' — Albert Camus

Introduction

Suicide is a major public health problem. Both attempted as well as completed suicides are a great source of distress to the families affected. Suicidal behaviors include suicidal ideation, attempts and completed suicide.

Suicide has a long-term impact on the individual, the family, and the community. Suicidal behavior varies across various age groups, gender, geographic region and socio-political groups, and is associated with a range of risk factors. Many cases of suicide can be prevented by timely intervention. Early recognition, enhanced knowledge and improved understanding of clinical, psychological, sociological and biological factors related to various aspects of suicide may enable the detection of high-risk individuals and assist in providing appropriate interventions.

Suicide can be defined as an act of deliberate self-harm with a fatal outcome. The word 'suicide' is derived from the Latin words *sui* and *caedere*, which together translate to 'self-murder'. Suicidal ideation, often called suicidal thought or idea, is a broader term used to describe a range of phenomena, like contemplation, preoccupation and wishes of death and suicide. Suicide attempts are included in the wider definition of self-harm, which means self-inflicted physical harm with or without an intention to die.

How Common is Suicide?

The WHO Global Burden of Disease study estimates that approximately 703,000 persons die by suicide globally every year. This counts to around one suicide every 40 seconds. The global age-standardized suicide rate was 9.0 per 100,000 people according to the census in 2019 and low- and middle-income countries accounted for 77% of suicides that occurred worldwide (Figure 1). Over one in every 100 deaths (1.3%) were due to suicide, making it the 17th leading cause of death in 2019.

The lifetime prevalence of suicidal ideations ranges between 14-18% and about 1 in 9 adults with suicidal ideations make a suicide attempt. The number of suicide attempts is considered to be 10–30 times higher compared to completed suicides. Pesticide ingestion is the method opted in around one-fifth (20%) of all suicides. Hanging and firearms are the other common methods of suicide.

Suicide and Mental Health

The prevalence of suicide is found to be at least 10 times higher in individuals with mental disorders than in the general population. Around 90% of the persons committing suicide suffer from a mental disorder with depression often in the background. Depression is also found in more than half of the individuals who attempt suicide. Substance abuse, specifically alcohol misuse, is also strongly associated with suicide risk, especially in older adolescents and young adult males. Alcohol

Global Suicide Mortality Rates

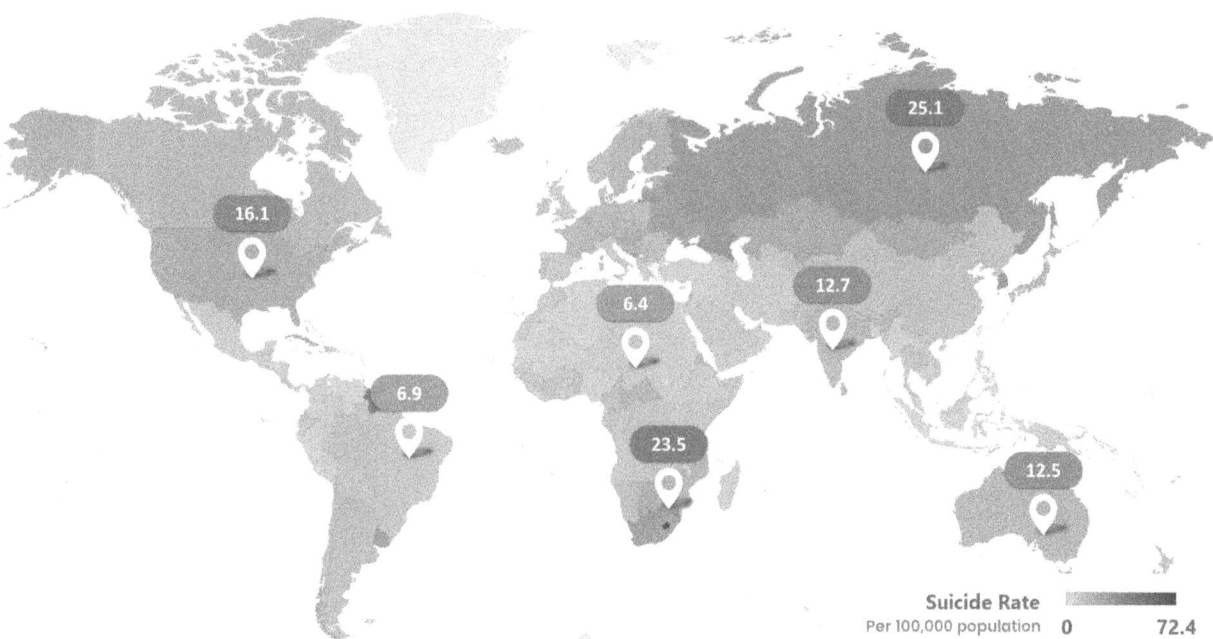

Figure 1. *Global Suicide Mortality Rates. Source: (Suicide Worldwide in 2019: Global Health Estimates, WHO 2021)*

intoxication increases suicidality, especially when related to adjustment disorders (e.g., bereavement) and depression. Around 30–40% of people who die by suicide have personality disorders, such as borderline or antisocial personality disorder. The risk of suicide is also high in patients with schizophrenia and bipolar disorder. In general, the comorbidities of mental disorders substantially increase suicide risk, especially the presence of mood and substance use disorders.

Risk Factors for Suicide

Social, physical and environmental factors

Social isolation and lack of adequate support from the community are associated with the increasing rates of suicide. Various cultural and religious views on suicide, such as considering suicide as a noble solution to problems, are seen in some societies. Traumatic events and interpersonal stressors occurring in adulthood are also found to

influence the rates. Financial and legal difficulties have also been found to be in the background of many suicides.

Physical illnesses, like chronic obstructive pulmonary disease (COPD) and asthma; cardiovascular diseases, such as coronary heart disease and stroke; or chronic diseases, like inflammatory bowel disease, migraine, epilepsy and brain injuries, are recognized to contribute to the risk of suicide.

The stigma associated with mental illness prevents people to approach mental health care providers. The lack of adequate availability and accessibility of these resources, especially in the low- and middle-income countries, adds to the problem. Migration and other changes in social structure have also been found to contribute to the increasing rates of suicide. Easy access to lethal means, such as firearms, medications and pesticides, further increases the risk for suicide.

Portrayals of suicide by the media by publicizing celebrity suicides and romanticizing suicides with little importance given to their association with

Risk Factors & Steps in Suicide

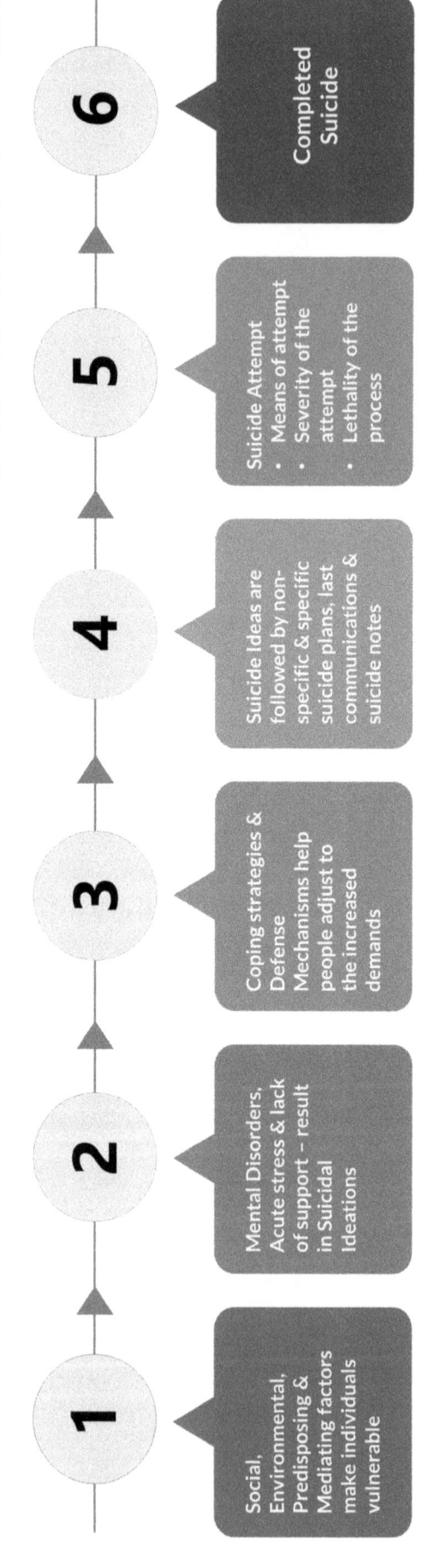

Social Factors
- Rapid societal change
- Social isolation
- Religious views
- Economic crisis
- Stigma
- Media Reporting

Environmental Factors
- Poor access to mental health care
- Easy access to lethal means
- Sunlight duration

Predisposing Factors
- Family history of Suicides
- Early life adversity
- Vulnerability to stress
- Genetic and epigenetic factors

Mediating Factors
- Chronic substance use
- Personality
- Cognitive deficits
- Increased vulnerability to stress

1
Social, Environmental, Predisposing & Mediating factors make individuals vulnerable

2
Mental Disorders, Acute stress & lack of support – result in Suicidal Ideations

3
Coping strategies & Defense Mechanisms help people adjust to the increased demands

4
Suicide Ideas are followed by non-specific & specific suicide plans, last communications & suicide notes

5
Suicide Attempt
- Means of attempt
- Severity of the attempt
- Lethality of the process

6
Completed Suicide

Figure 2. *Risk Factors and Steps in Suicide*

mental illness and its consequences on survivors also add to suicide rates, particularly among adolescents and young adults.

Individual factors

Several studies done over the years show that a history of mental illness, especially suicide in the family, serves as a definite risk factor for suicide attempts. Specific genes linked to suicidal risk are being identified, though the results are still elusive. Exposure to early life adversities is another well-acknowledged risk factor, which includes parental neglect, childhood physical, sexual or emotional abuse and chronic poverty. It may induce long-term effects through epigenetic changes in specific gene pathways.

Personality traits and cognitive styles have been noticed to mediate suicidal behavior. Impulsivity, aggressive behavior, conduct disorder, antisocial behavior and substance abuse are more prominent in adolescents and young adults with suicidal behavior. Negative affect and anxiety traits are also observed in those with a suicide attempt. A previous suicide attempt is the strongest risk factor for death by suicide. Cognitive deficits, such as poor problem solving, decision making and coping skills, also mediate the risk.

There is usually a temporal association between precipitating factors and suicide. The presence of psychopathology is an important predictor of suicide. Major depressive disorder, bipolar disorder, schizophrenia and personality disorders especially increase the risk of suicide.

In addition, other factors such as age, gender, marital status and geographic location also influence suicide. Suicide attempts are more often seen in the younger age group, particularly in females. However, the rates of completed suicides are over twice as high among men than among women. Suicide rates are high among vulnerable groups who are subjected to discrimination, including refugees, migrants, prisoners, indigenous people and individuals from the lesbian, gay, bisexual and transsexual groups. Figure 2 summarizes the risk factors and steps in suicide.

Levels for Suicide Prevention

Suicide prevention can be divided into three levels:

- *Primary:* Primary prevention aims to provide programs and services to prevent a suicide attempt. It focuses on reducing the risk factors and promoting the protective factors associated with suicide.
- *Secondary:* Secondary prevention aims to provide programs and services after an attempted or completed suicide. It addresses the short-term impact and effects of suicide.
- *Tertiary:* Tertiary prevention programs and services are long-term responses and plans to address the after-effects and consequences of suicide and suicide attempts, such as providing care for suicide survivors and the affected families, and regular follow-up to prevent further harm.

Box 1 summarizes the warning signs for suicide and Box 2 summarizes the protective factors for suicide.

Planning Suicide Prevention

Suicide prevention requires a comprehensive multi-centric approach that involves coordination across various systems, organizations, communities, cultures and environments to develop high-quality mental health care. Persons with suicide risk have an underlying mental health problem and need active intervention by mental health professionals.

Some of the strategies used for suicide prevention are discussed below (Box 3):

Raising public awareness: Awareness campaigns need to be conducted to improve public knowledge

---

Box 1.   Warning Signs for Suicide

Warning Signs
- ✓ Expressing suicidal feelings, well-formed plans
- ✓ Making preparations, such as making a will, putting affairs in order, giving away valuable possessions, suicide note
- ✓ Depression or other psychiatric illnesses
- ✓ Increased motivation after starting antidepressants
- ✓ Increased alcohol/drug use
- ✓ Marked hopelessness
- ✓ Feeling burdensome to others
- ✓ Strong feelings of guilt and shame
- ✓ Sense of entrapment
- ✓ Withdrawing from activities
- ✓ Isolating from friends and family
- ✓ Taking dangerous risks
- ✓ Recent trauma or life crisis

Box 2.   Protective Factors for Suicide

Protective Factors
- ✓ Positive social support
- ✓ Spirituality
- ✓ Sense of responsibility to family
- ✓ Children at home, pregnancy
- ✓ Life satisfaction
- ✓ Reality testing ability
- ✓ Positive coping skills
- ✓ Positive problem-solving skills
- ✓ Positive therapeutic relationship
- ✓ Availability of physical and mental health care

Box 3.   Strategies for Suicide Prevention

Strategies for Suicide Prevention
- ➢ Leadership by mental health professionals
- ➢ Public awareness
- ➢ Training general medical practitioners
- ➢ Gatekeeper training
- ➢ School-based interventions
- ➢ 24-hour helpline services
- ➢ Responsible media coverage
- ➢ Restriction of suicide means
- ➢ Proper screening, assessment and management
- ➢ Follow-up care

Policy measures: Legislations on decriminalizing suicide, setting regulations to prevent excessive use of alcohol and other substances, restricting access to lethal means, coverage of mental health conditions in health insurance policies and ensuring provision for adequate mental health care services are some proactive steps to prevent suicide.

Service development: The primary care setting and the emergency department are key areas where suicide screening must be implemented. Depression is often under-recognized and inadequately treated. Individuals with depression may present in these settings with complaints, like malaise, aches, fatigue and poor appetite. The associated psychosocial stressors often remain unidentified. Hence, sensitizing the primary health care staff to suicide risk detection would help in early identification and timely intervention. Emergency room doctors need to be trained for sensitive and empathetic handling of persons who have attempted suicide and to provide clear referrals to mental health services. Nurses and community health workers can also be included in the training to identify suicidal behaviors and provide immediate support to a person

about mental health and suicide prevention. This may change the attitude toward mental illness and help in better recognition of and accessing treatment services.

experiencing suicidal distress. The primary care setting and the emergency department are thus the key areas where suicide screening needs to be implemented.

Gatekeeper training: The term 'gatekeeper' refers to 'individuals in a community who have face-to-face contact with large numbers of community members as part of their usual routine'. As timely access to mental health professionals can be difficult at times, these individuals can be trained to identify persons at risk of suicide and refer them for appropriate management. Community, organizational and institutional gatekeepers, such as religious leaders, police officers, teachers, coaches, and those who work in prisons, juvenile detention, welfare centers, workplaces and homes for the elderly, can be trained. The gatekeepers can be educated about the suicidal burden, risk factors, warning signs, support system available, signs of depression, and communication and counseling skills to address the at-risk population.

School-based interventions: School mental health programs can go a long way via early identification of mental health issues and relevant interventions in school children. This can improve their mental well-being and also reduce the suicidal risk in long term.

24-hour helpline services: Access to 24-hour crisis care is one of the most important aspects of mental health service provision in the prevention of suicide. Telephonic and internet-based suicide hotlines are useful, where professionals/people with focused training can provide brief psychotherapy and crisis intervention. These services can allow time for the crisis to dissipate and provide appropriate referral pathways for further clinical assessment and intervention.

Impact of media: The influence of media has expanded over the years. Suicides are often sensationalized with explicit descriptions and details. Hence, media guidelines for reporting and portraying suicides should be followed. Media coverage can be done collaboratively between media professionals and mental health professionals for better dissemination and impact. Neutral and discreet reporting, keeping in mind the possible psychological harm to survivors is suggested. Public awareness of mental illnesses and suicide prevention can also be promoted with the help of the media. Providing knowledge, de-stigmatizing mental illness, and encouraging people to approach mental health professionals in time of need can be well-communicated through media.

Assessment and management: When an individual with suicidal behavior approaches a mental health care professional, a detailed assessment is conducted, focusing on:

➤ Suicide risk
➤ Clinical diagnosis
➤ Developing a treatment plan

Risk assessment. It involves building a therapeutic relationship and alliance with the patient, identifying risk factors and formulating the risk by clinical judgment. An individualized non-judgmental approach needs to be followed with warmth and empathy, along with consideration of the cultural factors. This helps in establishing a strong therapeutic relationship. The person can then be asked about suicidal ideation and plan.

Identifying the modifiable risk factors. The risk can then be stratified into low, medium or high risk and acute or chronic risk depending on the lethality, intentionality and inimicality of the suicide act. Modifiable risk factors are identified

Safety planning. It involves a set of strategies designed to help a person identify and cope when in a suicidal crisis. **'No suicide contracts' - making a commitment not to die by suicide until the next session** or that he or she will not enact suicidal behavior without first contacting the clinician - may be implemented. The person may need hospitalization depending on the degree of risk. The caregivers and family members are always involved in the process.

Effective treatment and long-term care for those with mental illness are likely to decrease the rates of suicide. The line of treatment varies according to the clinical diagnosis.

People who have made suicide attempts are at increased risk of making further attempts and of dying by suicide, especially in the first three months following a suicide attempt. Thus, it is important to keep the patient on regular follow up and the family members need to be cautioned about maintaining adherence to treatment and keeping the patient under constant supervision till full recovery.

Certain Policy Measures for Suicide Prevention

Restriction on methods to commit suicide is an effective strategy to reduce suicidal risk. Impulsivity is a component of suicide, and therefore, restricting access to lethal means can enable the suicidal thoughts to alleviate. It is a beneficial strategy to curb suicidal behaviors, as it addresses large populations including those in whom the risk remains undetected.

Some such measures include legislation restricting access to firearms, installing barriers at jumping hotspots (bridges, balconies in high rise buildings and towers) and CCTV at other prone sites, restricting the availability of pesticides and limiting over-the-counter availability of medicines and short duration prescriptions of high-risk drugs by doctors.

Public health measures can contribute to suicide prevention through the promotion of protective factors and environments. Financial and housing security issues must be addressed by the governments and community leaders. Social services and support can reduce isolation, promote life skills and provide practical support to vulnerable individuals and families to improve their quality of life. People from vulnerable communities can face additional barriers in accessing support, including language and cultural differences, experiences of discrimination, religious beliefs or concerns about confidentiality. Hence special attention needs to be given to these vulnerable individuals.

Suicide and the Media

The media has a paramount role in suicide prevention. The effect of media reports on increasing suicides is often referred to as the 'Werther effect', after the title character in Goethe's novel 'The Sorrows of Young Werther', who died by suicide, which, in turn, had a mass effect on the people who later committed the act. The terms suicide contagion and copycat suicide are common synonyms. Studies have demonstrated that it is not just the content of the news but its placement and prominence (defined as reporting inside special boxes, the news printed on the front page, and the word 'suicide' in the headline) can also influence copycat suicides.

The influence of the media, especially social media has increased manifold in the present era. Hence it is necessary that the media - print, visual and social - exercise caution and observe certain dos and don'ts.:

- There should not be sensational headlines, photos, video footage or social media links when reporting suicides.

- Details of methods, personal information, details of site or location, sensational details and repetition of the news should be avoided.
- The media should provide accurate information on where to seek help and educate the public on suicide prevention.
- Extreme caution should be exercised when reporting on celebrity suicides and when bereaved family members and friends are interviewed.

Are Suicides Preventable?

There is no doubt that almost all suicides are preventable. Hence, what should be the appropriate strategy based on available scientific evidence?

Eighty percent of people who commit suicide, do so due to emotional and mental problems. Depression is the single biggest cause of suicide. Depressive illness is treatable. Getting professional help, thus, remains crucial. The National Mental Survey of India of 2016 has reported that nearly 85% of the patients with depression remain untreated in India. Reasons include lack of awareness about the illness, stigma or lack of adequate mental health care facilities. Thus, creating awareness about mental health issues, the need for treatment and strengthening the mental health care systems remain important strategies for suicide prevention.

Statements expressing suicidal intent should never be taken lightly since these indicate a cry for help.

Conclusion

Suicide is a major public health problem and needs prompt preventive approaches with public participation. Educating community gatekeepers, like teachers, clergy and social workers, and promoting mental health in workplaces, prisons and offices is important. Providing help after a suicidal attempt, opening crisis intervention centers, suicide prevention centers and telephone helplines are all very useful. There needs to be a collaboration between schools, health services, social services and law enforcement agencies to provide health promotion and suicide prevention strategies among children and young people. Individual interventions and providing psychiatric treatment alone are not enough. Understanding human misery, poverty and denial of human rights, and finding a solution for these is going to be of long-term help. Increasing mental health literacy, increasing access to mental health care and reducing the stigma about mental health problems are important strategies. Undoubtedly, population-based interventions are the key to success.

KEY POINTS

➢ Most cases of suicide can be prevented.

➢ Mental illnesses, like depression, bipolar disorder and schizophrenia are associated with an increased risk of suicide.

➢ A suicidal attempt or expression of suicidal intent is a cry for help and should not be taken lightly.

➢ Persons with suicide risk or a history of suicide attempts need detailed psychiatric assessment and treatment.

➢ The media can play an important role by not publicizing the cases of suicide, especially regarding the methods used.

➢ Restricting access to methods of suicide has been found to be an effective strategy for preventing suicides.

REFERENCES

1. Suicide. https://www.who.int/news-room/fact-sheets/detail/suicide

2. Kallivayalil RA, Punnoose VP. Suicide Prevention: A Handbook for Community Gatekeepers. May 2009. National Alliance for Mental Health (NAMH) India

3. Self-harm in young people: for parents and carers. https://www.rcpsych.ac.uk/mental-health/parents-and-young-people/information-for-parents-and-carers/self-harm-in-young-people-for-parents-and-carers

4. Suicide Prevention. https://www.psychiatry.org/patients-families/suicide-prevention

CHAPTER 12

Stigma Due to Mental Ill-Health

Sathya Prakash

Introduction

The stigma surrounding mental ill-health is of great significance from the mental health care point of view. Understanding and acknowledging its presence, how it affects the path to good mental health and finding and implementing solutions to lessen the stigma are crucial.

What is stigma? The World Health Organization (WHO) defines stigma as 'a mark of shame, disapproval or disgrace that results in the individual being discriminated against, rejected and excluded from participating in different areas of society'.

Persons with mental illnesses and, by extension, their families, mental health professionals and mental health institutions may all be affected by stigma. The perception behind the stigmatizing attitude could take many different forms. Persons with mental illness may be perceived as 'aggressive or dangerous', 'odd or eccentric', 'inferior or weak', 'inauspicious or bringing bad luck' and so on. However, most of these assumptions are either completely untrue or vastly exaggerated or misinterpreted.

Figure 1 shows a pictorial representation of stigma.

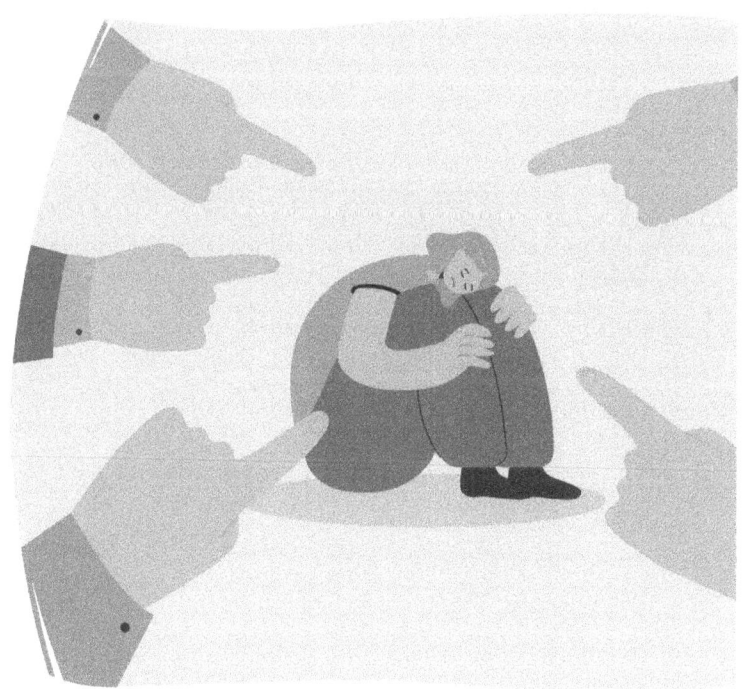

Stigma

The **World Health Organization (WHO)** defines stigma as 'a mark of shame, disapproval or disgrace that results in the individual being discriminated against, rejected and excluded from participating in different areas of society'

Figure 1. *What is Stigma?*

How Common is Stigma Related to Mental Health?

Stigma related to mental health is extremely common. Various studies have estimated that the prevalence of such stigma varies widely between 22-98%. Stigma may be subtle and not externally apparent or may be severe enough to result in overt discrimination. Studies from Nigeria have suggested stigma levels in the range of 20-30%, whereas those from Ethiopia and United Kingdom indicate levels of over 60%. Studies from India, Nepal, China and United States seem to suggest rates somewhere in between these. Stigma may be experienced at home, at work, in hospitals, institutions, on social media, social gatherings, in public discourse and so on.

Types of Mental Health Stigma

Stigma related to mental health can be classified in many ways. This includes stigma to the person with illness (self-stigma), stigma against family, stigma against the mental health professionals and institutions and stigma of illness vs medications (Box 1). These are briefly discussed below.

Self-Stigma

The persons suffering from mental illness often look down upon and stigmatize themselves. They may have internalized or imbibed how mental illness is commonly depicted and perceived by society.

Box 1. Types of Stigma

- Self-stigma
- Stigma against family
- Stigma against mental health professionals
- Stigma against mental health institutions
- Stigma against medicines used for the treatment of mental illness

---

Additionally, the low mood and poor self-esteem accompanying many mental health conditions further facilitate accepting such a view. Indeed, studies have found a strong negative correlation between self-stigma and self-esteem.

Repeated experiences of discrimination and rejection further cement such a view in the minds of the affected individuals. As stigma itself often results in no or unsatisfactory help-seeking, the person is caught in a vicious cycle of worsening mental illness and stigma, leading him/her to feel trapped. The power differentials between the affected people and the remaining population further perpetuate this process.

Certain studies have found that lower age at onset of the illness, frequent or multiple hospitalizations, female sex and longer duration of illness are all associated with greater degrees of self-stigma. Onset at an age lesser than 25 years has been associated with higher self-stigma. It has been hypothesized that this may be due to being impacted by the illness at an age where one is not fully equipped to deal with such adversity. Moreover, the illness itself may negatively influence the development of a healthy personality and coping abilities, especially when it develops at such a young age.

Women with mental illness probably suffer more stigma. This could be attributed to the cultural influences on expectations from women, their expected social roles and power differentials, which lead to a higher self-stigma in women. Mental illness may act synergistically with other sociocultural factors stacked against women, resulting in greater stigma.

Longer duration of illness and multiple hospitalizations, indicating greater severity of illness may lead to higher self-stigma. It has also been hypothesized that hospitalization might expose the individuals during a vulnerable phase to additional sources of stigma, such as health care staff, other patients and their relatives. Similarly, a long duration of illness may further lead to greater exposure to potentially stigmatizing scenarios and a waning ability to cope with such adverse circumstances.

Prior experience of trauma and the presence of other social, cultural, demographic and economic factors may put an individual at a disadvantage and, presumably, worsen the stigma. For example, a diagnosis of 'depression' attracts lesser stigma when compared to a diagnosis of 'schizophrenia'. While the latter attracts connotations of being 'dangerous and odd', the former attracts ideas such as 'being weak or needlessly seeking attention'. But broadly, both are often stereotyped as 'mental illnesses' regardless of the nature of the diagnosis.

The relationships of stigma with education, employment status, marital status and living arrangement are controversial and studies have yielded mixed results.

Stigma against the family

The immediate family of a person with mental illness may experience stigma within the larger family circle and friends. The family, in general, may be discriminated against by society. The fear of embarrassment may compel the family to hush up the matter, leading to a delay in seeking help. Often, fear of stigma leads to hurried marriages without communicating the presence of psychiatric illness, leading to turbulent marital life as well as illness exacerbation. Such acts may be associated with a sense of relieving oneself of, and passing on to someone else, the mark of shame. Associated ideas of marriage as a 'cure' for mental illness are sometimes in the background of such decisions.

Stigma against mental health professionals/ institutions

Mental health professionals may be seen by other health care professionals and society as being 'eccentric', 'dumb' or 'mentally ill' in some

way. Ideas that only people with some 'mental flaw' select this field or that constant exposure to persons with mental illness makes the health care provider mentally ill are highly prevalent. Mental health institutions may be seen as places that are dangerous and forbidden and are often the subject of jokes. References to mental illness/ institution/health care provider may be used interchangeably with abusive terms and in a casual manner.

Mental health history may be omitted or given less importance in a doctor's history-taking and evaluation. Symptoms of mental illness may be seen as imaginary, of one's own making, a product of stupidity and something that could be wished away if one tried hard enough, or because of the person's own 'fault'. But, at the same time, the presence of mental illness is seen as an invariable marker of poor prognosis. Other specialists may have a feeling of 'understanding psychiatry well enough' because of a falsely oversimplified view of it. Associated with this, sometimes, is an unsaid idea that not-so-serious attempts at treating psychological symptoms are okay. Symptoms of physical illness observed in persons with mental illness may not be evaluated as seriously as those of someone with similar symptoms, but not having a mental illness.

Stigma related to illness vs. stigma related to medicines

It has been observed that some persons may accept the idea of facing 'psychological difficulties' but are against the idea of taking medicines to 'deal with life difficulties.' This has been colloquially termed 'pill-shaming'. They consider how can life's problems be treated with pills? Such a view reflects a wrong understanding of the nature of mental illnesses as well as the nature and purpose of psychotropic medications. Sometimes, the same medications, when prescribed by a psychiatrist, are considered stigmatizing, but when prescribed by a physician or a neurologist, are not considered so.

Consequences of Stigma Related to Mental Health

Stigma related to mental health can be damaging in many ways. Some of the deleterious effects of stigma include delay in seeking treatment, neglect of physical health, poor life decisions, lack of opportunities and marginalization, low fund allocation for mental health and poor understanding by the public about mental health.

Delay in treatment-seeking

The symptoms of mental illness may be confusing to the patient and family. The patient may or may not have insight into the issue, and the family may not be aware of what is causing this or whether there is a problem at all or not. In such a scenario, the stigma results in the patient and the family not even discussing with others what to do about the issue, let alone consulting a mental health professional. Moreover, for many, the first and the final point of contact are not the same as far as the treatment of mental illness is concerned. So, even if a family does make contact with the first few rungs of what is perceived as the mental health care system, stigma makes the process difficult and many people drop out before the final or the desired point of contact is reached.

Neglect of physical health

A peculiar attitude of many, including that of the health care professionals, is that mentally ill persons, somehow, cannot be physically ill. This may represent a form of neglect or prejudice against the mentally ill and manifest as a lack of inclination to investigate the physical symptoms in those suffering from mental illnesses. The physical symptoms are dismissed as 'all in the mind' or are somehow seen as unworthy of being attended to. Ironically, several physical conditions, such as cardiovascular disorders, metabolic syndrome and malignancies, are more common in individuals with severe mental illnesses. Often, persons with mental illness may not be able to communicate their physical symptoms.

Poor life decisions

Stigma may directly or indirectly result in poor decision-making by the person suffering from the illness or by the family. The family, for instance, out of sheer desperation, might want to 'get rid of the burden' by marrying off the person. This, coupled with beliefs such as 'marriage cures mental illness', results in hastily done marriages, resulting in further destabilization and conflict. Needless to say, both the course of the illness as well as the stigma associated with it may only worsen in such a scenario.

Lack of opportunities and marginalization

Self-stigma may lead to the person with mental illness not actively reaching out to jobs or opportunities that the person might otherwise be qualified for. Similarly, employers may not consider hiring potential employees, when there is a possibility of the candidate suffering from mental illness. When any underlying mental illness of an already employed person comes to the knowledge of the employer, the employee may be removed from his/her job, citing other reasons on paper. Stereotyping often results in all mental health issues being put in one basket, regardless of the severity or nature of the problem, and its ability (or lack thereof) to potentially affect the person's skills required for the job. Thus, in the context of employment, stigma comes in many different shapes and sizes, leading, gradually, to the marginalization of persons with mental illness.

Less funding allocation and policy

Directly or indirectly, stigma may influence the judgment and decision-making ability of people in charge of allocating funds or approving policies. Stigma may result in mental health issues being seen as less/not important or not worthy of being allocated enough funds or resources. Similarly, mental health issues may be seen as 'not real problems' needing 'real solutions'. This only leads to a vicious cycle of further marginalization, more stigma and less policy attention.

Poor understanding by the public

When a topic is hushed up and not discussed openly, it becomes shrouded in mystery. This lack of clarity makes it further stigmatized, again leading to a vicious, self-perpetuating cycle. Poor understanding by the public further reinforces wrong beliefs about mental health issues, leading to various issues discussed throughout this chapter.

Less research interest

Researchers are often influenced by how fashionable a topic is to research. When a topic is seen as 'not fashionable' or 'mundane', it increases the likelihood of researchers not taking it up. The obvious downstream effects of this are the lack of innovative solutions to the existing mental health crisis.

Figure 2 summarizes the consequence of stigma.

Dealing with Stigma

Many strategies have been studied and tried to deal with the stigma surrounding mental health. They have yielded varying degrees of success. Some of the strategies and pertaining issues have been discussed below. Figure 3 summarizes these strategies.

Legislation

Legislation is a powerful tool to combat stigma, provided it receives support from other measures. Legislation must be comprehensive and inclusive yet sustainable to be able to ensure maximum impact and fairness. Once enacted, constant monitoring of the policy in terms of drawbacks, benefits and the overall impact is paramount. Periodic modifications, in part or in entirety, must be undertaken based on careful, regular and systematic monitoring. Funding and a proper enactment plan are the keys to making a real-world impact. It is well known that legislation and policy with respect to mental health is an often-neglected area, particularly with respect to funding.

Education and awareness

Any kind of forced intervention can only take things so far. Real, sustainable and meaningful change can only be observed when the need is understood, felt and enacted upon by the affected individual out of free will. Education and awareness are the key factors that bring about such a change. Involvement of key stakeholders, such as media, government, family, non-governmental organizations, educational institutions, famous personalities and youth, in general, are all meaningful goals to be pursued towards realizing this end outcome. 'Normalization' and avoidance of stigmatizing terms in public discourse, including social media, sets a role model as well as a minimum benchmark for people to follow. References to mental health issues should not be used as verbal abuse, subject matter of jokes, or to evoke a sense of horror, danger or shame.

Considering 'medicalization' as a form of normalization is controversial. Although, presumably, put forward with good intent, this approach may not be conceptually accurate for the entire gamut of mental health issues and may create other kinds of problems, including the generation

Consequences of Stigma

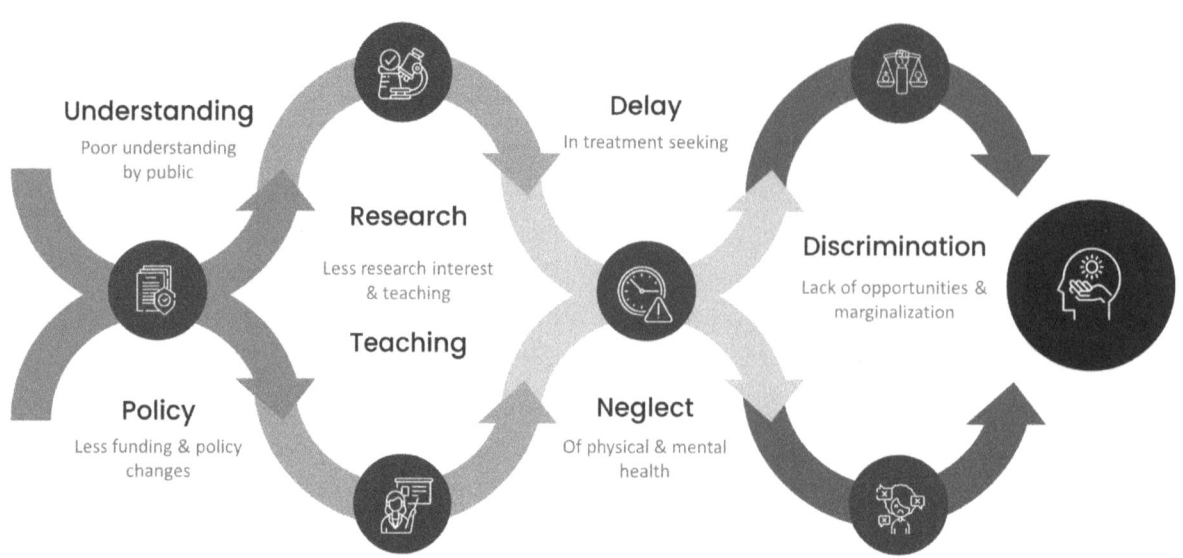

Figure 2. *Consequence of Stigma*

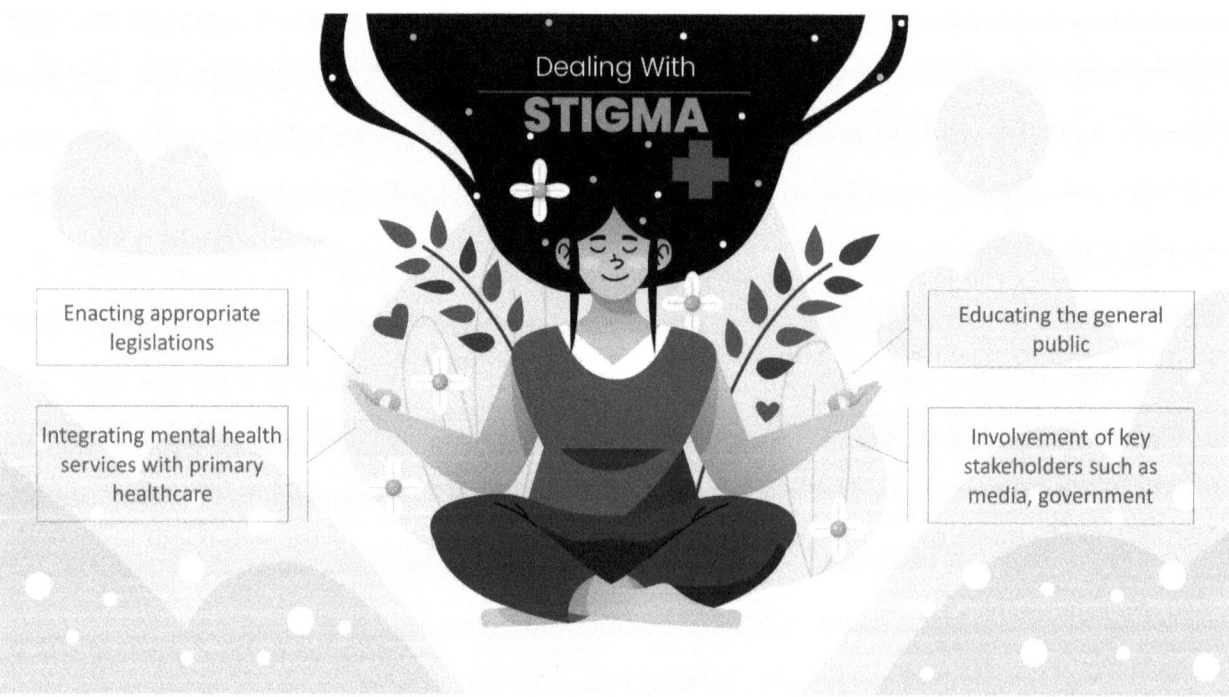

Figure 3. *Strategies for Dealing With Stigma*

of imperfect solutions. A biopsychosocial model perhaps best represents the conceptualization of mental health conditions. Mental illnesses are not to be seen as personal weaknesses, but as a complex interplay of biological, psychological and social factors at play. Medications, psychological interventions as well as social interventions all need to work in tandem to ensure the best possible outcome. Promoting only 'pill-popping' on the one hand versus 'pill-shaming' on the other extreme are both problematic. There must be a balance between educational and awareness messages.

Conveying the message that mental health issues are real, and not imagined or created by the affected individual, is crucial.

Capacity building and access to care

Improving capacity building and access to care are important for reducing the treatment gap for mental illnesses. Capacity building does not mean only increasing the number of psychiatrists, psychologists or social workers. Neither does it imply building new mental health institutions or departments. To be clear, the above is certainly important, but may not be sufficient to address the treatment gap. Untreated mental health conditions lead to a vicious cycle of increasing the stigma related to mental health, which, in turn, impairs the outcome for persons affected by these conditions.

Alternative models for reducing stigma include integrating mental health interventions as a part of primary health care and promoting community treatment rather than institutionalization or treatment at tertiary care centers. Sensitization of non-mental health care workers, including doctors of other specialties, nurses, technicians, pharmacists and other healthcare workers, is crucial.

Faith healers are often an important early point of contact for families of individuals suffering from mental illnesses. Innovative, culturally appropriate, respectful and non-alienating ways of utilizing this early point of contact not only serve to reduce stigma but also potentially improve the outcome.

Empathic, non-stigmatizing listening by friends and family is a huge reserve of both 'treatment' and 'anti-stigma intervention' that remains to be fully tapped into. As always, funding is an important issue that countries need to address in the context of capacity building. If basic, reasonable funding is not secured, how can even the most innovative idea make any impact?

Conclusion

Stigma related to mental health is an all-important topic. No amount of research and advances in the management of psychiatric disorders will be adequate if stigma is not properly addressed. Of what use is a wonder drug if the person in need is unable to reach out and ask for it, or, if he/she does reach out but does not want to continue taking it because of being looked down upon by others, or if he/she himself/herself looks down upon such an idea? The benefits and joy of recovery are significantly undercut if people around constantly look at the affected individual as if he/she will not, cannot or has not recovered. Stigma is very common and needs to be addressed comprehensively. Education, awareness, policy, legislation, capacity building and novel ways of delivering mental health care are all needs of the hour.

KEY POINTS

➤ Stigma related to mental health is very common and cannot be ignored.

➤ Types of stigma include self-stigma, stigma related to family and stigma against mental health professionals and institutions.

➤ Stigma results in delayed/interrupted treatment, neglect of physical health, inadequate life opportunities, poor decisions, less research, less funding and poor policies.

➢ Stigma can be addressed by way of legislation, awareness building, novel ways of care delivery and capacity building.

➢ Stigma research and alleviation need as much importance, if not more, as other areas of mental health research.

REFERENCES

1. Gaiha SM, Salisbury TT, Koschorke M, Raman U, Petticrew M. Stigma associated with mental health problems among young people in India: a systematic review of magnitude, manifestations and recommendations. BMC Psychiatry 20, 538 (2020). https://doi.org/10.1186/s12888-020-02937-x

2. Pescosolido BA, Halpern-Manners A, Luo L, Perry B. Trends in public stigma of mental illness in the US, 1996-2018. JAMA Netw Open. 2021 Dec 1;4(12): e2140202. doi: 10.1001/jamanetworkopen.2021.40202

3. Javed A, Lee C, Zakaria H, Buenaventura RD, Getkovich-Bakmas M, Duailibi K et al., Reducing the stigma of mental health disorders with a focus on low and middle-income countries. Asian J Psychiatry 2021; 58: 1-7.

CHAPTER 13

Mental Health Issues in Medical Illness

Vijay Krishnan and Koushik Sinha Deb

Introduction

The co-occurrence of mental health issues in medical illness is a norm, rather than being an exception. Yet, mental health issues are mostly ignored by the sufferer and are often missed or deprioritized by the treating physician. These mental health comorbidities are crucial, as they impact a person's overall functioning. Co-existing mental illness adds to the patient's suffering not only on its own but also by worsening the outcome of the primary medical illness.

Despite a wealth of academic literature testifying to the benefits of early treatment of such co-occurring mental illnesses, these conditions are seldom managed in the real world. A lack of awareness among general physicians and unavailability of specialized mental healthcare often contributes to lingering mental health issues and poor quality of life in patients. Psychosomatic medicine and consultation-liaison (CL) psychiatry are specialized branches of psychiatry, which have been specifically developed to understand and manage these complex interactions between medical and psychiatric conditions.

At the outset, it is important to understand that the dichotomous view of "medical" and "mental" is incorrect and often adds to the primary source of confusion. Mental illnesses are also medical conditions. Like any other medical condition, mental illnesses also occur due to changes in the physiology, structure and function of the brain and the mind. With modern research, genetic, molecular, receptor, protein and hormonal abnormalities have

now been discovered to be associated with most mental illnesses. Physical illnesses resulting from such genetic, molecular, receptor, protein and hormonal abnormalities are, therefore, expected to have associated mental symptoms too. Additionally, medical illnesses, surgical operations and treatment also alter the delicate chemical balance of the brain. Understandably, mental symptoms can be an emergent phenomenon of such biochemical fluctuations. Finally, all illnesses are associated with various life and economic stresses, which may be enough to precipitate mental health crisis in a patient.

There does not seem to be a single mechanism leading from medical illness to mental health issues, or vice versa. Instead, such presentations involve a complex interplay of factors, which derive from a patient's unique life conditions, current and past illnesses, and medical treatment. Thus, management of mental health issues in medically ill patients requires special considerations, skills and an integrated management approach combining the expertise of multiple branches of medicine.

Prevalence of Mental Health Issues in the Medically Ill

A range of mental health issues have been identified amongst patients in various medical settings. In primary or general healthcare settings, many patients present with mental health concerns. These conditions often include depression and anxiety, which are often mild or sub-syndromal and may be transient.

In specialist and inpatient settings, moderate or even severe mental illnesses become more common in comparison, and the morbidity of mental illnesses also increases significantly. Depression and anxiety, along with substance use disorders, remain the most common mental illnesses in both the primary and secondary care levels.

The pattern is somewhat different among patients in high-dependency, intensive care, geriatric, or palliative care settings. Depression and anxiety disorders still remain common in these populations; however, a substantial number of subjects suffer from conditions that are seen almost exclusively in this population - e.g., delirium, dementia or cognitive impairment.

Mental illnesses in the medically unwell are generally understood to be approximately two or three times higher than in the general population. Among hospitalized patients, the rates of depression and anxiety can be as high as 50%-70%. Several patient and illness-related factors have been suggested to increase the prevalence of mental illnesses in the medically ill. In general, the most common mental illnesses (depression and anxiety) are more likely to occur amongst patients with chronic medical conditions. Even within this population, diseases that place more restrictions on a patient's daily life, are more likely to be associated with mental illnesses, as compared to those that are milder. Similarly, illnesses that are progressive (diabetes, arthritis), stigmatizing (leprosy, HIV) or those requiring advanced medical care (dialysis in kidney failure, chemotherapy) are associated with higher rates of mental morbidity. Essentially, all illnesses are stressful, and depression and anxiety may often be the reaction to such chronic stress. Economic stability, education and family may play a protective role in preventing the development of mental disorders. Personality factors like resilience, meaningfulness in life, belief systems and hopefulness also protect individuals from developing mental illnesses in such situations.

By contrast, acute and severe medical illnesses tend to produce widespread physiological changes in blood chemistry, hormonal function, liver metabolism and kidney excretion. These alterations can induce a global impairment of cognition and awareness, resulting in confusional states or cognitive dysfunction. Children and older people are more often affected in this way, as their body reserves to counter alterations are generally less as compared to healthy adults.

Psychiatric symptoms may also occur as a result of medical treatment in certain cases. Treatment with steroid medications is the commonest cause of mood changes (either depression or mania) or psychosis seen at tertiary care centers. Similarly, chemotherapeutic agents often cause mental illness symptoms due to their widespread systemic toxicity. Some antitubercular medications like isoniazid cause mood elevation, while others like cycloserine can cause psychosis. In vulnerable patients, even commonly used antibiotics like ciprofloxacin can result in delirium. The list of such drug-mind interactions is essentially never-ending, and awareness and vigilance about them remain an essential skill for all physicians.

A final important consideration is that individuals with established mental illnesses also frequently experience multiple medical comorbidities. Obesity, diabetes, cardiovascular disease and substance use disorders are far more common in this group as compared to the general population. Decreased physical activity, prolonged disability, inability to perform daily activities as well as psychiatric medications have all been considered as contributing to these lifestyle disorders and these factors undoubtedly contribute to the higher all-cause mortality seen in the psychiatric patient population.

Figure 1 summarizes common mental health issues in mentally ill patients.

Common Mental Health Issues in Various Situations

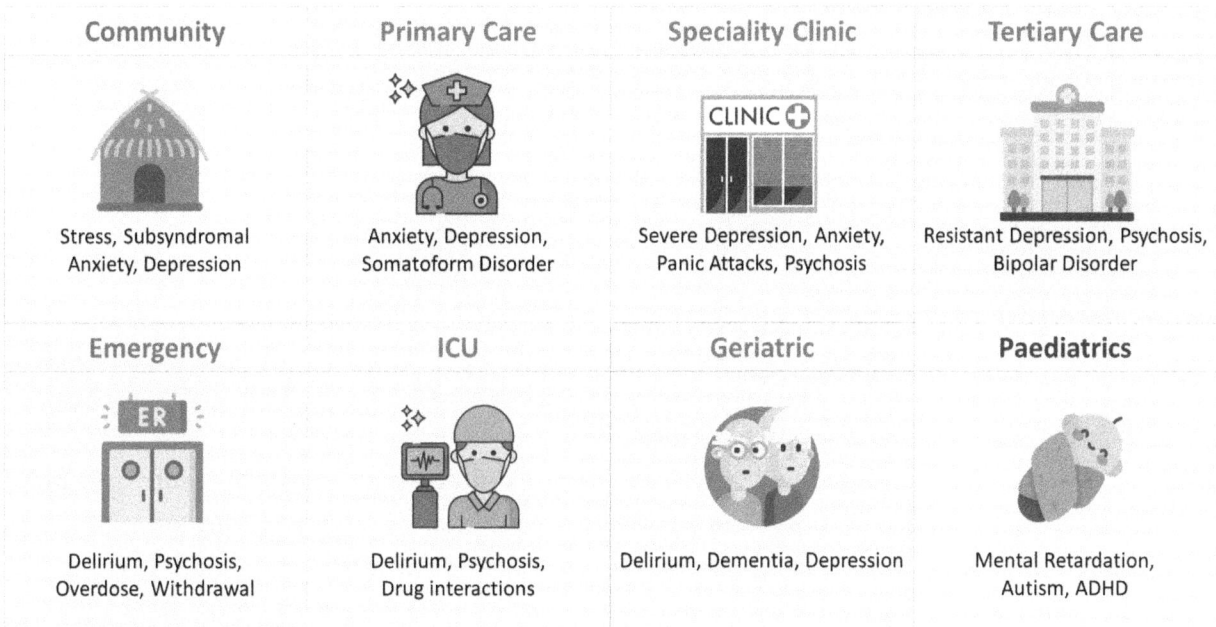

Figure 1. *Common Mental Health Issues in Mentally Ill Patients*

Importance of Mental Illness

Most mental illnesses are defined by their impact on thinking and behavior. Medically ill patients with psychiatric conditions are often unable to appreciate the severity of their illness, may not be able to communicate their symptoms and have difficulty following medical advice without significant supervision. Additionally, a preference for sedentary lifestyles, reduced socialization, reduced self-care and a global outlook of hopelessness and helplessness reduce an individual's quality of life and negatively impact the trajectory of any coexisting medical illness.

Specific alterations include late recognition of symptoms, inadequate treatment of illnesses and greater rates of alcohol and other substance use in the mentally ill. Mental illnesses can also place individuals in financial distress, making it difficult for them to afford adequate healthcare and nutrition. Due to the stigma experienced by persons with mental illness, they may also find it harder to access healthcare or to fulfill social roles such as marriage, employment or parenting. Many of these can be at least partially reversed by adequate treatment of the underlying mental illness.

Research shows that such outcomes are associated not only with well-described mental illnesses but also with "minor" symptoms, like anxiety, poor motivation or sleep disturbances, which may be characterized as "subsyndromal" mental health issues. These symptoms are liable to be missed during routine assessments and may thus persist or recur throughout an individual's lifespan.

For most hospitalized patients, diagnosis and management of co-occurring mental illnesses result in quicker remission, shorter hospital stays, less frequent re-hospitalization and better overall recovery. In patients suffering from chronic medical illnesses like diabetes and hypertension, management of mental health issues results in more physical activity, better adherence to treatment, tighter control of blood sugar or blood pressure and longer active life. In many chronic illnesses like rheumatoid arthritis, the requirement of pain-killer medicines is significantly reduced with proper mental health care. Finally, in patients with cancer, mental health interventions have resulted in reduced mortality and increased longevity, and an overall improvement in the quality of life experienced by the patients.

Suggested Mechanisms and Models of Mental Illness in the Medically Unwell

The relationship between mental and other medical illnesses is complex and bi-directional. Since the time that this association was first recognized, models have been proposed to encompass the various mechanisms.

1. **Direct physiological effects of medical illness:** Disease states are characterized by a wide range of physiological abnormalities. Global alterations arising from changes in the overall milieu (e.g. electrolyte imbalances), changes to the endocrine stress-response systems and changes in neurological functions can cause psychiatric symptoms. Other disorders, especially those directly affecting the central nervous system or the endocrine system can directly alter the functioning of identifiable brain regions. Examples include:
   • Electrolyte imbalances or metabolic changes such as hyperglycemia can present as confusional symptoms.
   • A tumor or defect in the frontal or temporal lobes of the brain can lead to depression or psychotic symptoms.
   • Disorders of the thyroid gland result in increased or decreased production of thyroid hormones, which, in turn, can cause severe anxiety or depression due to its effect on various bodily systems.

2. **Psychological reactions to being medically unwell:** Being diagnosed with a medical illness can entail a major change in a person's sense of self. Many diagnoses require modifications in lifestyle that may be difficult to sustain, making individuals dependent on social support and the healthcare system. Many find it hard to negotiate these changes and maybe demoralized or anxious about the impact of illness. Chronic diseases with a known impact on lifespan or with a significant impact on functioning are likely to be associated with such symptoms.

3. **Co-occurring medical and psychiatric illnesses:** Incidentally, medical illness may co-occur with any other illness. For example, a diagnosis of asthma has no medical association with a diagnosis of acute appendicitis, but a patient can suffer from both these conditions, purely by chance. Mental illnesses like anxiety and depression may occur in a substantial proportion of such patients.

4. **Medical presentations of psychiatric illnesses:** Certain psychiatric disorders present with physical symptoms only, often imitating a medical illness. For example, in panic disorder, a condition characterized by severe acute anxiety bouts, the condition is often mistaken as a heart attack by the sufferer. Similarly, dissociative disorders may present like seizures or a cerebrovascular stroke, and somatoform disorders are characterized by a variety of physical symptoms for which no medical cause can be found.

5. **Medical complications of psychiatric illness:** Psychiatric disorders themselves may result in a variety of medical complications that require attention. Severe depression often results in a stupor, a state where the patient lies statically unable to eat or care for self, resulting in risk to life. In mania, the patient can become excited to the point of dehydration and exhaustion.

In a condition called catatonia, the patients become stiff and rigid and cannot even eat or drink, resulting in an imminent threat to life. Most substance use disorders come with a host of medical complications. In long-term alcohol dependence, in addition to liver failure or cirrhosis, almost all organ systems are affected.

6. **Medical complications of psychiatric treatment:** Finally, like medical treatment resulting in psychiatric conditions, the opposite also remains true. Psychiatric treatment often results in medical conditions that need to be treated or addressed even before they develop. Most antipsychotic medications and mood stabilizers result in a condition called metabolic syndrome, characterized by hypertension, dyslipidemia, diabetes and weight gain. Antipsychotics can also cause acute side effects like dystonia and parkinsonian symptoms like tremors. Patients on lithium therapy may suffer from lithium toxicity, if they become inadvertently dehydrated, as in when having vomiting and diarrhea. Treatment of all illnesses, irrespective of being medical or psychiatric in nature, can result in adverse effects. Although this fact is often given undue prominence in the mass media, **one must understand that all modern medicines used for the treatment of mental disorders are safe, and the clinicians are well aware and well equipped to prevent the occurrence of such side effects. Avoiding treatment in the hypothetical fear of possible side effects becomes akin to not going out of the house in the fear of meeting with an accident.** The judicious and scientific use of pharmacotherapy has revolutionized modern medicine.

These mechanisms do not act individually or in isolation. Instead, medical and mental illnesses usually impact one another by means of multiple bidirectional processes that involve alterations caused by illness and the consequences of bodily adaptation to illness, encompassing both general physiology and the physiology of the nervous system.

Figure 2 summarizes the complex relationship between physical and mental illnesses

Models of Psychosomatic Disorders

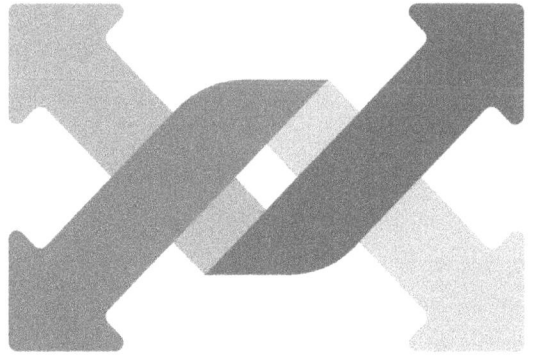

Mental Illness
Presenting as medical illness
Medical issue due to lifestyle
Illnesses having both components

Medical Illness
Physiological effects of illness
Reaction to medical illness
Comorbidity

Psychiatric Treatment
Metabolic Syndrome
Parkinsonism
Thyroid Abnormality

Medical Treatment
Drug induced psychiatric illness
Metabolic abnormality induced
Drug toxicity induced

Figure 2. *Models of Psychosomatic Disorders*

Barriers to Dealing with Mental Health Issues Amongst the Medically Ill

Despite mental health issues being common in medically ill hospitalized patients, they remain unrecognized in up to 70% of cases. This discrepancy has been extensively studied at the level of the patient, the medical practitioner and the health system. Dealing with these barriers can improve the identification and care of mental illnesses in patients who are being treated in general medical settings.

Patients often fail to recognize mental health issues, viewing them as moral or spiritual problems, and thus don't report to the doctor. Patients may also see these symptoms as personal failings and can feel embarrassed to discuss them. Even with symptoms that are recognized by patients and families, the stigma associated with psychiatric illness often makes them reluctant to seek treatment.

For all these reasons, mental health issues need to be elicited by the clinician, rather than being spontaneously discussed by the patient. However, clinicians often fail to ask about them, either due to a lack of formal training or due to sharing the stigmatizing views about mental disorders that exist in the community.

At the health systems level, the most significant barrier to recognizing or managing mental health issues includes the difficulties of access to competent mental healthcare. While many treatment options can be integrated with general medical care, their implementation is severely lacking. Thus, patients seeking care for psychological issues must put in additional effort and bear an additional cost as compared to most other medical illnesses.

The nature of the symptoms themselves may also act as a barrier. Many psychological and behavioral symptoms fluctuate in intensity and impact, making it difficult for the patients to attribute them to a coexisting mental health condition. The symptoms of depression make the sufferer hopeless about any possibility of recovery, robbing the patient of a will for treatment. Psychosis results in paranoia, where the patient believes that others are trying to harm him. Rather than seeking treatment, active resistance to treatment is seen even when family members have made the attempt. It has also been shown that symptoms of mental illness are far more variable and "atypical" as compared to physical illnesses, making the task of recognition difficult even for trained mental health professionals. Finally, the absence of any objective parameters and investigative proof often makes the diagnosis time-consuming and dependent on the clinical skill of the physician. The absence of such objective measures also creates doubt regarding the diagnosis in the minds of the patients and their care providers. Finally, the slow initial response pattern of psychotropic medications decreases the confidence in treatment, resulting in treatment discontinuity or multi-medication management.

Identifying Mental Health Issues in the Medically Ill

The first step in identifying mental health problems in medically ill patients is recognizing the fact that medically ill patients are indeed more susceptible to multiple psychiatric conditions, as compared to the general population. Therefore, strategies for systematic evaluation need to be actively implemented in such settings. These strategies should be focused on identifying the common mental illnesses in these populations, viz. depression and anxiety in the general medical setting, along with delirium in the intensive care setting. Such screening can indeed be undertaken without much additional effort. For example, it has been shown that just two questions ("Have you been troubled by feeling down, depressed, or hopeless"; "Have you experienced little interest or pleasure in doing things") can be effective in identifying patients who need further evaluation for depression. Similar short screening approaches have been developed for anxiety disorders, sleep disorders and substance use.

Further evaluation involves arriving at a definite diagnosis of mental illness, assessing its severity and assessing the urgency of treatment. With brief training, general physicians themselves can perform these assessments, at least for common mental disorders. Alternatively, a referral to mental health professionals can also be undertaken at this stage if primary care resources are inadequate or if the assessment is uncertain. Several structured questionnaires have also been developed, which patients can fill out themselves, with the intent to help them understand and make correct choices. Due to the constraints of time that most primary care physicians face, such self-guided screening strategies may be beneficial in increasing awareness and improving detection.

Treatment Options for Mental Illness

A range of treatment options exist, but treatment needs to be individualized, based on the nature and severity of symptoms, and the preferences of the patient. For certain symptoms, especially those of mild severity, careful monitoring may be the only intervention required. On the other hand, even mild, transient or self-limiting symptoms may require treatment if they impact a person's functioning or cause significant distress.

Treatment planning also requires a deep understanding of ongoing medical management. In some cases, the only intervention required may be the withdrawal or substitution of a drug used for the medical disease. Understanding of medical management is also necessary as psychiatric medications, when given in conjunction with other medications, may alter their metabolism and efficacy. Also, certain psychiatric medications might be safer in certain specific medical illnesses,

e.g., sertraline is safer in cardiac disorders, while quetiapine may be preferred as an antipsychotic in patients with neurological and movement disorders. Additionally, joint decisions are required in certain situations where, despite psychiatric side effects, the primary treatment needs to continue. For example, in certain cancers, if a particular chemotherapy regimen is considered to be essential, the treating team, in conjunction with the psychiatrist, might prefer to continue the same. The resultant mental symptoms arising out of chemotherapy can be managed subsequently by psychotropic medication by the psychiatrist in conjunction with the oncologist.

Patients who are already on several medications may be reluctant to take additional pills for the treatment of mental health issues and may appreciate non-pharmacological interventions. Patients might also prefer psychological interventions for a variety of other reasons, thereby making counseling and psychotherapy important tools in the management matrix.

The goals of treatment in this context also vary significantly. For self-limiting symptoms or those that are a direct consequence of a medical condition, the goal of treatment is often only to ameliorate distress or dysfunction, while the medical treatment improves the primary condition. Treatment targets in such situations may be limited to sleep disturbance management and problematic anxiety symptom management. Medications that are immediately effective and can be withdrawn after a short period, maybe preferred over agents that take time to exert their effects.

Long-term treatment may be required for patients with pre-existing mental illnesses that have shown worsening symptoms during a medical illness, or when mental health issues have persisted. In these situations, the treatment of mental illness is undertaken in the same way as in the general population, but with suitable modifications to account for the biochemical alterations due to the medical status of the patient.

Pharmacological management: Medications remain the mainstay for the treatment of psychiatric conditions in medically ill patients. However, understandably, such discussion is complex and beyond the scope of this chapter. However, certain general facts should be remembered when starting psychiatric medications in all patients. Sleeping medications should be used judiciously and only after ensuring proper sleep hygiene. Also, in most cases, sleeping pills should be used for temporary relief and should be stopped by the 4th to 6th week, except in certain cases as recommended by the clinician. Additionally, most psychiatric medications used to treat mood disorders and psychosis require some time to show response. As a general rule, around 10 to 14 days are required after the start of medicines for the patient and family members to perceive improvement in symptoms. It is important for clinicians to communicate this to patients to manage their expectations and to prevent unnecessary changes or addition of medicines. Side effects, when they occur with psychiatric medications, are generally mild (gastritis, nausea, etc.), and settle by the end of the first week. Long-term side effects do develop with some medicines but are generally manageable by drug and dose optimization.

Beyond pharmacological treatment: As discussed above, a scarcity of mental healthcare services forms a major barrier to providing adequate treatment. In this context, patients may be able to take some steps to manage symptoms themselves. These include making healthy lifestyle choices, developing a healthy routine, ensuring proper sleep hygiene, participating in physical and social activities and practicing mindfulness, relaxation or meditation.

Frequently used non-pharmacological intervention options that are likely to be useful for many patients in this population, are described in brief, below. Most of these can be used without

formal training and can have a substantial impact on the mental health of patients. At the same time, these steps should be considered to be preliminary measures that are generally useful but are not a replacement for specific psychological or pharmacological treatment that may be required for a substantial proportion of those with mental health issues.

1. **Patient education:** Being diagnosed with a medical condition is associated with a great deal of worry and uncertainty about the likely impact, effects on lifespan and treatment options. This is especially true for conditions that are likely to be chronic, and in which patients' self-management capacity may be modified by symptoms. It has been repeatedly shown that providing the patients with appropriate and adequate information about the likely course of illness and treatment reduces these impacts. Such education can be provided by specialized "health educators", or by nurses and even by the practitioners themselves. The major themes of such educational package include information about the nature and course of illness and the common warning signs of relapse; information about the need and duration of treatment; and logistic information regarding where and whom to contact in case of emergency. Additional lifestyle and functioning-related information, including daily activities, routine, work and leisure activities, might also be provided.

2. **Sleep hygiene:** Sleep is affected by a range of mental conditions, and lack of sleep can be disabling. "Sleep hygiene" refers to the way a person organizes their daily routine, which can affect the quality and amount of sleep that a person gets (Also discussed in Chapter on Sleep). By making practical changes to their routines, individuals can positively impact

their sleep duration and quality. The steps that are frequently taken include:

a. Keeping regular hours for sleeping at night and waking up in the morning

b. Leading a physically active life

c. Allowing for a period of relaxation in the hours before bedtime

d. Avoiding daytime naps

e. Avoiding the use of stimulants (e.g. caffeine, tobacco, etc.) close to the expected bedtime

f. Avoiding bright lights including phone screens very close to the expected bedtime

g. Avoiding "clock-watching" i.e. avoiding lying in bed waiting for sleep if it is delayed, or interrupted

h. Avoiding tasks that cause physical or mental arousal immediately before bedtime

i. Avoiding remaining in bed for extended periods after waking up

To help an individual achieve better sleep, clinicians would need to check for the presence of current problematic practices and suggest practical changes that the person can make in his/her daily routine.

3. **Problem-solving skills:** Poor coping with medical stresses, or other life difficulties, maybe a prominent contributor to psychological distress in medically ill patients. Clinicians can assist their patients to negotiate these difficulties by suggesting ways in which one can modify one's approach to deal with these problems. The steps that can be suggested include:

a. Breaking down difficult and complex problems into smaller chunks, some of which may be easier to solve

b. Distinguishing between problems that require immediate solutions, from those that do not, and addressing them first

c. Preparation for emotionally challenging situations, which may prevent them from becoming overwhelming or frightening

d. A systematic approach to making decisions that focus on both the benefits ("pros") and harms ("cons") that may arise from choosing a specific course of action

4. **Stress reduction:** A number of potential interventions have been suggested, that are generally useful to manage stress, irrespective of its cause. These interventions are mostly aimed at reducing physiological arousal and physical "tension" that may be distressing. Most of these stress reduction techniques involve practices that are most effective when they are undertaken regularly. Some suggested options include:

a. Breathing exercises: Deep and regular breathing to decrease heart rate and anxiety

b. Progressive muscle relaxation: A technique where each group of muscles from the toe to the head are voluntarily contracted (squeezed) and stretched, resulting in forced muscle relaxation.

c. Yoga or meditation practices: A variety of culturally accepted practices that focus on the body and mind to result in relaxation and form a sense of calmness.

d. Behavioral activation or "Externalization of interests" - Encouraging individuals to commence or resume hobbies or other pleasurable activities, which the patient has discontinued due to the current illness.

A consultation with a psychiatrist, psychologist or other mental health professional does not necessarily mean initiation of drug treatment but provides scope to the patient to explore possible interventions, and therefore, should be recommended despite initial reluctance from patients or their care providers.

Conclusion

The goal of all medical management is not merely the remission of symptoms but also ensuring a better life quality of the sufferer. It is being increasingly realized that a pure biological focus, although effective in symptom suppression, cannot address the issues of patient satisfaction and well-being. Therefore, researchers are increasingly focusing more on the role of holistic care, where the management of mental health forms an integral part of the overall treatment goal. Mental health issues during medical illnesses are common and need to be addressed for a better outcome of the index illness as well as for the well-being of the patient. Modern psychiatric medicines, when required, are safe and effective and have far greater patient acceptance as compared to drugs used even a couple of decades back. The current hurdle lies in developing services so that proper management reaches the sufferer in need at the time of greatest necessity.

KEY POINTS

➤ Mental disorders are also medical conditions and therefore treatable with modern therapeutics. The dichotomy between the mind and the body is artificial and illnesses in any one system can and will affect other systems too.

➤ Mental disorders are more prevalent in the medically ill as compared to the general population as illness induces a variety of physical, mental, social and economic stresses on the sufferer.

➤ Depression and anxiety are the commonest mental health conditions in chronic medical illnesses. Delirium and acute psychosis are very common in severe medical illnesses, requiring high support.

➤ Mental disorders are associated with medical illnesses through various bidirectional mechanisms, with one affecting the other through biological, social or psychological pathways.

➤ Identification of comorbid mental illnesses forms the greatest challenge, as mental health services of our country are often limited. Additional awareness and expertise of general medical practitioners might be a significant step to bridging the gap.

➤ Treatment of such mental comorbidities requires careful examination of the primary condition and its treatment, understanding the nature and severity of the psychiatric symptoms and developing a treatment plan in consultation with the treating physician.

➤ Even without medical management, certain psychological interventions like psychoeducation, relaxation, sleep hygiene and yoga may be practiced at an individual patient level to improve both mental and physical health.

REFERENCES

1. Coping after Physical Illness. https://www.rcpsych.ac.uk/mental-health/problems-disorders/physical-illness

CHAPTER 14

Disorders Related to Eating

Swarndeep Singh and Rakesh Kumar Chadda

Introduction

Disorders related to eating are not merely an odd or unusual pattern of eating in an individual and may represent mental ill-health. An excessive preoccupation with food, body weight and/or body shape, in combination with the maladaptive or disturbed thought process, emotions or perception related to eating, is a warning sign. Self-imposed severe and strict restrictions on food intake (in terms of amount and/or type of food consumed), episodes of food binging and indulging frequently in purging behaviors, like vomiting or over-exercising without any specific reason, are a common accompaniment. This behavior can lead to various medical problems, like nutritional deficiencies, electrolyte imbalance, being under- or over-weight with related complications, social isolation and anxiety or depressive illness. In many Western countries, there is a separate sub speciality of psychiatry taking care of disorders related to eating.

Eating disorders often remain unrecognized. Common eating disorders include anorexia nervosa (AN), bulimia nervosa (BN), binge eating disorder (BED), rumination disorder and pica.

This chapter is an attempt to sensitize the readers by identifying features of eating disorders and how a person with an eating disorder can be helped.

Identifying Eating Disorders

Anorexia nervosa (AN): A person with AN usually has an intense fear of gaining weight and/or perceives oneself as overweight (which is not true in reality). As a result, the person indulges in severe restriction of food intake leading to significantly low body weight for one's age, gender, height and developmental stage. Generally, a body mass index (BMI) of less than $18.5 \ kg/m^2$ is considered indicative of AN. (Figure 1)

There are two sub-types of AN: **Restricting type**, in which the person engages in self-starvation with or without over-exercising to lose weight, and **binge-eating/purging type**, in which the underweight person also engages in subjective binge eating episodes followed by significant psychological distress and purging behaviors, like self-induced vomiting, abuse of laxatives, diuretics or other drugs for weight loss. In women of the reproductive age group, amenorrhea or stopping of menstrual periods due to hormonal disturbances secondary to severe weight loss is a characteristic feature of AN.

Persons with AN often have an excessive preoccupation with thoughts of losing weight despite being underweight. They would often indulge in social media and internet use to explore ways of reducing weight or maintaining extremely low body weights, or frequently checking one's body shape or size in the mirror or in selfies.

Bulimia nervosa (BN): Bulimia nervosa (BN) is characterized by episodes of eating large amounts of food in an uncontrollable manner over a short period of time in a single sitting, followed by compensatory behaviors, such as self-induced

Anorexia Nervosa – Complications

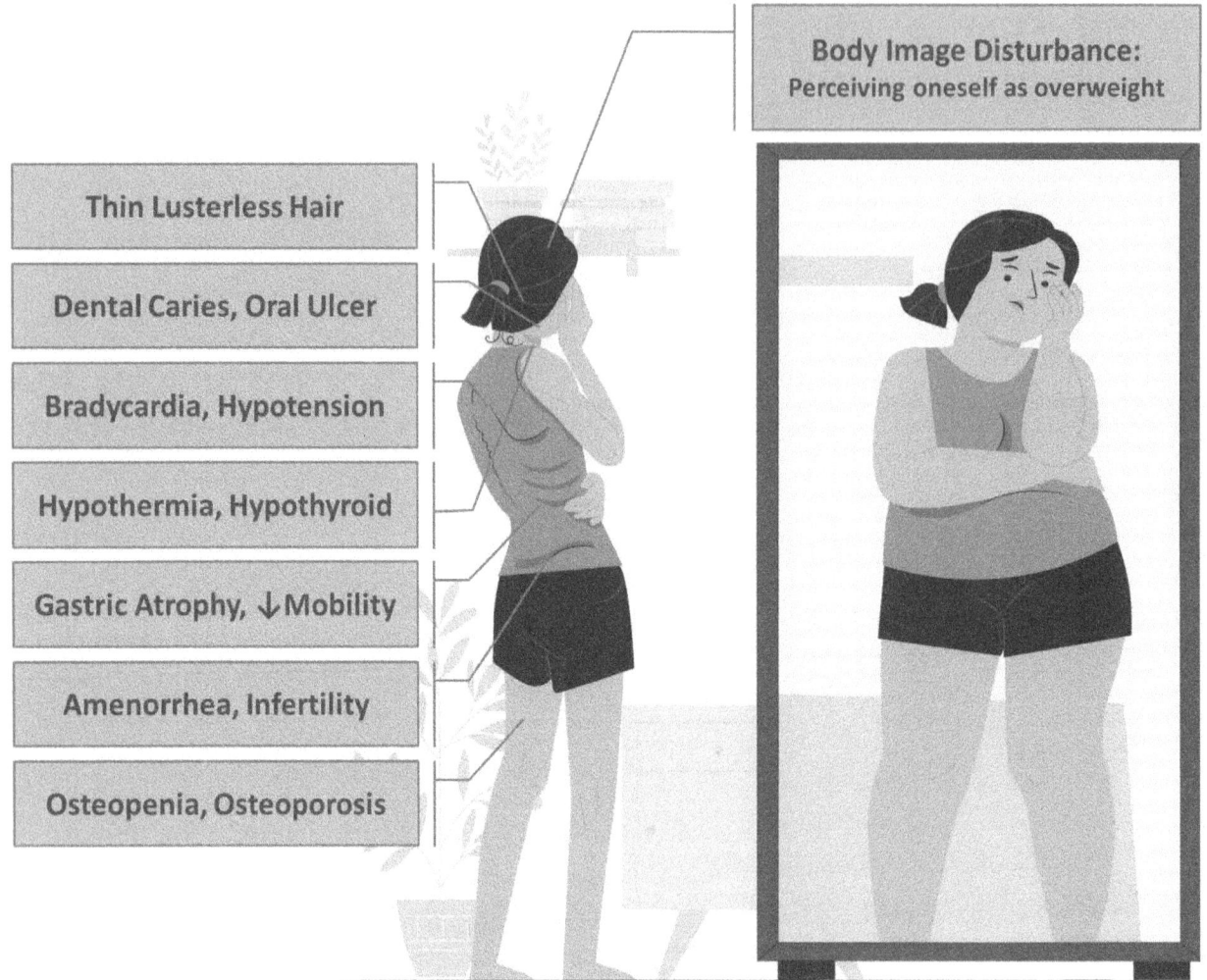

Thin Lusterless Hair

Dental Caries, Oral Ulcer

Bradycardia, Hypotension

Hypothermia, Hypothyroid

Gastric Atrophy, ↓Mobility

Amenorrhea, Infertility

Osteopenia, Osteoporosis

Body Image Disturbance:
Perceiving oneself as overweight

Figure 1. *Complications of Anorexia Nervosa*

vomiting, misuse of laxatives or diuretics, and deliberating over-exercising to prevent weight gain. The severity of BN is determined by the frequency of indulging in these inappropriate compensatory behaviors. These individuals are driven by negative self-evaluation or shame over one's body weight, shape or size. However, unlike people with AN, they are either normal or overweight as per their BMI. They often avoid checking their weight and wear oversized or loose clothes while going out in public places due to shame and/or distress experienced by them due to their body shape or size.

Binge eating disorder (BED): In binge eating disorder (BED), there occur episodes of binging, similar to that described in persons with BN. However, the episodes are not associated with inappropriate compensatory behaviors and don't have body image distortion. The person often binge eats at night or when alone, and experiences extreme guilt and distress over binging afterward. The severity of BED is determined by the frequency of indulging in these binge-eating episodes (at least once/week for three months is the threshold for making a clinical diagnosis). About 30-45% of individuals with BED are obese.

Box 1. Physical Complications Associated With Anorexia Nervosa

---

Cardiovascular: Bradycardia, Hypotension, Arrhythmias, Cardiomyopathy, Dizziness or fainting

Dermatological: Dry skin, Pruritis, Thin lustreless hairs, Hair loss, Cheilitis

Endocrine and metabolic: Electrolyte disturbances, Hypothermia, Hypothyroidism, Hypercortisolemia, Amenorrhea, Delayed or absent secondary sexual characteristics

Gastrointestinal: Delayed gastric emptying, Decreased intestinal mobility, Gastric atrophy, Constipation, Altered gut microbiome

Hematological: Anemia, Leukopenia, Thrombocytopenia, Pancytopenia

Neurological: Peripheral neuropathy, Brain atrophy

Oral: Dental caries or erosion, Tooth loss, Oral ulcers, Tongue atrophy

Skeletal: Osteopenia, Osteoporosis

Reproductive: Amenorrhea, Infertility, Reduced libido, Low birth-weight infant

---

Pica: It is generally seen in young children and sometimes may continue as one grows into adulthood. The person craves for and indulges in eating non-nutritive, non-food substances that are not developmentally appropriate or socio-culturally acceptable for a duration of at least one month. Commonly consumed non-food substances include dirt/soil, chalk, soap, paper, etc. The person may develop food poisoning, gastrointestinal infection or injuries, or nutritional deficiencies depending upon the consumed substance. The disorder may be associated with iron deficiency (anemia), malnutrition, pregnancy, intellectual developmental disorder or autism spectrum disorder.

Rumination disorder: In rumination disorder, the patient voluntarily regurgitates the food that was previously consumed and may either re-chew, re-swallow or spit out the regurgitated contents.

Effects on Health

Eating disorders, depending upon the type (anorexic vs. bulimic symptoms), duration and severity of symptoms, can cause harm to both the physical and psychological health of the affected person. In AN, almost all the systems of the body suffer physical harm due to severe self-starvation and purging or over-exercising behaviors. Similarly, overeating during binging episodes can cause an additional set of physical harms, apart from those associated with purging or over-exercising. Common physical complications associated with anorexic and bulimic eating disorders are summarized in Boxes 1 and 2, respectively.

Eating disorders are associated with low self-esteem and extreme shame or distress in relation to one's own body shape or size and eating behaviors. The person may also develop depression or anxiety disorders as a consequence of the primary eating disorder. Personality disorders are commonly seen alongwith with eating disorders.

What Causes Eating Disorders?

The exact cause for the development of eating disorders is not yet clearly established. There is a complex interplay between different bio-psycho-social factors in the genesis of an eating disorder. Table 1 summarizes some of the common biological, psychological and sociological factors that could act as predisposing and/or perpetuating factors for eating disorders.

Box 2. Physical Complications Associated With Bulimic Eating Disorders

---

Cardiovascular: Arrhythmias, Heart failure, Sudden cardiac death

Dermatological: Calluses on the knuckles or the back of the hand due to repeated self-induced vomiting

Endocrine and metabolic: Electrolyte disturbances, Metabolic acidosis (laxative abuse), Metabolic alkalosis (recurrent vomiting), Impaired glucose tolerance

Gastrointestinal: Constipation, Diarrhea, Peptic ulcer, Esophageal or gastric tear/rupture, Pancreatitis

Hematological: Leukopenia, Lymphocytosis

Oral: Dental caries or erosion

Renal: Renal stones, Acute kidney injury (from dehydration and purging)

Table 1. *Bio-psycho-social model for development and maintenance of eating disorders*

Biological factors	• Genetic predisposition
	• Female gender carries a higher risk
Psychological factors	• Temperament characteristics/personality traits (e.g. perfectionism, rigidity, intolerance to negative situations)
	• Body image disturbance or dissatisfaction
	• Pre-morbid high levels of anxiety
	• Low self-esteem
	• Child sexual abuse or neglect
	• Attention-deficit hyperactivity disorder or traits
Socio-cultural/ Environmental factors	• Sociocultural acceptability of thinness ideal
	• Peer pressure or problems (e.g. body shaming talk, bullying)
	• Problematic parental eating practices
	• Social isolation or poor social support
	• Social media exposure to pro-eating disorder content

Where to Seek Help for Eating Disorders?

Persons with eating disorders often do not realize that they are suffering from abnormal eating behaviors. Even when they do, most of them are very secretive about it and do not disclose or discuss the problem with others due to feelings of shame and self-stigma. Only about 20% of patients with an eating disorder receive specialized treatment ever and the median duration of untreated illness for most eating disorders is more than two years. Thus, family members and people close to an individual suffering from eating disorders can play an important role in recognizing possible signs and symptoms of eating disorders. Box 3 summarizes common warning signs of eating disorders.

A person with an eating disorder is severely distressed and often needs emotional support and sensitive handling by family and friends. Treatment can be initiated by consulting a general physician, pediatrician, gynecologist, gastroenterologist or a psychiatrist depending upon the most worrisome complaints and ease of availability.

Box 3. Common Warning Signs and Symptoms of an Underlying Eating Disorder

---

- Extreme changes in body weight (either loss or gain) over a brief period of time
- Restricting food or skipping meals to lose weight despite being normal or under-weight (as per BMI)
- Repeatedly eating unusually large amounts of high calorie or high sugar foods in a short period of time
- Repeated episodes of vomiting after having meals
- Eating secretly or while alone (e.g. at night)
- Going to the washroom during or immediately after a meal
- Excessive preoccupation with one's body weight or appearance (shape/size)
- Persistent worry about gaining weight or how to lose more weight to the extent that it hampers one's pursuit of personal (e.g. studies, work) and social (e.g. socializing with friends) activities
- Frequent checking of body weight or looking oneself in the mirror for fat
- Deliberate over-exercising or use of laxatives/other drugs to lose weight without any medical advice
- Expressing feelings of shame, guilt or distress over one's own eating habits

Treatment of Eating Disorders

A person with an eating disorder needs a detailed physical and psychiatric evaluation. Initial evaluation consists of detailed physical examination and laboratory investigations to rule out any serious medical condition (could be a complication of an eating disorder) requiring urgent intervention.

The patient and the family are educated about the suspected eating disorder he/she might be suffering from at the time of consultation. Treatment is generally provided by a psychiatrist along with dietary advice from a dietician. If there are some medical complications, advice from a physician is taken. Most patients can be treated as outpatients except the case where there are serious physical complications or eating behavior has resulted in very low life-threatening BMI or nutritional deficiencies.

The main goals of treatment for eating disorders include:

- Medical stabilization and prevention of serious physical complications

- Correction of nutritional deficiencies and body weight
- Reduction and preferably complete cessation of disordered eating habits and inappropriate compensatory behaviors (e.g. self-induced vomiting after meals, over-exercising to lose weight)
- Improving body image and correcting maladaptive beliefs about body shape/size or food
- Restoration of healthy eating habits
- Re-establishment of social engagement

Treatment includes psychotherapeutic interventions and medication management.

A. Psychotherapy: Cognitive behavioral therapy (CBT) and family-based therapy (FBT) have been found effective in the treatment of eating disorders. Principles of these treatments have been discussed in the chapters on Psychotherapy and Counseling and Family and Mental Health.

CBT focuses on maladaptive thoughts and emotional responses underlying the problematic eating behaviors in an individual and aims at restoring normal healthy eating with restrictions on binging, purging or other inappropriate compensatory behaviors. It also involves emotional regulation through teaching healthy ways of dealing with stresses of life, distress tolerance training, promoting body image satisfaction and improving interpersonal relationships.

In FBT, a manual-based therapy is delivered by a trained psychologist to the patient and his/her family members in separate as well as conjoint weekly treatment sessions. In this approach, the parents are usually trained to provide a supportive environment for the person with an eating disorder. The family can play an active role to help the patient re-establish healthy eating habits and restrict maladaptive behaviors (e.g. purging, binging, etc.).

Guided self-help is another possible strategy for effective management of bulimia spectrum of eating disorders (i.e. BN and BED). It is based on the principles of CBT and the patient goes through the educational material and instructional guidebook about eating disorders and their treatment on their own. The guidebook provides instructions for self-monitoring of eating habits and related behaviors and explains ways to learn and practice restoring healthy eating and stopping inappropriate compensatory behaviors.

B. Medication-based Treatment: Medications should be started under the supervision of a psychiatrist after completion of the initial assessment. Medications are often prescribed for providing nutritional supplementation to correct the associated vitamin or mineral deficiencies that occur due to maladaptive eating behaviors in eating disorders like AN. Certain medicines, like olanzapine (an atypical antipsychotic), have been shown to be helpful in initial weight gain and reduction of agitation among patients

with AN. Some antidepressants, like selective serotonin reuptake inhibitors (e.g. fluoxetine) and mirtazapine, have also been used for the treatment of eating disorders, for managing impulsivity and the coexisting depression. All medicines are to be taken only under strict medical supervision.

Long-Term Outcome and Prognosis

Eating disorders are a heterogeneous group of disorders with AN, BN and BED being the most commonly diagnosed eating disorders, requiring specialist treatment worldwide. In general, patients with pica and rumination disorder have better outcomes as compared to the other three eating disorders. For example, pica is a benign disorder with mostly a self-limiting course and resolution of symptoms in a few months. But patients with AN, BN and BED are at risk of suffering from significant physical and psychological harm if left untreated. For example, AN is associated with possibly the highest mortality rate among various mental disorders. The most common cause of death is due to physical complications associated with severe self-starvation and being underweight.

With appropriate treatment, more than half of the patients with eating disorders recover completely. Around one-third of patients with AN and BN may continue to experience significant symptoms and may require care by a multidisciplinary team comprising psychiatrists, clinical psychologists, physicians and dieticians.

Common Myths About Eating Disorders

Myth: Eating disorders are a matter of choice or lifestyle by people.

Fact: Eating disorders are mental disorders and occur as a result of maladaptive thoughts, emotions and perceptions about one's food intake, body weight and/or body shape. These are not a matter of personal choice and are caused by a complex interaction between various biological, psychological and socio-cultural factors.

Myth: Recovering from an eating disorder is just a question of eating properly.

Fact: Eating disorders are not just about food habits and are almost always associated with mental health problems, such as intense fear of gaining weight, body image distortion, low self-esteem, social withdrawal, etc. These manifestations need specialized treatment and consultation from a mental health professional.

Myth: People with an eating disorder are always underweight or extremely thin.

Fact: People with eating disorders can be underweight (AN), normal or overweight (BN, BED), depending upon the type, duration and severity of the eating disorder.

Myth: Eating disorders only occur in young females living in western countries.

Fact: Though commonly seen in adolescents and young females in their twenties, eating disorders can develop in people of all ages and gender. Further, due to westernization and increasing social media exposure to pro-eating disorder content online, eating disorders are now being increasingly reported in Asian countries like India as well.

Myth: Eating disorders are part of the adolescent 'phase' and will go away on their own without any intervention.

Fact: Eating disorders like AN or BN usually begin during the adolescent years of life and should not be ignored, since these do not necessarily go away with age. They can lead to serious physical and psychological complications, including death, if left untreated.

Conclusion

Eating disorders consist of a heterogeneous group of mental illnesses in which people characteristically develop an excessive preoccupation with their food, body weight and/or body shape due to maladaptive or disturbed thought processes, emotions or perception. The symptoms of self-starvation, binge eating or purging behaviors (e.g. self-induced vomiting) in people with eating disorders are associated with significant physical and psychological harm and can even cause death if left untreated. Eating disorders are caused by an interaction between biological and psychological vulnerabilities alongwith socio-cultural and environmental risk factors.

Family members or people close to those suffering from an eating disorder can play an important role in the early recognition of symptoms, initiation of appropriate treatment and supporting them during the recovery process. Most patients with eating disorders can be helped with treatment, which consists of both psychotherapeutic and medication-based management.

KEY POINTS

➤ Eating disorders include those associated with stoppage of eating (anorexia, nervosa) or excessive eating (bulimia, binge eating disorder).

➤ There is an excessive preoccupation with food, body weight and/or body shape due to maladaptive or disturbed thought processes, emotions or perceptions.

➤ The abnormal eating pattern can lead to significant physical and psychological harm, including death, if left untreated.

➤ Recognition of warning signs and symptoms of an underlying eating disorder by family members or general physicians is crucial for timely diagnosis and early treatment initiation.

➤ Treatments include psychotherapeutic and pharmacological interventions, often provided by a team comprising psychiatrists, clinical psychologists and dieticians.

REFERENCES

1. Anorexia and Bulimia. https://www.rcpsych.ac.uk/mental-health/problems-disorders/anorexia-and-bulimia. last accessed on 22nd February 2022

2. Eating disorders in young people: for parents and carers. https://www.rcpsych.ac.uk/mental-health/parents-and-young-people/information-for-parents-and-carers/eating-disorders-in-young-people-for-parents-and-carers. last accessed on 22nd February 2022

3. Eating Well and Mental Health. https://www.rcpsych.ac.uk/mental-health/problems-disorders/eating-well-and-mental-health. last accessed on 22nd February 2022

CHAPTER 15

Sexual Myths and Dysfunctions

Vaibhav Patil

Introduction

Sexuality plays a major role in human life and refers to the way in which we experience and express ourselves as sexual beings. People often experience and express sexuality through thoughts, fantasies, behaviors and relationships. It is perceived as the identity, feelings and behaviors associated with sex, and is determined by anatomy, physiology, culture, religion, ethics and developmental experiences. Sexual identity is based on the pattern of a person's biological sexual characteristics, whereas gender identity refers to the personal sense of an individual's own gender. Human sexuality has two aspects - procreative and recreational or pleasurable. The procreative aspect is the small part, while recreational aspects, intimacy and sexual activity form a more complex and major part of the sexuality. The human sexual response cycle comprises the subjective experiences and physiological changes that occur during intimacy

and sexual activity. When there is a problem in any phase of the sexual response cycle, which prevents an individual from attaining satisfaction from sexual activity, it is called **sexual dysfunction**. There are many myths and misconceptions related to sexuality, which need to be corrected.

This chapter discusses normal sexual functioning, sexual dysfunctions, myths and misconceptions associated with sexuality, and gender dysphoria.

Human Sexual Response

Human sexual response refers to a series of psychophysiological changes the body undergoes when becoming sexually aroused and engaging in sexual activity. This response is affected by various factors, such as psychosexual development, attitude towards sexuality, thoughts, fantasies, medication, emotional and physical well-being, etc. An individual may experience a sequence of

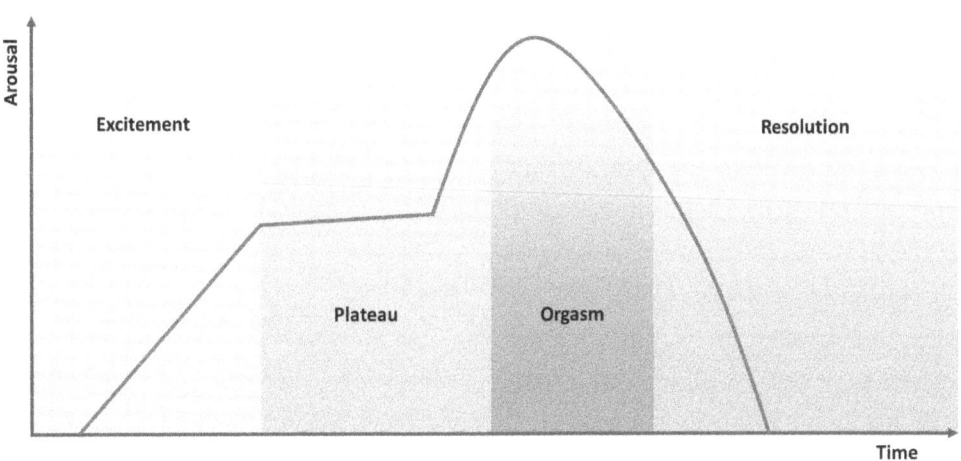

Figure 1. *Stages of Human sexual response*

physiological responses to sexual stimulation or to sexual desire as described in Figure 1 below (first described by famous sex therapists -William Masters and Virginia Johnson).

1. **Excitement** - This is the first phase of the sexual response. It refers to the initial physiological response to physical or psychological stimulation. It may last from several minutes to several hours. Initial changes include increased heart rate, blood pressure and respiration. In men, penile tumescence leads to erection while women have swelling of the clitoris, labia minora and labia majora along with vaginal lubrication. There is an increase in muscle tension and skin may become flushed. Continued stimulation leads to an increase in woman's breast size and man's testes. Nipples become erect or hard.

2. **Plateau** - Physiological changes that begin in the excitement phase are intensified in this phase. Heart rate, blood pressure and respiration continue to increase and stabilize. Muscle tension increases and may extend to the face, hands, feet and other parts of the body. The vaginal wall darkens and the clitoris becomes highly sensitive and retracts under the clitoral hood. In men, the testicles are drawn further into the scrotal sac. Few drops of secretions from the Cowper's gland in men and from Bartholin's glands in women are released in the respective tracts during heightened excitement.

3. **Orgasm** - Orgasm represents the peak of sexual excitement and is marked by involuntary, rhythmic contractions of the perineal muscles and pelvic reproductive organs along with the release of sexual tension. In women, orgasm is characterized by 3-15 contractions of the lower-third region of the vagina, along with strong sustained contractions of the uterus. In men, contractions of the muscles surrounding the base of the penis lead to the emission of semen. In addition, there is a rhythmic spasm of the prostate, seminal vesicle and vas deferens. It is the shortest of all the phases of the sexual response cycle, lasting a few seconds.

4. **Resolution** - This is the end phase of the sexual response cycle, whether an individual experiences orgasm or not. In this phase, the body returns to the pre-arousal state. There is a gradual decrease in muscle tension and blood pressure and respiration reach baseline levels. As blood flow to the genital region decreases, erectile tissues return to the previous state. This is followed by a refractory period in men wherein they cannot be stimulated or aroused for further orgasm for some time.

Common Sexual Myths and Misconceptions

Sex is a basic human drive, but talking about it is still considered a taboo subject. People avoid having a discussion on it. Due to lack of knowledge and awareness about sex and sexual health, the subject is associated with a wide range of myths and misunderstanding.

There are many misconceptions related to **masturbation and contraception**. There is a common belief that masturbation can lead to shrinkage of genitalia, and semen loss can lead to sexual inadequacy and physical weakness. Though the fact is that masturbation is a healthy practice that can be performed by both males and females, and it does not affect their performance while having sex. It does not lead to any physical weakness.

A belief that contraceptive pills prevent sexually transmitted diseases (STDs) is prevalent in many societies. However, contraceptive pills when taken correctly can prevent pregnancy but cannot protect from STDs like gonorrhea or syphilis. Physical

Table 1. *Common Myths About Sex*

All physical contact must lead to sex
Contraceptive use leads to permanent infertility
Women cannot become pregnant the first time they have sex
Only men who have sex with men can get HIV
HIV can be transmitted through any bodily fluids
Vasectomy or tubectomy decreases sexual potency
Circumcision may lead to sexual dysfunction
Women always experience orgasm with penetrative sex
Size of the penis determines sexual pleasure

Table 2. *Common Sexual Dysfunctions*

Low libido
Erectile dysfunction
Premature and delayed ejaculation
Absence of orgasm or delayed orgasm
Vaginismus
Priapism
Dyspareunia
Sexual dysfunction related to medication or substance use

barrier methods, like condoms, can protect from STDs.

Other common myths related to sex are stated in Table 1.

Sexual Dysfunctions

Sexual dysfunctions refer to disturbances in sexual functioning, which can occur during any phase of the sexual response cycle and interfere with experiencing satisfaction from sexual activity. These may lead to significant disturbance in the person's ability to respond sexually or to experience sexual pleasure during sexual activity. Sexual dysfunctions are quite common. Nearly 30-40% of people (both men and women) may suffer from some form of sexual dysfunction. The prevalence of such dysfunctions is slightly higher in women as compared to that in men. However, most individuals suffering from sexual dysfunction do not seek treatment, often due to a lack of awareness, and the dysfunction remains undiagnosed and untreated.

Table 2 summarizes various types of sexual dysfunction in men and women. Hypoactive sexual desire disorder is the commonest sexual dysfunction in women, whereas premature ejaculation is the commonest sexual dysfunction in men. Sexual dysfunctions can be lifelong or acquired and generalized or situational. Causes of sexual dysfunctions can be psychological, physiological or sociocultural, and may relate to physical health, medications, partner issues and relationship conflicts.

Management of Sexual Dysfunction

Sexual dysfunctions are managed by identifying and treating the underlying cause. While assessing a person with sexual dysfunction, it is important to identify the underlying causal factors. Assessment includes a detailed history and physical examination along with appropriate laboratory investigations. A person with sexual dysfunction may suffer from diabetes, cardiovascular diseases, endocrinal disorders, depression and psychoactive substance use which may be in the background of the sexual dysfunction. The person needs to be screened for these illnesses.

Steps in the treatment of sexual dysfunctions are summarized in Figure 2

Treatment for sexual dysfunctions includes:

1. **Education and communication:** Educating the individual or couple regarding anatomy of genitalia and normal sexual response and addressing their concerns and doubts about sexuality may help relieve anxiety related to sexual functioning. Establishing and improving communication with a partner may also help improve sexual functioning.

Treatment of Sexual Dysfunction

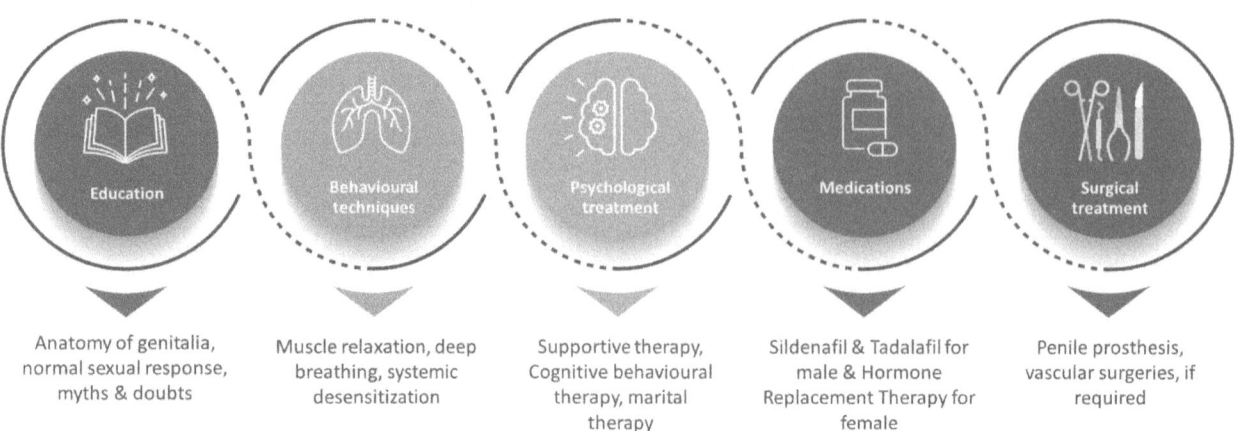

Education	Behavioural techniques	Psychological treatment	Medications	Surgical treatment
Anatomy of genitalia, normal sexual response, myths & doubts	Muscle relaxation, deep breathing, systemic desensitization	Supportive therapy, Cognitive behavioural therapy, marital therapy	Sildenafil & Tadalafil for male & Hormone Replacement Therapy for female	Penile prosthesis, vascular surgeries, if required

Figure 2. *Treatment of Sexual Dysfunction*

2. **Behavioral techniques:** Progressive muscle relaxation, deep breathing exercises or systemic desensitization can help relieve anxiety. Dual sex therapy is a specific behavioral treatment (conceptualized by Masters and Johnson), in which the couples with sexual problem are treated by the therapist.

3. **Medications:** Several medications, like antihypertensive drugs, antipsychotics, antidepressants and antiparkinsonian drugs, can cause sexual dysfunction. In such situations, a change in the medication might help. Drugs like sildenafil and tadalafil are used to treat male sexual dysfunction. For women, hormonal therapy such as estrogen and testosterone can be used if there is a deficiency of specific hormones.

4. **Psychological treatments:** Supportive psychotherapy, cognitive behavioral therapy and marital therapy can be helpful against sexual dysfunction. Psychotherapy can help resolve issues like childhood sexual trauma, guilt, anxiety, fear, and poor body image, which can help to improve sexual functioning.

5. **Surgical treatment:** Penile prosthetic devices may be used in patients with inadequate erectile responses who fail to respond to other

treatments and have a medically untreatable cause. Vascular surgery is indicated in patients with vascular insufficiency due to atherosclerosis or other reasons.

Dhat Syndrome

Dhat syndrome is a common clinical condition seen in young men in South Asia. Typical presentation includes a young male, usually in 20s, presenting with multiple physical complaints, such as fatigue, weakness, lack of appetite, burning micturition, body aches, numbness and psychological symptoms, like anxiety, dysphoric mood, sleep disturbances, poor concentration and guilt. Sexual complaints like premature ejaculation and erectile dysfunction are often present. The person attributes all the symptoms to loss of semen in nocturnal emissions or in urine and masturbation. There is a cultural belief in South Asia that semen is a precious fluid formed from ultra-condensation of food consumed and its loss may lead to weakness. There is a similar problem reported in young women, where various physical and psychological symptoms are attributed to a whitish vaginal discharge. This is also considered as the female equivalent of male dhat syndrome.

While treating a patient with dhat syndrome, it is important to provide sexual knowledge and clarify sexual myths. If there are clinically significant anxiety or depressive symptoms, specific anti-anxiety or antidepressant drugs need to be prescribed.

Paraphilias or Sexual Perversions

Paraphilia refers to an intense and persistent sexual interest in activities outside the realm of genital stimulation or preparatory fondling with physically mature, consenting human partners. There is a deviation from normal sexual behavior that can cause significant distress and dysfunction with serious social and legal consequences. In order to make a diagnosis, an individual must have a history of persistent and recurrent sexual interests, urges, fantasies or behaviors of marked intensity involving objects, activities, or even situations that are atypical in nature and are persistent for many months. Various types of paraphilic disorders along with their atypical sexual interest are listed in Table 3.

Paraphilia is more common in men than in women. Among all paraphilic disorders,

pedophilia is the most common. Various psychosocial factors such as childhood sexual abuse, arrested psychosexual development, difficulty in developing personal and sexual relationships and conditioning of non-sexual objects with sexual activity have been reported as causal factors. It is important to mention here that pedophilia is a criminal offence under Prevention of Children from Sexual Offences (POCSO) Act, 2012, and is to be reported to the relevant legal authorities. Non- consensual sexual activity of any kind with adults can have legal consequences.

Management of Paraphilia

Management of paraphilias includes psychological and pharmacological approaches.

1. **Psychological treatments:** The first step in treatment is to recognize and modify the deviant behaviors. Cognitive behavioral therapy aims at restructuring cognitive distortions. Other commonly used techniques are social skills training, sex education, relaxation techniques and imaginal desensitization.

2. **Medication:** Selective serotonin reuptake inhibitors (SSRIs) such as fluoxetine may

Table 3. *Various forms of paraphilia*

Type of Paraphilia	Atypical sexual interest
Exhibitionism	Recurrent urge to expose the genitals to a stranger or to an unsuspecting person
Fetishism	Non-living objects or non-genital body parts
Frotteurism	Touching or rubbing against a non-consenting person
Pedophilia	Recurrent intense sexual urges toward, or arousal by, children 13 years of age or younger
Sexual Masochism	Preoccupation with sexual urges and fantasies involving the act of being humiliated, beaten, bound or otherwise made to suffer
Sexual Sadism	Sexual arousal from physical or/and psychological suffering of another person
Voyeurism	Observing unsuspecting persons who are naked or engaged in grooming or sexual activity
Transvestism	Fantasies and sexual urges to dress in opposite gender clothing

help decrease the compulsiveness associated with paraphilia and reduce the number of deviant sexual fantasies and behaviors. Anti-androgen drugs help reduce sexual drive and the frequency of mental imagery of sexually arousing scenes.

3. **Treatment of comorbid conditions:** If the paraphilic disorder is associated with any other psychiatric illness, like schizophrenia or depression, treatment with antipsychotics or antidepressants may be helpful.

Gender Dysphoria

Gender dysphoria refers to feelings of distress and discomfort that a person experiences when his/her assigned gender does not match his/her gender identity. An individual may feel distressed about the conflict between his/her sexual characteristics and what he/she feels and thinks about him/herself. The affected person has a desire to remove primary or secondary sexual characteristics, to have sexual characteristics of the opposite gender or desire to be treated as the opposite gender. In children, it is manifested as dressing like the other gender, preference for other gender roles during the play, preference for other gender toys, games or stereotypes, or dislike of one's own anatomy. In general, the person experiences discomfort or distress over the role assigned to him/her based on their birth gender.

The exact cause of gender dysphoria is not known. There may be an association with childhood physical and sexual abuse, maltreatment and neglect. Many cases remain unidentified due to stigma and social reasons.

Management of Gender Dysphoria

Before formulating the plan of management, it is important to conduct a detailed psychiatric assessment, physical examination and appropriate laboratory investigations. Based on assessment and the person's need, an individualized treatment plan is formulated.

Conclusion

Sexuality is an important and central part of every human being and sexual functioning adds to the quality of human life. It is important to understand the normal sexual response and associated dysfunction. Sexual dysfunctions, paraphilia and gender dysphoria are prevalent in the general population. They are associated with significant distress and have a negative impact on day-to-day functioning. Due to a lack of awareness and associated myths and taboos, an individual suffering from these dysfunctions rarely seeks treatment. A range of management strategies are available for sexual dysfunctions. Myths and misconceptions associated with sexuality need to be corrected.

KEY POINTS

➢ Sexuality and sexual functioning are important aspects of human life.

➢ Sexual dysfunction, paraphilia and gender dysphoria are associated with significant distress and dysfunctions.

➢ There is a lack of awareness regarding sex due to associated myths and taboos.

➢ Increasing awareness and early seeking of treatment may help reduce associated distress and dysfunction.

REFERENCES

1. Gender Dysphoria. https://www.psychiatry.org/patients-families/gender-dysphoria accessed on 14th March 2022.

2. Grover S, Avasthi A, Gupta S, Hazari N, Malhotra N. Do female patients with nonpathological vaginal discharge need the same evaluation as for Dhat syndrome in males? Indian J Psychiatry. 2016 Jan-Mar;58(1):61-9.

3. Masters WH, Johnson VE. Human Sexual Response. Boston: Little, Brown; 1970

4. Rao TSS. History and mystery of Dhat syndrome: A critical look at the current understanding and future directions. Indian J Psychiatry. 2021 Jul-Aug;63(4):317-325.

CHAPTER 16

Disorders Related to Sleep

Ravi Gupta

Introduction

Sleep is an important and necessary physiological need of all living beings. On average, an adult spends around one-third of life sleeping, yet we do not pay much attention to its importance, necessity and functions. In modern times, for worldly pleasures and responsibilities, if anything is sacrificed, sleep comes on the top of that list. The most probable reason for it is the absence of basic knowledge regarding the need and functions of sleep. Further, societal, personal, health-related and economic impacts of sleep disorders are also largely unknown to the general population.

This chapter introduces the readers to sleep and common sleep disorders.

What is Sleep and How is it Important?

'Healthy sleep' is defined as one that follows a natural circadian rhythm, with adequate duration and good quality, contributing to the growth and repair of the body.

Sleep has multiple vital functions:

- Rejuvenating and repairing functions of sleep occur through the secretion of hormones, viz. growth hormone and adrenocorticotropic hormones.
- Sleep is tightly linked to immunity. Suboptimal sleep enhances the risk of catching infections.
- Sleep provides a chance to take rest to the body organs. Both heart rate and blood pressure

decline during 'healthy sleep' and thus it reduces the chances of high blood pressure and heart attacks. Sleep provides rest to muscles and bones, and helps in their repair. Sleep also provides rest to the gut, liver and kidneys to name a few.

- Sleep plays an important role in regulation of metabolism, especially that of glucose, by controlling the secretion of hormones, like insulin and glucagon. Blood sugar rises after cutting down sleep for as short as one to two nights. In long term, sleep deprivation increases the chances of the development of diabetes mellitus through complex mechanisms. Inadequate sleep increases the chances of weight gain, which is minimally influenced by a portion of meals taken during forceful awakenings.
- Sleep is important for the brain as healthy sleep enhances the clearance of waste material from the brain through the 'glymphatic system' and reduces the aging of the brain. Memory consolidation occurs during sleep and through this process, information gathered throughout the day shifts to the long-term memory. Sleep plays an important part in the regulation of emotions and cognition, as well. Sleep deprivation enhances negative emotions, such as irritability, impulsivity, sadness and anxiety, and causes cognitive impairment, including inattention, impaired concentration and poor decision making.

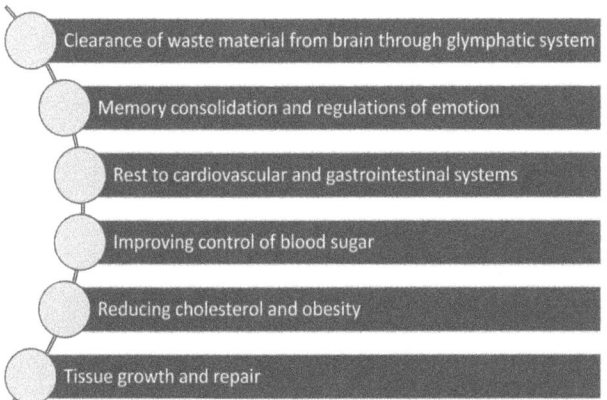

Figure 1. *Functions of Optimal Sleep*

Functions of sleep are summarized in Figure 1.

Unfortunately, people in the 'modern' world are cutting down their sleep for other pleasures, e.g., enjoying the nightlife, watching television, use of computers and spending time on social media, to name a few.

Why do we sleep?

The sleep-wake cycle is regulated by two interdependent processes known as the homeostatic process and the circadian process.

- **Homeostatic process** regulates the duration of sleep in response to sleep pressure. Sleep pressure increases with the duration of wakefulness and reduces when we take a nap or sleep.
- **Circadian process** is regulated by exposure to light and dark. In humans, exposure to darkness (as in night) stimulates the release of melatonin that induces sleep. Co-occurrence of sleep pressure and melatonin at night makes us fall asleep. Melatonin secretion reduces by morning along with a reduction in sleep pressure after a good sleep.

Any disturbance in the synchrony and amplitude of these processes can cause sleep disorders.

How Much Sleep is Enough?

This is the most common question asked by people. However, the answer to it is not straightforward. This is because:

- Natural duration of sleep alters with age.
- Sleep duration varies across days even in healthy people.
- There is variation in natural sleep duration across individuals.

The duration of time spent in sleep in a given day reduces from infancy till one attains adulthood and then becomes constant till the age of 65 years. Beyond that age, it may reduce further (Figure 2).

Some people are short sleepers and some are long sleepers. Short sleepers spend less than 6 hours a day sleeping, yet do not feel sleepy during the day. Long sleepers require at least 10 hours of sleep each night to function optimally during the day. On an average, 7-8 hours of sleep is considered optimal for an adult.

Largely, one is considered to have an adequate amount of sleep if after waking up one remains active and alert before the next scheduled time for sleep. By late adolescence, the 'daily requirement of sleep' is established. However, a change in the required sleep (increased or decreased) compared to one's usual pattern could indicate a sleep disorder.

When Should I Sleep?

Nature has designed human beings to sleep after dusk and to rise before dawn. A change in sleep-wake time, i.e., shift to later bedtime and waketime has been observed since the invention of electricity and different kinds of screens despite traditional teaching advising 'early to bed and early to rise'. **To ensure that the natural sleep-wake cycle**

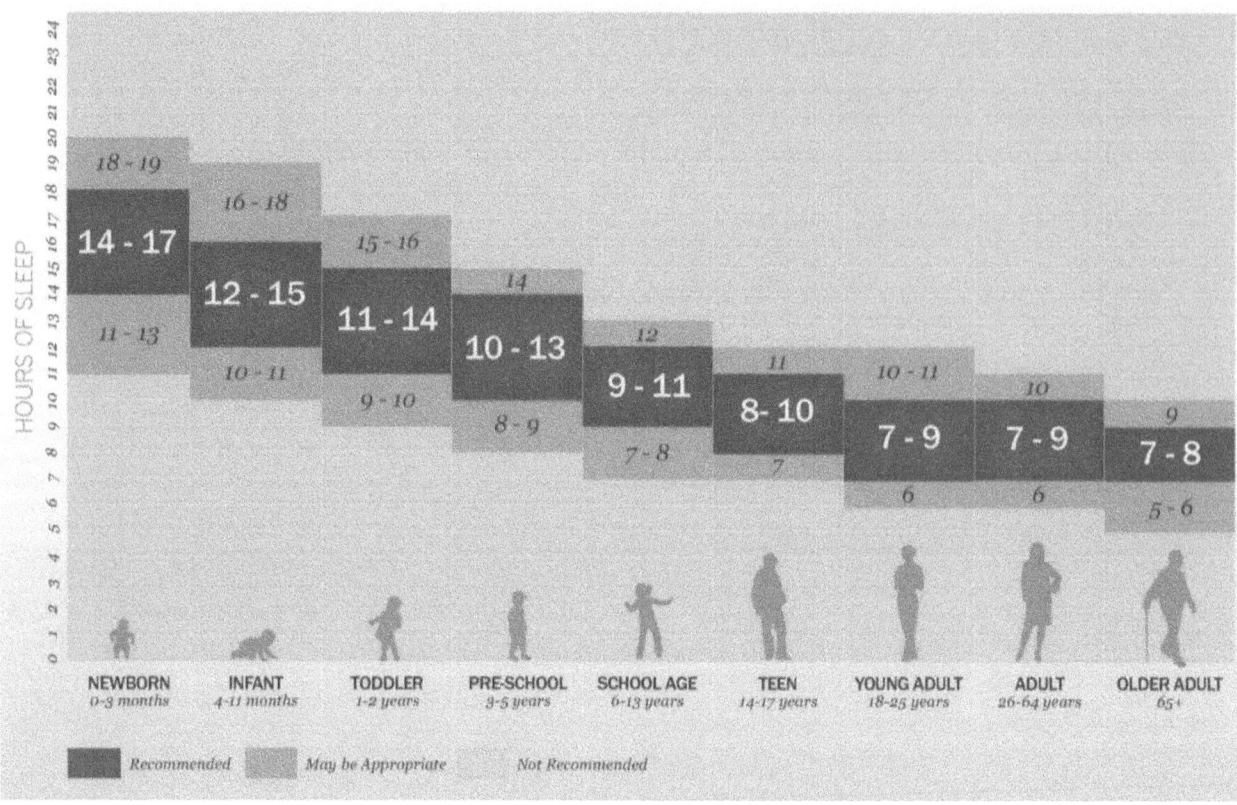

Figure 2. *Recommended Duration of Sleep Across Age Groups**

*Adapted from Sleep NSF; Creative Commons Attribution-Share Alike 4.0 International license; Available at https://commons. wikimedia.org/wiki/File:NSF_Sleep_Duration_Recommendations_Chart.jpg; Last accessed 31 Jan 2022

is followed, our ancestors attached religious practices with sleep-wake time. In Hindu and Islamic cultures, the first prayer of the day is offered well before dawn and the last prayer soon after dusk.

During darkness, the pineal gland in the body secretes melatonin, a hormone that induces sleep. Contrarily, the presence of light, especially in the violet to blue range (424-460 nm wavelength), which is emitted by most of the electronic screens, suppresses its secretion. Not only the wavelength, but the intensity of light is also important for suppressing melatonin. Even the dim indoor light (50 lux, irrespective of wavelength) is enough to suppress the secretion of melatonin in sensitive individuals.

Later bedtime and high variability in bedtime both have been found to increase the risk of obesity, metabolic syndrome, heart problems, cognitive dysfunction, diabetes and depression. **Social jetlag** (curtailing sleep on workdays and sleep extension on holidays) also has similar adverse effects on health. Exposure to light at night has been found to enhance the risk of breast cancers in women and prostate cancer in men. Thus, it is important that the timing of sleep-wake should be in concordance with what nature has designed us for.

It is also important to mention the **quality of sleep** here, which refers to a subjective feeling of freshness and energy after waking up. Sleep quality is perceived as 'good' when enough time is spent in sleep, sleep-wake time is in synchrony with nature and, lastly, factors interfering with the maintenance of both sleep and wakefulness are absent. Poor sleep quality has also been found to worsen the overall health and increase the risk for other disorders.

Common Sleep Disorders

Common sleep disorders include insomnia, obstructive sleep apnea, hypersomnia, restless leg syndrome, parasomnia and circadian rhythm sleep disorders.

Insomnia:

Insomnia is the most common sleep disorder and affects approximately 10%-15% of the adult population, with prevalence further increasing with age. People with insomnia experience both night-time and day-time symptoms. Night-time symptoms include trouble falling asleep or staying asleep or waking up earlier than the desired wake time despite adequate opportunities for sleep. Daytime symptoms of insomnia include irritability, headache, impulsivity, poor attention and mood disturbances. Due to daytime symptoms, it can often be mistaken for psychiatric disorders, e.g., depression or anxiety, even by specialists. If symptoms occur three or more times a week, it needs consultation with a specialist.

Some people may develop insomnia after exposure to a precipitating factor, usually acute stress, or an illness. This is known as acute insomnia (if symptoms are present for lesser than 3 months) and it may fade away as soon as the precipitating factor terminates. However, some persons develop dysfunctional beliefs and practices that are sleep defeating; for example, they start worrying excessively about insomnia and its consequences; extend the time spent in bed to fall asleep; consume stimulants (caffeine, nicotine, etc.) during the day to remain alert; use the bed for work besides sleep and sex, e.g., watching TV; mentalize or plan while unable to sleep. These factors perpetuate insomnia, making it chronic (lasts >3 months).

Diagnosis of insomnia is primarily based on clinical information and no laboratory test is usually required. However, cases of chronic unexplained insomnia may require sleep study (polysomnography) to rule out other sleep disorders, e.g., sleep apnea, periodic limb movement disorder and sleep-related seizures to name a few. These sleep disorders may either co-exist with insomnia resulting in inadequate response to insomnia treatment or may masquerade as insomnia. Actigraphy and a sleep diary may help clarify the diagnosis in such a situation. Actigraphy is a watch-like instrument that is worn on the non-dominant wrist for at least 14 days for the diagnosis and, thereafter, throughout the course of management to collect objective data regarding improvement.

Acute insomnia is usually treated by hypnotics. However, for chronic insomnia, a combination of multi-model cognitive behavior therapy for insomnia along with hypnotics is required. Following the sleep hygiene guidelines (Box 1) helps maintain good sleep.

Obstructive sleep apnea (OSA):

Snoring is a common problem and many middle-aged adults snore. In Indian culture, snoring is considered to represent deep and good quality sleep. However, scientific evidence suggests that snoring is not good for health as it represents a partial obstruction in the upper airway (nose and throat) that makes breathing difficult while sleeping. In many snorers, obstruction turns complete leading to the cessation of breathing. If this cessation continues for at least 10 seconds in one go, it is considered obstructive sleep apnea (OSA). Careful observers and bedpartners can report a lack of chest and abdominal movements during these periods. During apnea, the body tries hard to breathe, resulting in increased effort of breathing. This results in sweating on the scalp, around the neck and on the chest. The enhanced effort also

Box 1. Sleep Hygiene Practices

Dos	Don'ts
• Follow a fixed sleep-wake schedule • Sleep should also be a priority • Have around half an hour to unwind before bedtime • Dim lights in bedroom • Exercise in the morning • Have dinner at least two hours before scheduled bedtime • Make bed and bedroom environment sleep facilitatory	• ...take naps in the afternoon and evening • ...use screens at least one hour from intended bedtime • ...use caffeine or caffeinated beverages after the evening • ...smoke in evening or later • ...use the bed for any activity other than sleep and sex

increases the pressure in the chest leading to the production of excessive urine at night. Hence, voiding at least two times a night could be a sign of sleep apnea. Some people may breathe from the mouth during sleep because of difficulty breathing from the nose, leading to dryness of the mouth and increased thirst. Sleep-talking is another sign of OSA and occurs because some parts of the brain wake up recurrently to support the effort of breathing.

Nearly one-third of patients complain of non-refreshing sleep and feel tired or sleepy during the day, especially when they are sitting idle or engaged in monotonous work, e.g., driving, watching TV or in class. Other third patients experience only non-refreshing sleep and the remaining do not experience any symptoms. In the Indian population, nearly five to nine adults among every 100 adults suffer from OSA. Diagnosis of OSA requires an attended sleep study under the guidance of an expert.

Patients with mild OSA require only lifestyle management. Mandibular advancement devices that pull the lower jaw forward have also been found effective in patients with mild to moderate OSA.

For those with moderate to severe OSA, positive pressure airway (PAP) therapy is the gold standard. PAP devices blow the air with a pressure that works as a splint and keeps the upper airway open. There are three types of PAP devices - automatic (APAP), which keep changing pressure all night, and fixed pressure devices, like continuous (CPAP) and bilevel (BPAP). Some patients may need surgical treatment, which is generally done by ENT surgeons.

Restless legs syndrome (RLS):

Restless leg syndrome (RLS) belongs to the category of sleep-related movement disorders. RLS is characterized by an urge to move the legs that is often accompanied by abnormal sensations, e.g., tickling, stretching, bubbling or pain, usually in the muscles of legs and thighs and in some cases, in the muscles of arms. These symptoms usually worsen by evening and at rest. Movement of legs, viz., repeated stretching of foot, walking and massage, provide relief in symptoms. RLS interferes with sleep onset and is often mistaken for insomnia.

Nearly 2% of the Indian adult population suffers from RLS. Prevalence is higher among patients suffering from iron deficiency anemia, chronic kidney disease, rheumatoid arthritis, and Parkinson's disease. Pregnancy also increases the risk for RLS among genetically predisposed people.

Reducing intake of tea/coffee/in the evening, and avoidance of nicotine and heavy exercise in the evening also help reduce the symptoms. Some patients may need medical treatment.

Parasomnia:

Parasomnia is a group of disorders where goal-directed complex movements are observed during sleep, but the sufferer often does not have any recall for the same. Night terror and sleep-walking are examples of parasomnias.

Night terror and sleepwalking are common among children till the age of 5-6 years and result from the incomplete and partial maturation of the brain. Till this age, they may not require any intervention unless disabling. A child suffering from night terrors usually wakes up from sleep, screams, cries and is often inconsolable. This could be in response to a bad dream, however, the recall for the same is either partial or none. During sleep-walking, the person leaves the bed with open eyes and navigates the house. The person may perform complex activities during the episode but does not have any recollection after the episode is over.

Continuation or appearance of these problems during adolescence and adulthood often indicates the presence of some sleep disorder and should be thoroughly investigated by a sleep specialist.

Some parasomnias, e.g., REM sleep behavior disorder (RBD), appear in late adulthood or old age. These are characterized by complex movements, e.g., shouting, screaming, punching, fighting, running and/or kicking within the bed or after getting up from the bed, usually in response to a bad dream. This often results in significant injury to either the bed partner or the patient himself/herself. People can recall their dream. RBD could antedate neurovegetative diseases, like Parkinson's disease or dementia, by 10 years.

Diagnosis of parasomnia may require a long-term, attended, video synchronized sleep study (polysomnography-PSG) that differentiates it from other sleep disorders. PSG also helps diagnose other sleep disorders that can precipitate parasomnia and thus helps in the optimal planning of treatment.

Hypersomnia:

Hypersomnia is characterized by increased time spent in sleep. The most common type of hypersomnia is insufficient sleep syndrome. This occurs after voluntary sleep deprivation that may be acute or chronic resulting in increased sleep pressure and daytime sleepiness. It can be improved by opting for the premorbid sleep-wake schedule.

Idiopathic hypersomnia usually starts during adolescence. The persons often sleep for most of the day and despite spending excessive time in sleep, do not feel fresh. Narcolepsy, another type of hypersomnia, also starts around this time with similar symptoms. However, it has additional symptoms, viz., **sleep-paralysis** (waking up from sleep and not be able to move any part of the body for a few seconds), **cataplexy** (loss of muscle tone resulting in drooping of eyelid, bucking of knees or drooping of the jaw associated with sudden emotions, such as while laughing) and episodes of irresistible desire to fall asleep during the day. Actigraphy and PSG are often required for the diagnosis of these disorders. Hypersomnia is treatable and can be managed by scheduled naps and medications.

Circadian rhythm sleep disorders (CRSD):

Circadian rhythm sleep disorders (CRSD) are characterized by a mismatch between the subjective day-night cycle (internal circadian-rhythm) and an environmental day-night cycle. CRSD can arise

Box 2.   Circadian Rhythm Sleep Disorders

Diagnosis	Clinical Presentation
Delayed Sleep Wake Phase Schedule (DSWPD)	Common among adolescents and in modern society. Persons go to bed late at night to wake up late. If they are allowed to follow their own schedule, they remain asymptomatic. Often mistaken for either insomnia or hypersomnia.
Advanced Sleep Wake Phase Schedule (ASWPD)	Common among elderly. Persons go to bed early in the evening to wake up early in the morning. If they are allowed to follow their own schedule, they remain asymptomatic. Often mistaken for either insomnia or hypersomnia.
Non-24-hour Sleep-Wake Rhythm Disorder	Persons experience a delay of 30-60 min in sleep and wake schedule each night. Thus, for a few days, their sleep-wake schedule is synchronized with the environmental day and night. On a few days, it mimics insomnia, and on other days, hypersomnia. Common among visually impaired persons and those having neurodevelopmental disorders.
Irregular Sleep Wake Rhythm Disorder	Persons do not have any regular period of sleep and wakefulness. Sleep and wakefulness are in short bouts interspersed throughout 24 hours that keep on changing on day to day basis.
Shift Worker Disorder	Because of constantly changing shifts, there is a mismatch between the environmental and circadian rhythms. One finds it difficult to sleep after night shifts and often feels sleepy during the work shifts, especially night shifts.

because of dysfunction in internal rhythm or by extrinsic factors, viz., having a sleep-wake schedule that does not match with the environmental day-night cycle, as seen among shift-workers (Box 2). Their prevalence in the community is not known.

Detailed medical history, actigraphy and sleep diary are required for the diagnosis of CRSD. Treatment includes timed melatonin, chronotherapy and timed bright light therapy.

Conclusion

Sleep disorders are highly prevalent in the community. However, these often remain undiagnosed, untreated or poorly treated. Healthy sleep is important for the optimal functioning of not only the brain but also of other systems of the body. Sleep regulates functions of other organs and organ systems through endocrine, immune and autonomic nervous systems. Many of the sleep disorders are preventable by adopting a healthy and active lifestyle and following measures to ensure a healthy sleep. The absence of a healthy sleep (of adequate duration, optimal timing and good quality) or untreated sleep disorders results in multiple health issues and poses an economic burden (through direct and indirect costs) (Figure 3).

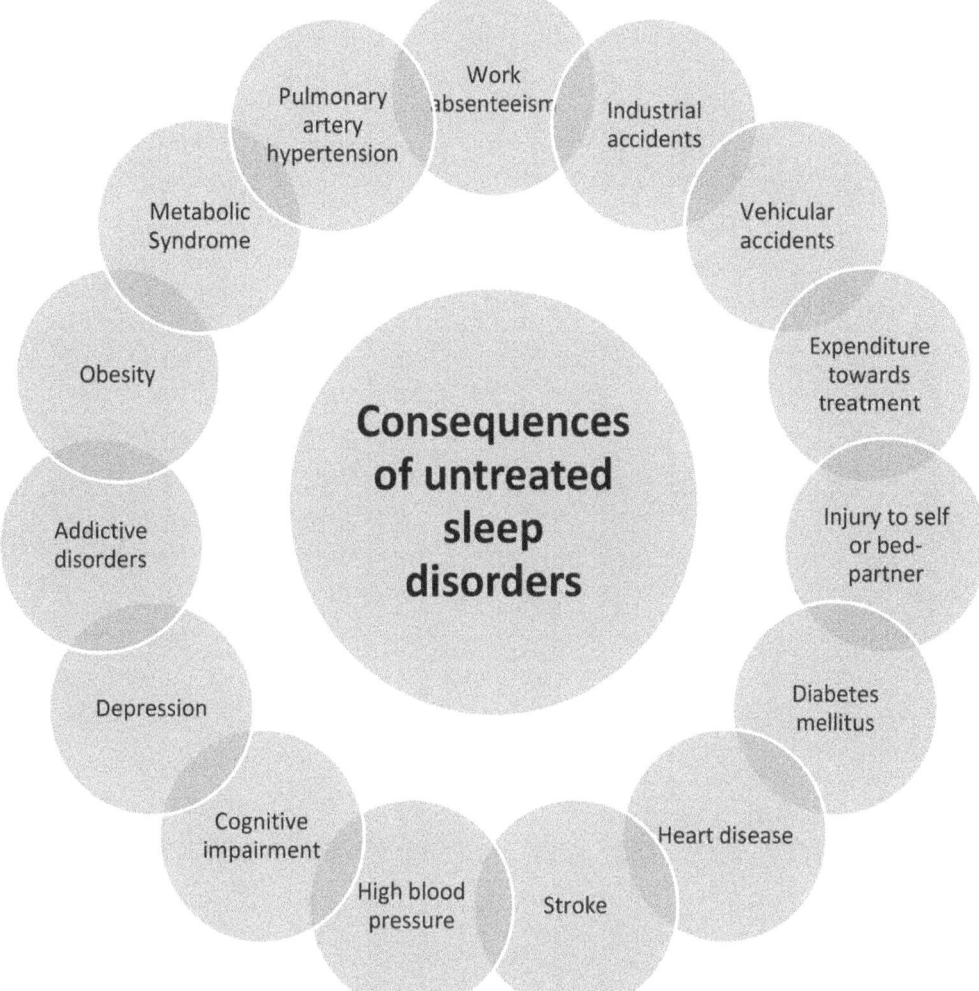

Figure 3. *Consequences of Untreated Sleep Disorders*

KEY POINTS

➢ One should follow a regular sleep-wake schedule.

➢ Taking adequate sleep is important for maintaining good health.

➢ Societal changes have been a major contributor to sleep-related disorders.

➢ Disorders, like sleep apnea, should not be ignored.

REFERENCES

1. Chaput JP, Dutil C, Featherstone R, Ross R, et al. Sleep timing, sleep consistency, and health in adults: a systematic review. Appl Physiol Nutr Metab. 2020;45(10):S232-47.

2. Phillips AJK, Vidafar P, Burns AC, et al. High sensitivity and interindividual variability in the response of the human circadian system to evening light. Proc Natl Acad Sci U S A 2019 Jun 11; 116:12019-12024.

3. Sleeping well. https://www.rcpsych.ac.uk/mental-health/problems-disorders/sleeping-well. last accessed on16th February 2022

4. Tähkämö L, Partonen T, Pesonen AK. Systematic review of light exposure impact on human circadian rhythm. Chronobiol Int. 2019 Feb;36(2):151-170. doi: 10.1080/07420528.2018.1527773. Epub 2018 Oct 12. PMID: 30311830.

CHAPTER 17

Recognizing Mental Health Issues in Growing Children

Rajesh Sagar and Swarndeep Singh

'The child is the father of the man'
– William Wordsworth

Introduction

Childhood and adolescence have been regarded as the most critical periods for the development and maturation of the human brain and personality. This is also a period of particular vulnerability, as adverse events or deviations during this stage of of development can have a profound and long-lasting impact on the overall well-being of the person, even into adulthood. This period can be divided into different stages, such as infancy (0-1 year), toddler (1-3 years), pre-school (3-5 years), childhood (5-10 years), adolescence (10-19 years) and youth (15-24 years). For the sake of convenience, in this chapter, the word child or children refers to all individuals below the age of 18 years, unless specified otherwise. This chapter discusses the importance of ensuring good mental health in children.

Mental health in children is not merely the absence of mental illness but a complete physical as well as psychological well-being of the child with the attainment of age-appropriate developmental milestones in the behavioral, emotional, social and cognitive (e.g., critical thinking and logical reasoning ability) domains.

All children are not the same in terms of their social skills, coping, problem-solving ability and overall quality of life or functioning. Mental health in children includes the following characteristics:

- Ability to experience a different range of emotions, such as happiness to anger to sadness, in an appropriate manner (with respect to both context and intensity)
- Ability to achieve developmentally appropriate emotional, social and cognitive skills needed to interact with self, family, peers and community members
- Ability to develop and maintain meaningful interpersonal relationships (e.g. friendship, love, etc.) with other people and function productively
- Ability to develop good self-esteem and show respectful behavior towards other people
- Ability to learn new skills and develop healthy ways of coping for dealing with new problems or undesirable situations
- Ability to play with others and also enjoy 'me time' or solitary activities (i.e. self-regulation)

Importance of Mental Health in Children

Identifying mental health issues in children is extremely important since children with poor mental health are likely to experience problems in navigating successfully through different developmental stages of childhood. More so, children might not be able to fully comprehend or communicate about their mental health problems like adults. Children with mental health problems are on average three times more likely to have poor physical health, achieve lower academic achievement scores (e.g. failure in a grade, drop-out from school, etc.) and develop unhealthy or risky health behaviors, such as alcohol or drug use. Children with mental health problems are also six times more likely to experience suicidal ideation and indulge in self-harm behaviors. Untreated mental health problems experienced during childhood have several detrimental and long-lasting consequences on the physical and mental well-being, continuing even as they become adults. It is important to mention here that about half of the mental illnesses emerge by the age of 14.

As in adults, there is significant stigma attached to mental health problems and treatment-seeking in children too. This is coupled with a relative lack of knowledge and sensitivity required for the identification of mental health problems in children among parents, teachers and even health care professionals (e.g. primary care doctor, community nurse, pediatrician, gynecologist, etc.), who are in a position to facilitate early detection and treatment of such issues. Thus, it is essential to create awareness among different stakeholders about the importance of recognizing child mental health problems and also an early intervention. Figure 1 summarizes the importance of mental health in children.

Mental Health Issues Among Children

Mental health problems among children could present either as non-specific symptoms (e.g. frequent stomach aches, sleep disturbance, etc.) or sub-threshold behavioral/emotional disturbances. Alternatively, these symptoms, if untreated or not adequately managed, might increase in frequency or severity and give rise to a mental illness. Common childhood mental illnesses can be broadly divided into the following broad groups:

A. Developmental disorders: These are due to some delay or deviation or regression in developmental milestones attained by the children in one or more domains (e.g., motor, language, social, etc.). For example, intellectual disability (mental retardation), specific learning disability (SLD), autism spectrum disorder (ASD), etc.

B. Emotional disorders: These are also referred to as internalizing disorders since manifestations of maladaptive thoughts and/or feelings remain inside one's own mind or body. For example, depression, anxiety disorders, etc.

C. Behavioral disorders: These are also referred to as externalizing disorders since maladaptive

Importance of Mental Health in Children

Children with mental health problems are

- Three times more likely to have poor physical health.
- Achieve lower academic achievement scores
- Indulge more in substance use disorders
- Six times more likely to experience suicidal ideation and indulge in self-harm behaviors.
- About half of the mental illnesses emerge by the age of 14

Figure 1. *Importance of Mental Health in Children*

thoughts and/or feelings are manifested outwards towards people or things in the surrounding environment. For example, attention deficit-hyperactivity disorder (ADHD), conduct disorder, oppositional defiant disorder, etc.

D. Other disorders: This group comprises mental disorders that cannot be classified in any one of the above three categories. For example, psychotic disorders, eating disorders, etc.

Identification of Mental Health Problems in Children

It is often easier to identify and assess children suffering from some physical health problem, as physical illnesses have distinguishing signs or symptoms that are usually evidently observable from the outside to people around the child as well as general health professionals (e.g., cough, fever, a tumorous growth visible on the body/imaging report, shortness of breath due to respiratory disease, etc.). This is unlike symptoms of a mental illness, which is often experienced by the individual internally in his/her own subjective space and is often not spontaneously observable to others from the outside (e.g., persistent sadness due to no apparent reason, excessive difficulty in reading or learning despite child's best efforts, etc.). Further, children might not be able to recognize or communicate the symptoms of mental illness.

Box 1. Common Warning Signs and Symptoms of Mental Illness in Children

- Persistent sadness or loss of interest in previously pleasurable activities for more than two weeks
- Spending most of the time alone and avoiding participating in social activities or interaction with family or friends
- Engaging in deliberate self-harm behaviors (e.g. cutting of wrist or burning of skin) or reporting thoughts about dying or killing oneself
- Excessive temper tantrums or extremely irritable behavior
- Dramatic changes in mood and behavior
- Marked changes in sleeping (e.g. feeling sleepy throughout the day or decreased need for sleep) or eating habits (e.g. reduced appetite leading to weight loss or increased consumption of sweets)
- Increased difficulty in studies or decline in academic performance
- School refusal behavior
- Frequent complaints of headache or stomach-ache or other physical complaints without any diagnosable medical cause
- Smoking, drinking alcohol or consuming other drugs of abuse
- Fidgety child with difficulty in sitting still in one place (except watching a TV show or playing a video game of their choice)
- Difficulty in performing tasks requiring sustained attention (e.g. organizing books according to school timetable, listening to a lecture, etc.)
- Lack of interest in playing with other children or difficulty in making friends. Poor eye contact and communication skills
- Frequent lying, truancy, stealing, cruelty towards animals, disobedience and/or vindictive behaviors
- Repetitive actions (e.g. washing hands) or checking things many times at a stretch
- Reports false firm beliefs about someone trying to harm him/her or hear sounds that other people around him/her cannot hear

Thus, it is important for parents, teachers and healthcare professionals usually involved with treating children (e.g., pediatrician, primary care doctor, etc.) to be observant of the signs and/or symptoms of possible mental illness in children. Box 1 mentions some of the common warning signs that could be used for the identification of children with possible underlying mental illness, requiring mental health consultation or assessment.

Burden of Mental Ill Health in Children

According to global estimates, at least one in every five children experiences some mental health problem or issue during their childhood and about one in every 10 children suffers from a clinically diagnosable mental health disorder. The National Mental Health Survey of India (2015-16) reported that 7.3% of children aged 13-17 years suffer from a diagnosable mental illness with the prevalence comparable between boys and girls. Children account for 41% of the total population of India. Thus, a significantly large number of children need active intervention by child mental health services.

It is estimated that only about 1% of children with mental health issues receive appropriate treatment in India. This huge treatment gap could be partly explained by the relative neglect of child mental health in the overall framework of health and mental health services planning and delivery. It is unfortunate to say that in India, less than 1% of the total health budget is allocated to mental health, and a further minimal percentage of that is spent on activities aimed at improving child mental health. There are a very limited number of child psychiatrists in India with usually adult psychiatrists providing treatment for mental health issues in children. Only about 1% of the total in-patient psychiatric treatment beds available in India are earmarked for children. Thus, there is a huge demand-supply mismatch for child mental health services in India.

Mental Health Impact of COVID-19 Pandemic on Children

There has been a significant direct (e.g., fear of getting ill or spreading COVID-19, death of loved ones, etc.) as well as indirect impact (e.g., disruption of daily routine due to containment measures, non-access to classrooms or playgrounds, etc.) of COVID-19 pandemic on the psychological well-being of children. Younger children are also likely to lack the developmental maturity required to understand the concept of death and fully grasp the irreversible, inevitable and/or untimely nature of the loss of their loved ones during the COVID-19 pandemic. All these factors are likely to produce psychological distress and lead to mental ill-health, and also worsen the pre-existing mental health problems in children. The commonly described emotional and behavioral problems among children include symptoms of depression, anxiety, panic disorder, fear of getting or spreading COVID-19 infection, feelings of loneliness/boredom, increased irritability or clinginess, sleep disturbances and increased sedentary behaviors. The prevalence rates of clinically significant anxiety and depressive disorders among children are estimated to have doubled as compared to the pre-pandemic period. Lastly, the COVID-19 pandemic has also led to the disruption of already scarce mental health services for children due to the repurposing of facilities and the diversion of human resources to take care of patients with COVID-19. This has led to a double whammy with a significant rise in the demand or need for child mental health care services on one hand and a decline in the availability of already limited child mental health care resources on the other.

Treatment of Children with Mental Illness

There is an inadequate number of child mental health professionals and services to manage the existing burden of child mental ill-health and high levels of prevailing stigma attached to mental health-related treatment-seeking among children and the society. Thus, it is important to create awareness about common signs of mental ill-health and available treatment options for parents and teachers. This chapter is also an attempt in this direction. As in adults, treatment approaches include psychotherapeutic and pharmacological interventions.

A. Psychotherapy (Talk Therapy/Counseling):

It is a process in which a usually trained mental health professional (therapist) interacts with a child experiencing mental health problems with the objective of helping him/her. Additionally, this may also include a parent or another person involved in providing care to the child. There are different types of psychotherapies available for the management of childhood mental illnesses. Some common psychotherapeutic approaches are listed below:

i. **Cognitive behavior therapy (CBT):** The therapist elicits the underlying maladaptive cognitions (thoughts) and emotions responsible for causing symptoms of mental illness. During CBT, the therapist and the child gradually work together towards either correcting or replacing these maladaptive thoughts, feelings and behaviors with positive or desirable ones. CBT is a structured, manual-based therapy with a large body of evidence supporting its efficacy for the treatment of depression and anxiety disorders. It has also been used with some modifications for the treatment of other mental illnesses.

ii. **Parent skills training:** The therapist tries to strengthen existing positive parenting practices

and introduce parent(s) or caregiver(s) to new practices or skills, which would be helpful in handling problem behaviors in the child and promote a reduction in problem behaviors gradually by using principles of learning and habit formation. The exact techniques taught or suggested may vary depending upon the type of mental health problem and the ability or willingness of the parent to adopt certain techniques.

iii. **Supportive psychotherapy:** The therapist tries to help children to deal with their emotional distress and problems in life, identify helpful and harmful coping strategies, and improve their self-esteem. It involves a combination of various common-sense practical methods, such as comforting, reassuring, patient and active listening, explaining behaviors, advice and encouragement or praising, among others.

iv. **Play therapy:** The therapist employs play-based techniques (e.g., using art or drawing, playing with dolls, playing hide-and-seek, etc.) to help younger children usually aged between 3-12 years process their emotions and articulate their mental health issues to the therapist or parents.

v. **Eclectic therapy:** It involves a combination of different psychotherapeutic techniques depending upon the expertise and comfort of the health professional and the child. For example, delivering psychoeducation about the nature of the disease and teaching simple techniques for relaxation (e.g., deep breathing, humming or listening to soothing music or song, etc.) and anger management (e.g., serial subtraction, writing down what is bothering you and rip it up, etc.), among other things.

B. Pharmacotherapy (Medications): Medications are an effective treatment option for the management of severe or psychotherapy-resistant childhood mental illnesses. Also, they are often used as a first-line treatment option for certain common mental illnesses, when psychotherapy is not feasible (mental health professionals capable of providing psychotherapy are not available or the child is not comfortable with psychotherapy). Further, the available scientific literature suggests that a combination of pharmacotherapy and psychotherapy treatment produces the best results as compared to either of them given alone. Some examples of common pharmacotherapeutic treatments are as follows:

i. **Selective-serotonin reuptake inhibitors:** These are used for the treatment of depression and anxiety disorders (e.g., panic disorder, agoraphobia, obsessive-compulsive disorder, etc.). These have excellent safety profiles and can also be prescribed by a pediatrician or a primary care physician, trained in the assessment and management of children with mild-moderately severe depression or anxiety disorder.

ii. **Medications for ADHD:** These are divided into stimulants (e.g. methylphenidate) and non-stimulants (e.g. atomoxetine) and are used for symptom management of ADHD in children.

iii. **Antipsychotics:** These are the mainstay treatment for psychotic disorders. Also, low-dose atypical antipsychotics, like risperidone or aripiprazole, are used for symptomatic management of irritability/aggression or problematic behaviors in children with ASD or intellectual disability.

Common Myths Associated with Child Mental Health

In this section, we describe some of the common myths associated with mental illnesses of children and their treatment currently prevalent among the public.

Myth: Children do not experience any mental health problems. They are either moody or are just going through a rough stage/phase in life.
Fact: Some degree of mood swings, aggression, temper tantrums and acting out or defiant behavior may be explained by normal developmental changes in the brain and hormonal changes experienced by growing children and adolescents during puberty, but when these behaviors are associated with significant distress and/or dysfunction; it is likely to be a part of a mental illness. About 10-20% of children experience some mental health problems during childhood.

Myth: Most children tend to grow out of their mental health problems with advancing age.
Fact: Children are less likely to 'grow out' of their mental health problems if left untreated and are more likely to 'grow into' more severe mental illness. About 50% of adult mental illnesses have their first onset of symptoms in childhood prior to the age of 14. With early recognition and initiation of appropriate intervention, there are greater chances of faster and complete recovery from the mental health problem.

Myth: Children who get good grades and have a lot of friends cannot have mental health problems because they have nothing to be depressed about.
Fact: Depression is one of the most common childhood mental illnesses and can affect anyone regardless of their socio-economic status or intelligence level. Like all mental illnesses, it results from a complex interaction between several different biological, psychological and social or environmental factors in an individual. For example, a child with good grades might feel pressured to continuously excel in studies to maintain his friendships and might experience anxiety due to this. Alternatively, he/she might have experienced physical or sexual abuse at home or had a strong

genetic risk for developing depression without any apparent stressors or difficult situations in life.

Myth: Mental illness in children occurs because of bad parenting.

Fact: Parents and early home environment do play an important role in the development of a child, with parental violence or parental alcohol or drug use and lack of a loving parent reported as risk factors for several mental health problems. But these factors are unlikely to produce mental health problems among children in isolation (i.e., they are neither necessary nor sufficient to produce mental illness in children). Mental illness is a result of a complex interaction between several different biological, psychological and social or environmental risk factors in an individual. Further, certain childhood mental illnesses like ADHD, ASD and intellectual development disorder are strongly dependent on biological factors and cannot be caused by bad parenting. Thus, a child's home environment and the kind of relationship with parents could exacerbate symptoms of an underlying mental illness, whereas positive parenting practices play a significant role in promoting the mental health of children and reducing symptoms of mental illness.

Myth: Mental illness in children is a sign of weak character/personality or attention-seeking behavior.

Fact: It is important to emphasize here that most of the mental illnesses in children are not due to any character or personality flaw in children. Some emotional and behavioral disturbances, like impulsivity, anger outbursts out of proportion to the said provocation or restlessness, may be explained by certain character or temperament/personality traits in children. Further, some of the dramatic or shocking presentations of mental illnesses, such as deliberate self-harm attempts or abrupt onset dissociative symptoms, are usually a cry for help, and not attempts at seeking attention.

Myth: A child can overcome symptoms of a mental illness through his/her willpower.

Fact: Though children are often not able to fully understand or communicate the severity of their mental illness, it is associated with a significant amount of distress and dysfunction. A mental illness is not caused by weak willpower and one cannot expect children to overcome these overwhelming conditions on their own. On the contrary, early recognition of mental illness and initiation of appropriate treatment can help the child to recover from symptoms of mental illness and lead a productive and happy life.

Myth: Nothing can be done to protect children from developing a mental illness.

Fact: The chances of developing mental illness can be reduced by increasing the number of protective factors (e.g. presence of a loving, caring and stable relationship with an adult, good problem-solving skills, positive peer relationships, etc.) and removal of modifiable risk factors (e.g. poverty, experiencing bullying, lack of engagement with education, etc.). There is an increasing interest in mental health promotion and primary prevention of mental illnesses. For example, teaching life skills to adolescents through school-based mental health programs or having special support programs to provide additional emotional and social support to vulnerable children such as children of parents with mental illness, children with a history of sexual abuse are likely to improve the mental health of children and reduce the chances of them developing mental illness.

Conclusion

Mental health problems in children are associated with significant physical and psychological negative consequences in life. About one in five children have at least one significant mental health problem or disorder and only 1% of them receive appropriate treatment for them. This is due to a combination of several factors, such as poor recognition of mental illness in children, high level of stigma to mental illness and a lack of easily accessible child mental health services.

It is vital to create awareness about the importance of good mental health among children, common signs of mental illness in children and availability of effective pharmacological and psychological treatment options for childhood mental health problems among the general public, teachers and community healthcare workers.

Child mental health also needs to be promoted through school mental health programs (e.g. life-skills training, screening of children for common mental illnesses by teachers, etc.). Community participation and inter-sectoral coordination (e.g. housing, nutrition, sanitation, education, etc.) must be encouraged to provide conducive home and community environment for healthy child development.

KEY POINTS

➤ Good child mental health does not mean the mere absence of mental illness. It refers to the attainment of developmental milestones in social, emotional and cognitive domains, developing coping and problem-solving skills and engaging in age-appropriate activities and learning new things.

➤ About one in five children have at least one significant mental health problem or disorder and about half of all adult mental disorders emerge by the age of 14 years.

➤ Common mental health disorders in children are depression and anxiety disorders, conduct and oppositional defiant disorder, attention-deficit hyperactivity disorder, autism spectrum disorder, intellectual developmental disorder, specific learning disorders and psychosis.

➤ There are effective psychotherapy and pharmacotherapy-based treatments available for the management of child mental health disorders.

➤ There is a need to create awareness about common signs and symptoms of childhood mental disorders, especially among gatekeepers (i.e. parents, teachers, community health workers, primary care doctors, pediatricians, etc.) of child health to facilitate their early detection and treatment.

REFERENCES

1. Help With ADHD. https://www.psychiatry.org/patients-families/adhd

2. Help With Autism Spectrum Disorder. https://www.psychiatry.org/patients-families/autism

3. Help With Intellectual Disability. https://www.psychiatry.org/patients-families/intellectual-disability

4. Help With Specific Learning Disorder. https://www.psychiatry.org/patients-families/specific-learning-disorder

CHAPTER 18

Aging and Mental Health

Bichitra Nanda Patra and Mandeep Kaur

'It is not enough for a great nation merely to have added new years of life - our objective must also be to add new life to those years.'
— *John F Kennedy*

Introduction

Aging is an inevitable part of human life. Aging can be defined as a persistent decline in the age-specific fitness components of an organism due to internal physiological deterioration. It is associated with a decline in physical strength and functioning due to changes in various bodily systems with increasing age. Therefore, it is important to know about various factors that might impact this process of aging. It is estimated that by 2050 there will be more people aged 60 or over than adolescents and youth aged 10–24 years (2.1 billion vs. 2.0 billion) globally. The number of people at very advanced ages is increasing too – the global population aged 80 years and above is projected to grow from 125 million in 2015 to 202 million in 2030 and to 434 million in 2050. Recent advance in health sciences is a major reason for an increase in life expectancy in many parts of the globe. With aging, a number of mental health issues emerge specific to the elderly people. This chapter discusses important mental issues relevant to old age.

Importance of Mental Health in the Elderly

During the last few decades, society has been going through many changes associated with urbanization, such as intra-country and inter-country migrations and advances in information and communication technology. The movement of the population from the rural ancestral dwellings to faraway cities in search of employment and economic gains has led to disintegration in the family setups leading to neglect of the older people in the family often left back home in the native place. Moreover, the altering of the social setups of society in the name of modernization affects personal and social relationships in a negative way. The demographic change not only increases the number of older adults but also leaves them without much psychosocial support back home. Elderly population is highly prone to psychiatric morbidities. This could be attributed to physical inactivity and problems with physical health, leading to dependency on others for their activities of daily living; socio-economic factors, such as decrease in economic independence due to retirement and loss of income; and breakdown of the family support system. Due to aging of the brain, memory may decline too. In addition, if one has lost his/her spouse or friend, which is more likely in old age, then the likelihood of encountering a psychological disorder increase. Disorders such as dementia and depression also affect judgments as to whether or not physical illness can be managed at home or needs outside help. Cognitive decline further affects the ability for self-care and the capacity to perform activities of daily living. Absence of formal family support and a decline in the ability for self-care increases the need for long-term residential care or increased expenditure in domiciliary services, which are often either not available or unaffordable for most of the population in low- and middle-income countries. As the number and proportion of elderly individuals are on the rise, there is a need to be aware of the mental health issues occurring in old age and their workable solutions.

Mental Health Issues and Illness in the Elderly

Aging is a progressive decline in physiological function, leading to an age-dependent decrease in the rates of survival and reproduction. As aging is a process, it includes a period of transition rife with various challenges owing to the changes taking place. Such changes and challenges often affect the social and mental well-being of the elderly. Thus, mental health also faces challenges, as people age. Whether or not someone develops mental illness is based on a number of factors, such as genetic loading, environmental influences and individual characteristics. Emphasizing the importance of mental health in elderly, we should not overlook how certain older people are able to remain resilient in life despite multiple adversities such as the loss of a friend or a relative, loss of status and dignity, the declining nature of their health and many more such events. Nearly 15% of people aged 60 and above suffer from a mental illness. Moreover, elderly people are more prone to experience multiple medical problems at the same time due to aging and physical decline. There are also many other significant contributory factors in old age that lead to disability, such as absence of family and social support, lack of social security and financial problems. Older people staying in controlled family systems, with restricted personal autonomy, financial dependency and poor family support, are more prone to mental and behavioral disorders.

In addition to the already existing mental health issues, the COVID-19 pandemic has brought further suffering for older people across the world. Elderly people often had to handle the entire emotional toll related with the death of their spouse or peers of the similar age group. These factors have been escalated by elderly abuse during the pandemic. Complete shut-down in the world with social distancing increased the loneliness in elderly people. And the idea that older people are more prone to get infected with the corona virus pulled the community even further away from communicating with them (an attempt to protect them from infection added to social isolation). Many elderly people, especially in later age groups, were not very comfortable in adapting to the latest technology, social media and various online platforms to communicate with their near and dear ones, which were used extensively throughout the COVID-19 pandemic. This would make them feel lonely and have worrisome and depressive thoughts, further adding to the fear and insecurity during the pandemic.

Mental illness in old age can be either new onset or an exacerbation of a preexisting psychiatric illness. The preexisting illness could be any like depression, anxiety disorder, bipolar disorder or psychosis. New onset depression is also common in old age, but neurocognitive disorders, like dementia, generally occur in this age group.

Prevalence, Burden and Treatment Gap

The prevalence of mental disorders is high among the elderly compared to the other age groups due to various reasons as discussed earlier. Around 20% of people aged more than 60 years suffer from mental health or neurological problems. This accounts for a total of 6.6% people in the elderly group having a disability. Mental and neurological disorders in older people account for 17.4% of the Years Lived with Disability (YLDs). The National Mental Health Survey of India of 2016 also found that weighted lifetime prevalence and the current prevalence of psychiatric morbidity are higher in the older adults than in the younger adults (15.1% vs. 13.4% and 10.9% vs. 10.5%, respectively).

The treatment gap for mental health problems is much wider in the elderly people compared to the young people for various reasons. As the elderly people are often dependent on others due to their physical ailments or financial dependency, they can't go for treatment on their own in most of the cases. This further adds to the problems and suffering and makes them more disabled and their illness more difficult to treat.

Common Mental Disorders in Old Age

Dementia

Dementia is classically an illness of old age. The illness has a chronic and often progressive course. There is a significant decline in cognitive functions in one or more areas that include memory, thinking, orientation, comprehension, calculation, learning capacity, language and judgment. Impairment of cognitive function is commonly accompanied, and occasionally preceded, by deterioration in emotional control, social behavior or motivation. In the early stages, the illness starts with forgetting small things of daily activities, losing track of time and becoming lost in familiar places. In the initial stage, when the symptoms are less severe, it is called as minimal cognitive impairment (MCI). When it progresses, the person may start forgetting recent events and names of people and may be confused. There may be difficulty in communication and behavior changes, such as wandering tendency. In the later stages, memory disturbances become more pronounced and the person may even become unaware of the time and place and has difficulty in recognizing relatives and friends. There also occur behavioral changes, like aggressive behavior, disorganization and complete neglect of personal care. Dementia/neurocognitive disorder can occur due to several causes, including

Alzheimer's disease, vascular diseases/stroke, head injury, substance/medication-induced or multiple etiologies. As the disease progresses, there is a need for assisted care. Figure 1 shows common identifying features of dementia.

Old age depression

Depression is the commonest mental illness of old age and contributes substantially to medical, economic, and social burden. Often, it is associated with physical illness and also adds to suicidal risk. Depression is a treatable illness, but unfortunately, it may remain unrecognized and the person might not seek treatment. Common symptoms of depression are given in Box 1.

Depression in old age is linked with greater disability and more neuropsychological abnormalities and is associated with more stressful life events as compared to depression in the younger age group. Usually, it presents with irritability, disturbances of sleep and appetite, loss of weight and aches and pains and may be accompanied by guilt and psychotic symptoms (delusion/hallucination). Sometimes, forgetfulness and other cognitive deficits are the presenting symptoms, which resemble dementia (pseudodementia).

Box 1. Symptoms of Depression

- Sadness of mood, continuing throughout the day and in all situations
- Losing interest in previously pleasurable activities
- Feeling fatigued with minimal effort
- Decreased attention and concentration, leading to forgetfulness
- Ideas of hopelessness, helplessness and worthlessness
- Wish to die, suicidal thoughts
- Negative views of self, ideas of guilt
- Lack of sleep, change in appetite

Dementia: Major Features

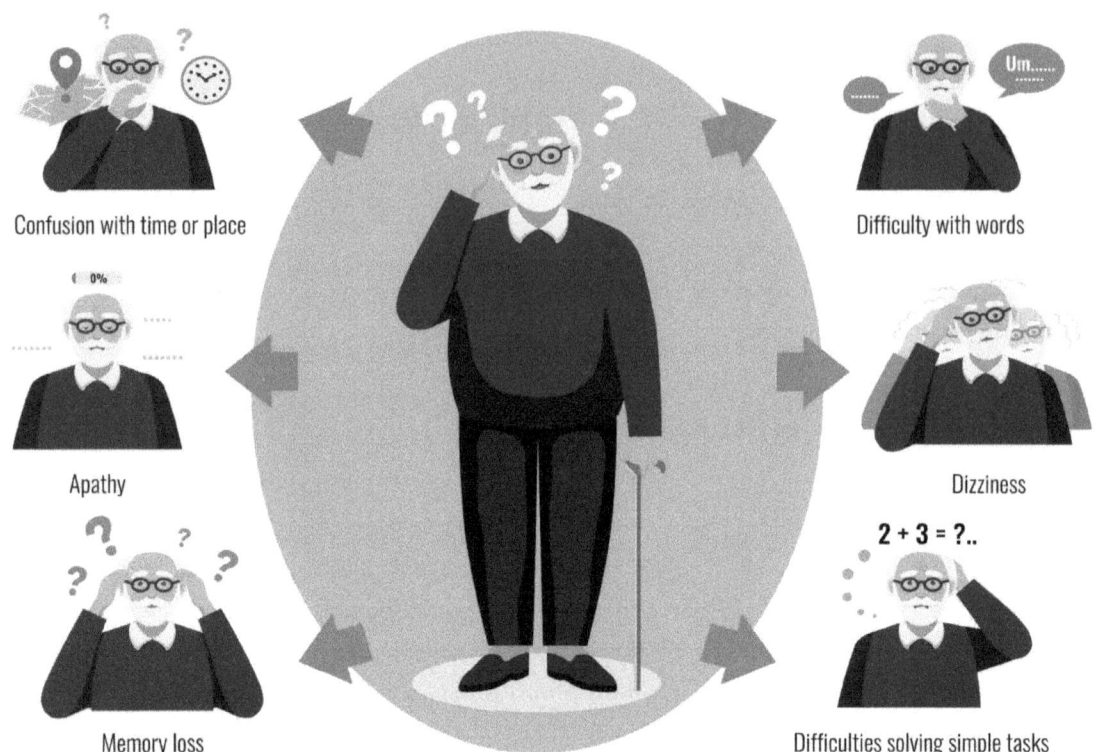

Confusion with time or place

Apathy

Memory loss

Difficulty with words

Dizziness

Difficulties solving simple tasks

Figure 1. *Dementia: Major Features*

The illness is treated with antidepressants and psychotherapy.

Anxiety disorder

Anxiety and worrying are a part of life, as discussed in previous chapters. But in older age, it can become more troublesome. Anxiety may lead to difficulties in sleep, body aches and headache. Anxiety disorders occur more commonly in old age. In old age, symptoms of anxiety can also arise due to medical illness, e.g., uncontrolled hypertension, coronary artery disease, necessitating examination and investigations. It is important to conduct a detailed assessment and screen for depression as well as psychosocial stressors. Sometimes, there may be an unidentified physical illness, which may be presenting as anxiety.

Psychosis

Psychosis in old age can be a continuation of an early illness or a new onset. Schizophrenia and bipolar disorder have an onset at an early age in life and can continue in old age. In old age, there can also be relapse of these disorders. There may be new-onset psychotic symptoms, like delusions of persecution and hallucinations. Sometimes, these occur in the background of a hearing deficit. Neurological illnesses, like parkinsonism, can also be complicated by psychotic symptoms. Delirium, an acute confusional state with altered sensorium, disorientation to time and place, and hallucinatory behavior is very common in old age. Delirium often occurs in the background of a medical illness or poor oral intake. Delirium is a medical emergency that warrants immediate medical attention.

Table 1. *Myths and Facts About Aging and Mental Health*

Myths	Facts
Depression and loneliness are normal in older adults.	Depression and loneliness are not a normal part of aging. Studies indicate that people aged 60 and above have more contented and satisfying relationships leading to positive emotional and mental health compared to the younger population.
There is no need to see a professional for mental health issues in older adults.	Mental health issues should be detected early, regardless of the age group. Older adults may experience mental health symptoms ranging from mild to severe; these may worsen and become disabling with time if not treated. Thus, it is important to seek help from a professional at the earliest.
Mental health is not important in older age.	Mental health issues are just as important in elderly people as in any age group. Mental health issues should not be considered part and parcel of the normal aging process.
Mental illnesses, such as dementia, are an inevitable part of aging.	Dementia is an illness, seen in a small percentage of the elderly population. It is not an inevitable part of aging
Elderly people are a burden to society's healthcare costs.	If we make sure to keep the healthcare system updated, then spending money on the mental health of the elderly will be an investment and not a burden.
Aging is an illness and synonymous with mortality.	Old age is not always associated with disease.

Myths about Mental Health in Old Age

There are some myths and misconceptions about mental health issues in old age, related to age group, the aging process and the illnesses. Because of a society that is preoccupied with its youth, we have all absorbed such a pessimistic and downbeat outlook about aging; therefore, older people may come across many stereotypical labels and beliefs. Table 1 summarizes myths and facts related to mental health issues in old age.

Whom/Where to Approach?

Almost two-thirds of the elderly people with a mental illness are unable to obtain the needed services. Whenever any mental illness is suspected, it is better to seek treatment at the earliest. This is because the symptoms of mental illness can be a manifestation of serious physical illness in the elderly. Family members or caregivers should be proactive in initiating the treatment process because of the limitations in mobility due to physical illness or in some cases due to impaired judgment or poor comprehension in the elderly. To begin with, one needs to approach the nearest healthcare facility when one notices any change in behavior. This can be a primary health care setting or a specialty mental health care setting. Any common mental disorder with less severity can be managed by a general physician. People requiring special care and those with more severe illnesses may need to go to a physician, a psychiatrist or a neurologist, depending on the kind of symptoms.

Available Treatments

The aim of treatment is to restore health, improve the quality of life, reduce disability and protect autonomy. Early detection and intervention help in improving prognosis as well. After the diagnosis, the intervention can be pharmacological (with medications) or non-pharmacological (psychological).

Pharmacotherapy: Most of the illnesses in the elderly are treated by the medications used for young adults. For depression and anxiety disorders, commonly selective serotonin reuptake inhibitors (SSRIs) are used, such as escitalopram and sertraline. Psychosis is treated with antipsychotic medications, such as haloperidol, risperidone and olanzapine. Dementia or cognitive impairments are treated with medicines like donepezil, rivastigmine or memantine. Most of the patients can tolerate the medications well for prolonged periods of time. Sometimes other medications can be used for symptomatic relief, e.g., benzodiazepines (e.g. lorazepam) for sleep disturbances and anxiety symptoms. These are usually prescribed for a short duration (2-4 weeks) to avoid dependence. In most cases, even after the improvement of symptoms, the psychotropic medications need to be continued for a few weeks to months depending on the illness.

Psychological interventions: Psychological interventions are used alone when the illness is less severe. In some patients, psychological interventions are combined with medication for an optimum outcome. Some of the specific non-pharmacological measures used for dementia are as follows:

- **Behavior therapy:** Behavioral approach entails a detailed assessment of triggers, behaviors and reinforcers (antecedents, behaviors and consequences- ABC). Further interventions are centered significantly on these assessment results.
- **Reality orientation:** In this approach, patients with memory loss are oriented to their surroundings with the help of various tools and activities. This often includes regular usage of various memory aids to help the orientation process, such as notices, signposts, etc.
- **Validation therapy:** Therapists/clinicians make an empathic effort to interact with patients with dementia by attending to their feelings and emotions, which are unknowingly masked behind their confused speech and behavior. The focus is more on the emotional content of the conversation rather than the patient's current orientation.
- **Reminiscence therapy:** Patients with dementia are asked to relive their past experiences, mainly the good ones, which have had some positive impact on them, such as family holidays and gatherings. Reminiscence therapy is seen as an attempt to level up the well-being of the individual and to provide pleasure and cognitive stimulation as well.

Taking Care of Mental Health During Old Age

As we have already discussed, good mental health is of utmost importance in old age. Some of the strategies for good mental health in old age are as follows:

- Good diet/nutrition
- Adequate sleep
- Regular exercise/yoga to stay physically fit
- Take care of physical health and follow a daily routine
- Maintain social relationships and stay in touch with family and friends
- Spirituality/religious activity: These have a potential to increase resilience and provide opportunity for group participation.
- Develop an optimistic and positive attitude
- Develop an attitude of gratitude
- Involve in mentally challenging tasks/exercises, e.g., chess, puzzle or cultivating a new hobby and spending time in recreational activities can keep oneself mentally fit
- Stop smoking and alcohol abuse
- Active engagement with life by involvement in community membership, volunteering, caring for friends/family (grandchildren) and social activities

Conclusion

Mental health problems are common in old age. With the increasing elderly population, mental illnesses in the elderly have become a major public health problem. Common mental illnesses in old age include depression, anxiety disorders and cognitive decline progressing on to dementia. There can be a new onset of mental illness in old age, or a preexisting mental illness can worsen or relapse. Mental health issues in old age should not be ignored since these can be highly disabling. Mental health care for the elderly should be incorporated with general healthcare so that psychological morbidity gets treated at an early phase.

KEY POINTS

➢ Old age is not always associated with disability or depression.

➢ It is important to recognize and start timely intervention for mental health issues in the elderly.

➢ Services should be made available in places, which the elderly people visit frequently, such as basic health care settings, collective meal and senior-citizen centers, residential settings, libraries and other community areas.

➢ With a good lifestyle and self-care, old age can be more satisfying and meaningful.

REFERENCES

1.   Addressing violence against children, women and older people during the covid-19 pandemic: Key actions. https://www.who.int/publications/i/item/WHO-2019-nCoV-Violence_actions-2020.1, last accessed on 31st Jan 2022.

2.   Dementia. https://www.who.int/news-room/fact-sheets/detail/dementia, last accessed on 12th Feb 2022.

3.   Memory problems and dementia. https://www.rcpsych.ac.uk/mental-health/problems-disorders/memory-problems-and-dementia. last accessed on16th February 2022

4.   Mental health of older adults. https://www.who.int/news-room/fact-sheets/detail/mental-health-of-older-adults. last accessed on 31st Jan 2022.

CHAPTER 19

Women and Mental Health

Shalini Singh

Introduction

Women's reproductive cycle and their compromised socioeconomic position in the community make them more vulnerable toward certain mental health problems. However, their superior abilities to emote feelings, build deep interpersonal bonds and exhibit higher resilience play a protective role toward their mental well-being. Gender equality and woman empowerment are being championed in most parts of the world today. Still, women with mental health problems suffer more stigma and psychosocial complications than men.

Mental Health Across a Woman's Lifespan

Adolescence and women's mental health: Adolescents deal with several psychological issues, such as body shaming, low self-esteem and preoccupation with their image projection on social media. The rate of clinically significant depression among adolescents ranges between 17.3% and 25%. Mental health problems at this tender age lead to higher rates of self-harm, interpersonal difficulties, poor coping skills, substance misuse and adult-onset psychiatric disorders. Participation in sports plays a protective role by fostering peer support and a healthy body image. Other protective factors include positive parenting, having good role models, a sense of self-efficacy, being emotionally stable and being extroverted. Risk factors include exposure to childhood adversity, trauma, a perception of precocious puberty, poor

body image, less involvement in school and mental disorders in parents.

Women's mental health during young adulthood: Young women face increasing pressure to balance their professional aspirations and domestic duties while dealing with relentless misogynistic microaggressions. They are more likely to experience an imposter syndrome, feel stressed over the accomplishment of future goals and receive subdued encouragement from family to pursue their career goals. Each of these issues can act as potent psychological stressor.

Mental wellness of a mother: While motherhood brings immense joy, it can be an isolating experience of intensive caregiving, loss of one's old identity and disconnect from the rest of the world. New mothers should be encouraged to focus on self-care and prioritize mental wellness so as not to lose their psychological resilience during this transition. Policies for the provision of child-care support to mothers that validate the all-consuming job of a parent and help them create supportive networks should be a priority for employers and communities.

Women and mental health during old age: The prevalence of delirium and dementia is higher in women due to greater life expectancy. Aging women tend to continue with their role as caregivers in their family, which increases the mental burden and

146

Mental Health Issues Across Life Span of Women

Adolescence	Menarche	Young Adulthood	Mid-life
Body shaming, low self-esteem, self-harm, interpersonal difficulties, substance misuse	PMS & PMDD Symptoms: mood swings, pain, bloating, impaired cognition	Pressure to balance professional & domestic duties, pressure of future goals without much encouragement	More vulnerable to mental health problems; Raised exposure to abuse and trauma; Reduced help seeking

Family	Pregnancy	Menopause	Old Age
Exposure to violence: major cause of psychiatric illness; Women with mental illness suffer abusive relationships	Postpartum blues (baby blues): 3-10 days after childbirth; Perinatal depression: 1-12 months after delivery	Hot flashes followed by an aura of anxiety and panic attacks; Increased risk of anxiety and depression	Increased risk for late onset depression; Triple stigma: mental illness, old age and woman

Figure 1. *Mental Health Issues Across the Life Span in Women*

can cause burnout. Female gender and menopausal changes are a major risk factor for late-onset depression. An aging woman with mental illness is dealt the triple blow of stigma: mental illness, old age and woman. This lowers the possibility of early diagnosis and adequate treatment.

Figure 1 summarizes the mental health issues in women across the life span.

Mental Health Problems Specific to Women

Menstruation: The trigger for peri-menstrual disorders is an increased sensitivity towards monthly fluctuations of estrogen and progesterone levels due to lower serotonin levels in the brain. There is a component of genetic preponderance too. These disorders range from a mild premenstrual syndrome (PMS) to the more severe pre-menstrual dysphoric disorder (PMDD). Symptoms include mood swings, impaired cognition, pain and bloating. They occur in the second half of the

cycle with relief upon the start of the period. Usually women in their 20s and 30s report more distressing symptoms, which worsen following childbirth. The subjective threshold of discomfort, perception about menstrual cycle, cultural beliefs about menstruation (a woman becomes 'impure' while menstruating) and co-morbid psychiatric and medical disorders modulate presentation. Treatment includes adopting a healthier lifestyle. Antidepressant medication is helpful in severe cases.

Pregnancy and childbirth: The potential mechanisms for perinatal disorders include rapidly shifting levels of stress hormones, estrogen and progesterone during pregnancy and after childbirth. Risk factors include history of mental illness in family and self, sleep disruption, ambivalence towards pregnancy, exposure to stressful life events, lack of social support, history of psychological trauma in past and poor physical health.

Three common perinatal mental health disturbances are:

- Postpartum blues (baby blues) usually occur between day 3 and day 10 after childbirth. The woman presents with tearfulness, restlessness, lack of sleep and feeling overwhelmed.
- Perinatal depression shares clinical features with regular depression. It occurs within first month post-delivery but can occur at any point within the year after delivery.
- Perinatal anxiety commonly presents as generalized anxiety, specific phobias (including fear of delivery), panic disorder and post-traumatic stress disorder (PTSD).

Management begins with counseling during pregnancy so that the expectant mother and her caregivers are prepared. The **NEST-S** program – getting adequate **N**utrition, **E**xercising regularly, getting adequate **S**leep and rest, dedicating **T**ime for self, building **S**upportive social networks and fostering healthy relationships – is advised in all cases. Correction of vitamin and mineral deficiencies (especially Vitamin B6, calcium and magnesium), bright light treatment (exposure to bright light for 30-90 minutes per day) and psychotherapy are useful for milder cases. Medications such as low-dose antidepressants and hormonal therapy that suppresses ovulation are prescribed in moderate to severe cases. Detailed evaluation is essential to rule out underlying medical conditions.

Postpartum psychotic disorders are less common. Due to nature of presentation and threat to life of newborn, these disorders are considered as a medical emergency. Risk factors include past history of mental illness, discontinuation of treatment following pregnancy, family history of psychotic illness, younger age at delivery and first and/or unplanned pregnancy. Treatment is the same as for psychotic disorders during any other time.

Menopause: It is characterized by a drop in hormone levels, which leads to marked physical and psychological changes. These changes coincide with more intensive caregiving roles for both growing children and aging parents. Hot flashes during menopause are often preceded by an aura of anxiety and panic attacks. The risk of depression and anxiety doubles during this period and a resurgence of past symptoms are common leading to a more severe presentation. For milder psychological symptoms, building a support system, monitoring mood to identify avoidable triggers and remembering their temporary nature helps. Expert advice should be sought in case of severe presentation.

Gender-based violence: The relationship between women's mental health and their experiences of violence is bi-directional. In most cases, the exposure to violence occurs first and then follows depression, suicidal tendencies, anxiety disorders, PTSD and later substance misuse or self-medication of these symptoms. Other related mental health problems include low self-esteem, isolation, attempts to self-harm and physical symptoms, such as chronic pain and insomnia. Women with mental illness (especially substance misuse and psychotic disorders) are more likely to suffer abusive relationships. At individual level, steps include individual or group psychotherapy, support groups and feminist-based counseling. Health system interventions include universal screening for violence and integration of gender violence screening into reproductive health services. Women availing non-medical support against violence should be screened for mental illness. From a policy perspective, steps must be taken to reduce the gender disparity and promote women's rights.

Gender gap and women's mental health: Gender gap has resulted in lower socio-economic status of women, greater exposure to abuse and traumatic experiences, reduced help-seeking behavior and unequal division of household and parenting responsibilities. These factors interact with biological factors unique to women and make them more vulnerable to mental health problems. In orthodox cultures, women are celebrated for their sacrificing and submissive nature. Given this narrow spectrum of acceptable behaviors from women, any heterogeneity or exaggerated emotional or behavioral responses are likely to be labeled as pathological. Clinicians tend to either over-diagnose or under-diagnose women with mental illness and often prescribe them only mood-altering agents. For the longest time, research in mental health excluded female participants since their menstrual cycles and pregnancies were deemed too inconvenient. This has widened the treatment gap and research gap and perpetuated some myths about women's mental health (**Table 1**).

Table 1. *Some Common Myths and Counter Facts Surrounding Women's Mental Health*

Myth	Fact
Women are more likely to over-report psychological distress and physical symptoms, such as pain.	There is an implicit sexist belief that women are overly emotional and irrational. As a result, doctors tend to under-diagnose women's reports of pain and psychological distress.
Women are psychologically weak due to which they experience more mental health problems.	Women are more likely to experience psychological distress due to bio-psycho-social risk factors. However, due to their emotive nature, they are more likely to share their psychological problems and seek emotional support, which plays a protective role.
Medications used to treat psychiatric disorders should be avoided by women as they affect fertility and pregnancy.	None of the medications used to treat psychiatric disorders have a direct deleterious impact on fertility. Most psychiatric drugs either don't harm the unborn child or the absolute risk may be acceptable. It is better to modify but continue treatment as the illness might be exacerbated in the postpartum period.
During pregnancy and motherhood, a woman is in a state of bliss, and therefore no distress is experienced.	Pregnancy and motherhood are stressful life events. Mental health problems are common (20%) during pregnancy and early motherhood. They can negatively impact the mother, the unborn child and the baby's development if they are ignored.
Postpartum mental illness develops when the mother doesn't love her baby.	Postpartum depression occurs due to hormonal changes in the body. It is not related to attachment with the child.
Postpartum depression is rare and resolves spontaneously.	One in every 10 mothers suffers from postnatal depression, which, if untreated, can progress to major depression. Treatment is important to improve outcomes.
Postpartum depression only affects women who have given birth.	It can also affect an adoptee mother.
Pre-menstrual syndrome (PMS) is not a real condition.	Nearly 3/4th of women experience PMS with wide variation in clinical presentation.
Eating disorders are a lifestyle problem of wealthy young women.	These are serious mental disorders that require treatment in form of medications and therapy. If not treated, these can have serious consequences.
Substance use disorder is only seen in men.	Women are prone to substance use disorders and show a shorter and more devastating clinical trajectory as compared to men.

Prevalence and Burden of Mental Illness in Women

Nearly 20% of women suffer from common mental disorders, such as depression and anxiety. Both depression and anxiety disorders are two to three times more common in women as compared to men. Depression is more persistent in women and they are more likely to suffer atypical features, such as chronic pain, lack of energy, increased appetite and weight gain. Depression is associated with impaired functioning, higher risk of medical co-morbidity and an increased risk of suicide. In case of anxiety disorders, there is a higher risk of co-morbid depression and a more severe presentation. Perinatal depression occurs during pregnancy in around 10% of women, and in 13% of women, it occurs within the first year of childbirth. Overall, postpartum blues and mood and anxiety disorders occur in nearly 85% of women, and in around 20-25% women it progresses to major depression.

PTSD is twice as likely to occur in women. Women represent 90% of all cases of eating disorder. The prevalence of severe mental illness, such as schizophrenia and bipolar disorder, is independent of gender. Women with schizophrenia have better prognosis as compared to men but experience more stigma and abuse. Women with bipolar disorder have more frequent depressive episodes and rapid cycles and are more severely impacted by the seasonal pattern of mood disturbances. They are more likely to present with thyroid disorder, migraine, obesity and anxiety disorder.

Women are three times more likely to attempt suicide and deliberate self-harm. In regions where women are exposed to dowry harassment, domestic violence, sexual abuse and strained ties with in-laws, the rate of completed suicide is higher than in men. More than 2/3rd of married Indian women experience domestic violence. Sexual abuse is reported by nearly a third of Indian women.

There is a huge economic burden of untreated psychiatric morbidity and medical co-morbidities in women. High rates of mental illnesses also result in reduced treatment compliance and blunted response for other diseases.

Figure 2 summarises the burden of psychiatric illness among women

Identification of Mental Illness

Clinical presentation of some common mental health conditions in women is described below:

- **Depression:** This illness is characterized by persistent sadness, which impacts all aspects of life. It is accompanied by low self-confidence, pessimism, inability to derive pleasure and poor sleep and appetite. Symptoms should persist for more than 2 weeks.

- **Generalized anxiety disorder:** It is characterized by a constant feeling of excessive worry and anticipation of some unpleasant event, such as injury, humiliation, etc. The patients also experience restlessness, breathlessness, fidgeting, trembling, palpitations, stomach upset and sweaty palms and feet. Symptoms should persist for at least 6 months.

- **Obsessive compulsive disorder:** Obsessions refer to an uncontrollable stream of unwanted thoughts, images, actions and impulses that cause discomfort and lead to an urge to do certain actions to get relief.

- **Panic attacks:** Panic attacks are episodes of a heightened sense of dread and impending doom, accompanied by breathlessness, fidgeting, trembling, palpitations, dizziness, fainting, heaviness in the chest and upset stomach.

- **Eating disorder:** It is characterized by an unhealthy preoccupation with food, and body

Burden of Psychiatric Illnesses Among Women

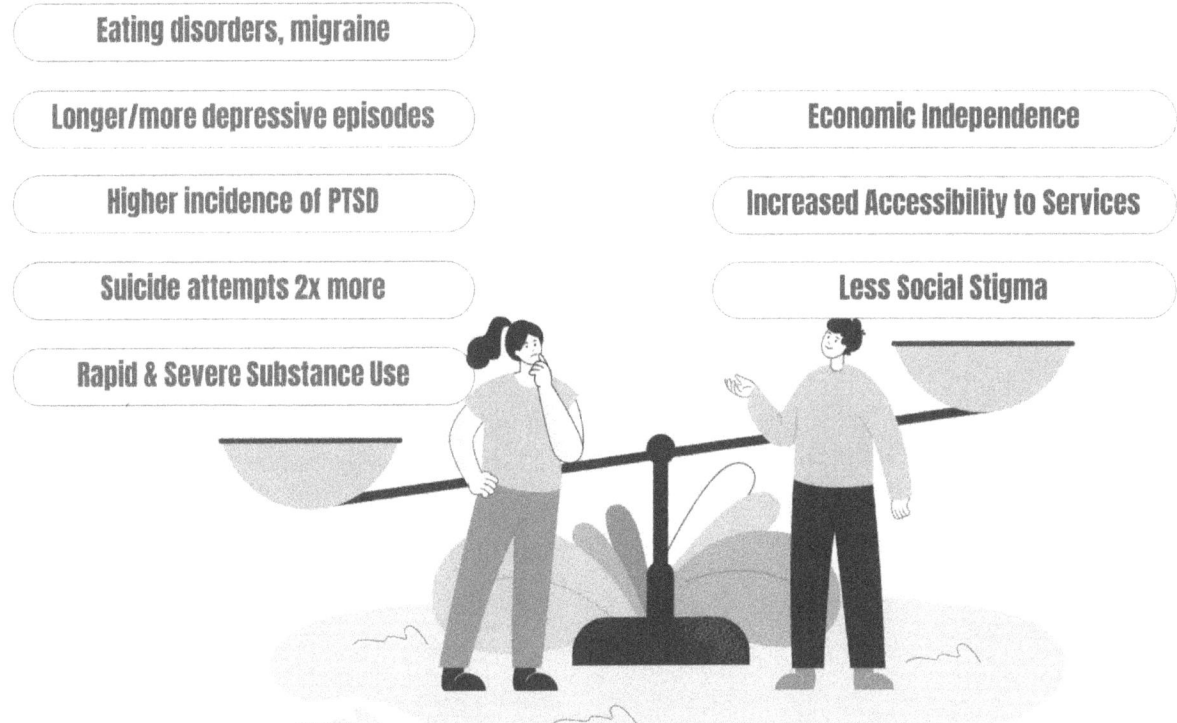

Eating disorders, migraine

Longer/more depressive episodes

Higher incidence of PTSD

Suicide attempts 2x more

Rapid & Severe Substance Use

Economic Independence

Increased Accessibility to Services

Less Social Stigma

Figure 2. *Burden of Psychiatric Illness Among Women*

shape, size and image that leads to excessive restriction or purging after eating.

- **Post-traumatic stress disorder (PTSD):** A trauma triggers excessive thoughts about the event, avoidance, flashbacks, nightmares, anger outbursts and an increased preponderance of depression and anxiety. Symptoms usually appear within 6 months of exposure to a major trauma of exceptional severity.

- **Borderline personality disorder:** It is characterized by the development of a malfunctioning viewpoint of the world and adopting unhealthy coping mechanisms leading to unstable emotions and relationships that generally develop during adolescence or early adult life itself.

Sexual dysfunction: It is widely prevalent and affects 41% of women in the reproductive age group. The dysfunction may be related to arousal and pain during sexual intercourse, and usually has a bio-psycho-social etiology. A detailed psychological and medical evaluation precedes therapeutic planning.

Substance use: Women are quickly becoming the fastest-growing demographic of substance users. They usually exhibit an accelerated progression from use to addiction. Gender-specific prevention and treatment programs that address trauma, medical and psychiatric co-morbidities, and mobilize social support are more likely to succeed.

Management of Women-specific Mental Disorders

Increasing accessibility

Mental health problems in women should be diagnosed as early as possible. For this to happen, women should feel comfortable discussing their mental health status with their loved ones. They should have social networks both offline and online to be vocal about stressful life events, menstruation, pregnancy and childbirth. Research indicates that women are more likely to seek mental health care from non-mental health personnel. This highlights the key role that integrated health services can play in providing treatment. Public health campaigns can spread awareness about common symptoms of mental illnesses.

Treatment strategy

The common elements of the treatment process are assessment, diagnosis and management.

Assessment comprises detailed history and physical and mental state examination. Information about the menstrual cycle, pregnancies, childbirth and history of endocrine and gynecological illness is recorded. Personal history should include sexual history, history of abuse (e.g., intimate partner violence) and a detailed evaluation of socio-cultural background, family structure and strength of existing support system.

Management needs to be tailored to the needs of the woman and should be recovery-oriented. It must be integrated with care provided by other specialties (both medical and non-medical). The approach must be empathetic and value her autonomy. Her loved ones must be made a part of the process and should be encouraged to provide adequate support such as help with domestic work.

Special issues, such as stigma and apprehension towards pharmacotherapy, must be addressed during psychoeducation sessions with the affected woman woman and her family members.

Initiating and continuing treatment

In women with mental illness, initiating and continuing treatment is an uphill task due to multiple reasons. Box 1 highlights the specific barriers to adequate care for women and some solutions.

General line of treatment for various mental health problems in women is on standard guidelines as discussed in various chapters in this book.

Conclusion

Women are vulnerable to mental illness throughout their life span. There are several risks and protective factors unique to women that impact the onset and progression of mental disorders. These vary based on the age group and local culture, but the gender disparity, high prevalence of trauma, violence and abuse in girls and women and the risks related to women's reproductive and menstrual health are key risk factors. The improvement of women's mental health at individual and community levels needs a collaborative effort of women, health care professionals and communities. The women's mental wellness programs must be recovery-oriented and integrated into all medical specialties that come in contact with treatment seekers.

Box 1. Specific Barriers to Adequate Care for Women and Some Solutions

Barriers

Women:
- Poor self-recognition of symptoms
- Low willingness to seek formal help
- Fear and stigma of being labeled with mental disorders
- Fear of being started on medications due to apprehensions about the impact on fertility, pregnancy, etc.
- Tough logistics for getting an appointment and attending an appointment due to domestic responsibilities
- Anticipation of hostile/judgmental reaction from the health care provider
- Nature of mental health problems, such as anxiety

Community:
- Missing support from family and partners
- Not letting the women make decisions regarding her treatment
- Limited accessibility to a mental health care facility

Health care system:
- Lack of training and sensitization of health care professionals towards mental health problems in women
- Lack of screening for mental health problems at a primary health care level
- Lack of referral services and follow up support
- Lack of coordinated services between various health care providers
- Lack of research on women's mental health due to exclusion of women from clinical trials

Solutions:
- Public health programs should sensitise the community about mental health problems in women and reduce stigma, misunderstandings and unfounded fears.
- Public health campaigns on the menstrual cycle, pregnancy, childbirth, protecting women against domestic violence and gender disparity
- Generating data on the extent of women's health problems and studying the impact of both individual and environmental factors

- Evidence-based digital help-seeking options: Internet forums and community blogs, support groups on social media platforms to aid recognition of symptoms and provide encouragement to seek support
- Training and sensitization of health care staff on how to universally screen for mental health problems, stress and abuse in women
- Assurance by health care professionals of a non-judgmental and empathetic approach to women
- Improving accessibility through phone/online consultations
- Increasing availability of integrated care to treatment-seeking women
- Provision of childcare services during an appointment
- Removing barriers to seeking legal recourse against gender-based violence
- Promotion of civic action for women by women to improve social, political and economic status in the community

KEY POINTS

➤ Gender-based variation in mental health can be partly attributed to the impact of estrogen and progesterone on brain function and stress response. Gender disparity, lower social status and higher exposure to poverty, abuse, violence and trauma also play a role in precipitating and perpetuating mental illness.

➤ Mental disorders such as depression, anxiety disorders, panic attacks, obsessive compulsive disorder, eating disorders, post traumatic stress disorder and borderline personality disorder are more common in women than in men.

➤ Poor mental health in women increases inter-generational risk of mental illness and family dysfunction since women are the primary caregivers in most households.

➤ The premenstrual mental problems include premenstrual syndrome and the more severe pre-menstrual dysphoric disorder.

➤ Perinatal disorders include postpartum blues, postpartum depression and anxiety and postpartum psychosis.

➤ Management of women with mental illness should be recovery-oriented and integrated with other specialties.

REFERENCES

1. Fisher J, Mello MC, Patel V, Rahman A, Tran T, Holton S, Holmes W. Prevalence and determinants of common perinatal mental disorders in women in low-and lower-middle-income countries: a systematic review. Bulletin of the World Health Organization. 2012; 90: 139-49.

2. Kendall-Tackett KA, Ruglass LM, editors. Women's mental health across the lifespan: Challenges, vulnerabilities, and strengths. Taylor & Francis; 2017 Mar 16

3. Kohen D, editor. Oxford Textbook of Women and Mental Health. Oxford University Press; 2010 Mar 18.

4. Niaz U, Hassan S. Culture and mental health of women in South-East Asia. World Psychiatry. 2006 Jun;5(2):118.

CHAPTER 20

Looking After Students' Mental Health

Pratap Sharan and Rahul Mathur

'When educating the minds of our youth, we must not forget to educate their hearts.'
– Dalai Lama

Students are often vulnerable to a variety of mental illnesses. Attending a school, college or university can be a stressful experience for some students and might predispose them to develop a mental illness. It is estimated that about 75% of those with mental disorders exhibit their first symptom in childhood and adolescence. Mental health issues can lead to academic underachievement, family problems, drug abuse, etc., which, in turn, might exacerbate the underlying mental illness, thus forming a vicious cycle. Therefore, it is critical that we work for the prevention and management of mental illnesses in this age group.

Mental Health Issues in School Children

Schools play a key role in healthy development and functioning of children. According to a study by the Indian Council of Medical Research, 1 in 5 Indian school children suffer from emotional, behavioral or learning problems. Some studies suggest that mental disorders in school going children are rising in India with prevalence varying from 10-20%. This matches with the global data, which suggests that 13.2% children and adolescents between 10-19 years of age suffer from a mental disorder. Among various disorders, depression and anxiety disorders are the most common among school children followed by attention deficit hyperactivity

disorder (ADHD), conduct disorder, bipolar disorder, autism spectrum disorder, etc. It has been observed that there is a direct relation between a sound mental state and academic success. Thus, mental health issues early in academic career can undermine students' achievements later in life.

Various risk factors associated with developing mental illness in school are listed in *Box 1*.

In school, mental health promotion and prevention are equally important. Mental healthcare services have now moved on from the more traditional models (health care locations) to places like schools for increasing access and early recognition and treatment of mental health problems. This makes the role of parents, peers (in high school), teachers and school administrators very crucial. Intervention at an early age is likely to not only improve the well-being of children but would also lessen the burden on parents and society.

Role of Teachers and Counselors in Mental Health Care at School

Teachers play a crucial role in the development and mental well-being of students. They can also act as gatekeepers for wellness services and interventions. Mental illnesses in childhood and adolescence differ in symptomatology from those of adults. For example, an adolescent might not exhibit classical symptoms of depression but instead may display symptoms like irritability, absenteeism or a rapid decline in academic performance. Teachers and

Box 1. Risk Factors Underlying Mental Illness in School Children

Individual-related
- Male gender
- Younger age
- Low IQ
- Birth related complications
- Poor general health

Parental/Family-related
- Parental mental illness/psychopathology
- Low maternal education
- Strict physical punishment
- Childhood sexual abuse
- Substance use history (cannabis, alcohol, etc.)
- Broken home
- Poor parental supervision
- Poor communication between ward and parents

School-related
- Bullying by peers
- Low academic achievement
- Peer rejection
- Poor relation/communication with teachers

Box 2. School Mental Health Services/ Programs

International School Mental Health Services/ Programs (SMHS)
- Positive Behavior Interventions and Supports (PBIS)
- FRIENDS
- Promoting Alternative Thinking Strategies (PATHS)
- Skills for Life
- Mind Matters
- Good Behavior Game (GBG)
- Cognitive-Behavioral Interventions for Trauma in Schools

Indian Programs/Services
- Life Skills Education and Mental Health Awareness Program, NIMHANS
- The Adolescent Reproductive and Sexual Health (ARSH)
- Zippy's Children
- Clean Campus, Safe Campus
- Cascade Model of Life Skills Education
- Teachers' Orientation Program
- Student Enrichment Program

various educators must be trained to recognize these danger signs at the earliest. This doesn't mean that a teacher should be a therapist – rather, it means responding to warning signs with proper referrals before crisis situations, like self-harm, arise.

Teachers are the central point of any school-based intervention program. Early intervention can help an adolescent to better cope with academic stress and can result in improved emotional well-being, resulting in positive long-term consequences both academically and personally. It is well known that intervention at school level with coordination between teachers and parents can have positive effect on mental health of child or adolescent.

Various school mental health services are listed in *Box 2* and some are described in *Table 1*.

Numerous studies have looked at the evidence supporting various school mental health services in the western setting. A meta-analysis of more than 40 randomised control trials indicated that intervention at primary school level is associated with better long-term outcomes. The Positive Behavior Interventions and Supports (PBIS) is known to have maximum effect size. In India, a comprehensive national program to deal with children and adolescent mental health at school level does not exist; however, a few programs are delivered as a part of other national programs. DISHA, a collaborative effort of National Health

Table 1. *Evidence-Based School Mental Health Services/Programs*

Program/Service	Objective	Target group	Intervention
Positive Behavior Interventions and Supports (PBIS) **US Department of Education**	A multi-tier framework to prevent disruptive behavior and enhance the schools' organizational climate, thereby improving students' social, emotional and academic performance.	All school students	**Tier 1 (*All students*)** • Teaching appropriate behavior • Regular progress monitoring • Preventing unwanted behaviors • Identifying high-risk behaviors • Intervening early before unwanted behaviors escalate • Use research-based, scientifically validated interventions whenever possible • Using data to make decisions
			Tier 2 (*At Risk students*) At this level, the focus is on students who are more prone to developing a more serious behavioral problem before it escalates. • Enhanced social skills • Increased parent and teacher supervision • Enhanced academic support • Easy accessibility • Adequate referral services
			Tier 3 (*Individualized*) Meant for students with developmental disabilities, autism and emotional and behavioral disorders More intensive and individualized interventions
FRIENDS Program	To enhance children's and adolescents' ability to cope with stress and worry by enhancing social and emotional skills and simultaneously promote resilience and preventing development of anxiety and depressive disorders across the lifespan.	Students till 6th grade (8-11 years of age)	• Increasing ability to recognize and regulate one's own emotions, thoughts and behavior • Relaxation exercises • Attention training • Enhancing resilience • Importance of self-rewarding
Promoting Alternative Thinking Strategies (PATHS)	To promote social and emotional capabilities of school students aged between 5-12 years with the help of teachers and counselors.	Primary-middle school students	Teaching students scientifically derived lessons aimed at improving: • Emotional intelligence • Self-control • Social skills • Enhancing relations with peers • Interpersonal problem-solving skills

Program/Service	Objective	Target group	Intervention
Mind Matters	A mental health guidebook aimed at improving health, educational and social outcomes in the life of secondary school students	All students	Training of teachers, families and students Organizing face-to-face events, webinars and other events
Good Behavior Game	It aims at the management of classroom behaviors that rewards children for displaying appropriate on-task behaviors during instructional times.	Primary school students	Delivered by class teachers to a group of students with group activities enhancing pro-social behaviors and discouraging disruptive behavior • Prevents antisocial behavior • Reduction in suicidal ideation • Reduction in lifetime drug abuse
Promotive Mental Health and Well- Being NIMHANS, Bengaluru	To enhance positive mental health and enhancing resilience among students.	Middle-secondary school students	Module based on various themes, delivered by school teachers • Prevention of suicide • Mental health awareness • Exams and school-associated issues • Self-image • Parents-related issues • Awareness about sexual health • Gender-related issues
Life Skills Education and Mental Health Awareness Program	To sensitize parents and teachers for early identification of learning and developmental disorders. To develop life skills in older students to improve their coping skills.	Primary school students, till 10 years of age Middle school students	• Training of teachers and parents for identifying early warning signs • Students as 'peer educators' to develop essential life skills proactively
Clean Campus, Safe Campus Home Department, Govt. of Kerala, India	To decrease the high rate of substance use among students and cut down the availability of drugs around the school area.	Higher secondary schools (in Kerala)	• Psychoeducation to students about the harmful effects of drugs and negative long-term consequences • Vigilance by Police around the school campus to ensure the non-availability of drugs
The Adolescent Reproductive and Sexual Health (ARSH) Health Department, National Rural Health Mission, India	Outreach program that aims at developing essential coping skills in adolescents to deal with emotional issues.	School going adolescents	• Life skills training • Enhancing problem-solving skills

Mission and Department of Health and Family Welfare, offers round the clock telephonic support for students to alleviate academic stress. The Help Desk Program, which is part of the Sarva Shiksha Abhiyan, aims at training school staff and teachers in the early identification of warning signs and psychological issues in children, especially girls. Under this program, a drop box is provided in schools in which students needing help can submit their messages in private.

In India, school mental health services are still in the early stages of development. Lack of adequate financing of mental health programs, lack of trained professionals/counselors at school level, stigma among parents, lack of awareness about early childhood mental health issues and lack of effective public private partnerships are some of the reasons for India's limited progress in this regard.

Mental Health Issues in College and University Students

Transition from school to college is a major life event. College life opens new challenges both in academics as well as personal life. Frequent examinations, extensive syllabus, rank-based system, problems with teaching and learning methods and difficulty adjusting to the academic transition are some of the factors responsible for mental health issues in college or university students. Though most individuals with mental disorders exhibit their first manifestation by adolescence, many remain undetected till later in life due to lack of awareness or reluctance in seeking mental health services. Fear for privacy, embarrassment in reaching out to a mental health professional, and concern about long term consequences of treatment or medications are some of the barriers that restrict the students from seeking professional assistance.

Anxiety disorders are among the most common mental health conditions among college students, with prevalence rates varying from 10-15% across studies. Among anxiety disorders, social phobia, panic disorder and generalized anxiety disorder are very common. Indian studies also show that anxiety and depressive disorders are common in college students across different genders, streams and semesters, with about 30% reporting some degree of depression. Suicide is a leading cause of death among college students. A study on over five thousand college students found that more than 1.5% reported having suicide plans and another 0.5% reported having attempted suicide at least once in the past year. Surprisingly, most of these students did not seek help from any mental health professional. This illustrates the importance of training gatekeepers (peers and educators) for screening and referral and awareness-raising programs during the college years to enable students to access services for early interventions.

The use of various drugs, like cannabis and alcohol, is also very common among college students. The age of onset of substance use is generally adolescence and early adulthood (college years). The prevalence of problematic substance use varies from 20-50% across college samples with alcohol, tobacco and cannabis use being common in this population.

Interventions:

In addition to individual counseling offered at dedicated student wellness centers, the following mental health interventions may be highly effective during the college years:

Student awareness: Treatment seeking among college students continues to be low due to a lack of adequate understanding of mental illnesses, leading to low identification, perceived stigma and poor recognition of need for treatment. This makes it important to provide adequate knowledge to students with the help of counselors, webinars, role-play activities, etc., so that they seek help early and motivate their peers for seeking help if need arises.

Parental education: Even though parents might not be there with students in college, they are still important for promoting mental health among college students as only they can ensure continuity. Thus, their participation should always be encouraged.

Faculty education: As discussed earlier, the role of a teacher is very crucial in any student's life. Teachers can help with the early identification of warning signs with a prompt referral. Training of faculty/teachers is central to taking care of mental health issues in colleges.

Web-based CBT: Now-a-days, there are many online platforms that provide free counseling to students. These platforms can help overcome the issue of perceived social stigma related to seeking care in the mental health professional sector as well as issues of time and distance and unavailability of local resources. It is seen that more than 70% of students use web as the medium for receiving health-related information. Many studies have reported positive outcomes with web-based CBT and other psychotherapeutic interventions. Some of the freely available online resources are offered by

- CIMS (Centre of Mental Health Solutions) https://cimhs.com and;
- iCALL https://icallhelpline.org/what-is-icall/, started in 2012 by School of Human Ecology, TISS – Mumbai

Group therapy on coping with stress: These can help with the identification of risk factors related to stress, stress-related cognitions and enhancing one's ability to better cope with stressful situations.

Peer counseling and support: Peer counseling carries the potential to tackle barriers in accessing mental healthcare. Students with mental health issues are known to feel comfortable in reaching a peer counselor for help than to a professional counselor or 'a person of authority'. Peer counselors have usually had some similar issues in the past, thus the help-seeking students can learn from their experiences and solve problems more efficiently.

Challenges to Mental Health in Educational Institutions

Individual challenges

An Indian study estimated that more than 50 million children have some mental health issue and only 1% of them seek treatment from specialists. A survey of twenty thousand students by UNICEF and Gallup (2021) showed that only 41% of young people aged 15-24 years in the Indian sample believed that it is good to seek help for mental health problems, compared to more than 80% in samples from 23 other countries. Only a small proportion of respondents considered reaching out to others for mental health issues as necessary, compared to about 90% in other countries.

Stigma about mental illness is a big hindrance to treatment-seeking, not only among students but also among parents and teachers. It is seen that parents do not allow their children to seek help from a mental health professional because they feel embarrassed due to the negative attitude of society. Even when students seek help, retention in treatment is low because of negative experience with help providers or perceived ineffectiveness of treatments.

Structural challenges

- Providing efficient and quality care is important for healthcare. In India, there are very few mental health professionals. For instance, there are only 0.75 psychiatrists per 1 lakh people, which is very low as compared to other nations.

- Not many universities and schools hire trained counselors on regular basis, and if present, they are often overutilized and underpaid.
- Most teachers are not trained in the identification of mental health issues.
- Even though mental disorders are among the highest contributors to global morbidity, mental health continues to be neglected with less than 1% of the health budget in India allocated for mental health.

Creating Resilience

Kintsugi is an ancient Japanese art that means 'join with gold'. In this art form, scattered pottery is gelled with help of lacquer imposed with gold. As a result, a broken pot is converted into splendid motifs. Similarly, students, too, can be taught to overcome the effects of trauma and redesign their lives to make it meaningful and fruitful. Resilience is an individual's tendency to cope with stress and adversities. Considering the ability to regulate one's emotion as a positive attitude and seeing failures as a form of positive feedback are important components of resilience.

The American Psychological Association has made some important suggestions for developing resilience among college students (Box 3).

Conclusions

Mental illnesses are on the rise among students at all levels. Interventions at the school level can greatly reduce morbidity among students in

---

Box 3. Resilience Building

- Staying connected with friends, family and others
- Positive attitude towards stressful events
- Acceptance that not everything is in one's control
- Having more rational and achievable goals and taking gradual steps towards them
- Enhance decision making in crisis situations
- Continuous self-exploration
- Developing self-confidence
- Focusing on long-term consequences and viewing tough situations with a wider view
- Maintaining a positive outlook and having clear goals in mind
- Understanding one's own feelings while taking care of one's mind and body

---

later life. There is a need for collaborative efforts from various stakeholders involving students themselves, peers, parents, teachers, school boards, government and private sector to enhance the mental health of students. Having a strong human capital is essential for any country to succeed. Students are indeed the future of every nation and thus, it is time to make adequate efforts to improve the mental health of students. Immense efforts are needed from all stakeholders to improve access to quality healthcare and narrow the intervention gap.

KEY POINTS

➢ Mental disorders are highly prevalent among students and negatively affect their academic performances and personal lives.

➢ Early diagnosis and intervention at the school level can reduce rates of anxiety and depressive disorders as well as lower the rates of suicide among students.

➢ Teachers training programs, involving parents in treatment and establishing students' wellness centers in universities/schools could enhance access to mental healthcare.

➢ Use of online platforms and technology can increase the dissemination of mental health resources among students

➢ Involving students in creating awareness, providing peer support and developing essential life skills and wellness proactively can help in promoting mental health .

REFERENCES

1.   Kessler RC, Wang PS. The descriptive epidemiology of commonly occurring mental disorders in the United States. Annual Review of Public Health. 2008 Apr 21;29:115-29.

2.   Malhotra S, Patra BN. Prevalence of child and adolescent psychiatric disorders in India: a systematic review and meta-analysis. Child and Adolescent Psychiatry and Mental Health. 2014 Dec;8(1):1-9.

3.   Sharan, P, Sagar R. Mental health policy for children and adolescents in developing countries. Journal of Indian Assoociation for Child and Adolescent Mental Health 2007; *3*(1): 1-4.

4.   Kuppili PP, Nebhinani N. School Mental Health Program: Scenario in India. Journal of Indian Association for Child and Adolescent Mental Health. 2020;16(1):1-2.

5.   Sanchez AL, Cornacchio D, Poznanski B, Golik AM, Chou T, Comer JS. The effectiveness of school-based mental health services for elementary-aged children: A meta-analysis. Journal of the American Academy of Child & Adolescent Psychiatry. 2018;57(3):153-65.

6.   Deb S, Banu PR, Thomas S, Vardhan RV, Rao PT, Khawaja N. Depression among Indian university students and its association with perceived university academic environment, living arrangements and personal issues. Asian Journal of Psychiatry. 2016;23:108-17.

7.   Downs MF, Eisenberg D. Help seeking and treatment use among suicidal college students. Journal of American College of Health 2012;60(2):104-14

CHAPTER 21

Treatments for Mental Ill-Health

Rohit Verma

Introduction

A wide variety of treatments are available for mental disorders, including medications or drug treatments, physical methods of treatment and psychological methods or psychotherapies.

Till the middle of the last century, very few medications were available for the management of mental illnesses. In the 1950s, the first medications to be discovered for use in mental illnesses were lithium, chlorpromazine, imipramine and chlordiazepoxide. Over the next few decades, many new drugs were discovered and used in clinical practice. In the 1990s, newer molecules with lesser side effects like serotonin reuptake inhibitors and atypical antipsychotics were discovered. The medications used to treat mental illnesses are also called psychotropics.

After it is discovered that a drug molecule may have a role in the management of a mental illness, it is not straight away used in clinical practice or prescribed to patients. The use of that drug molecule in clinical practice is determined by conducting clinical trials. The clinical trials are usually conducted in four phases to establish the right dosage, side effects, safety and effectiveness. It is approved for use by the drug regulatory agency of the country. Guidelines are then formulated for the use of a particular drug in clinical practice.

This chapter focuses on psychotropic medications and physical methods of treatment. Psychotherapies are discussed in detail in Chapter 19.

Pharmacotherapy (Drug Treatment)

A large number of medications are available to treat various mental illnesses, which are grouped as under:

- Antipsychotics
- Antidepressants
- Anxiolytics
- Mood stabilizers
- Medications for insomnia
- Psychostimulants
- Medications for dementia
- Medications for substance use disorders
- Others

Principles of pharmacotherapy

It is important to understand the important principles of pharmacotherapy.

Pharmacokinetics is the study of how the body handles a drug after it is ingested. For example, a drug taken orally gets absorbed through the gut and then released in the blood, crosses the blood-brain barrier and acts on the different receptors or sites in the brain to produce its action. After this, the drug is metabolized in the body, especially in the liver and excreted through feces, bile and urine. Thus, when a medication is taken, it takes time to reach its peak concentration. Half-life is an important concept that guides the dosage schedule of a drug. The half-life of a drug is the time taken for one-half of a drug's peak plasma level to be metabolized and excreted from the body. If a drug's half-life is short, it needs to be taken twice or thrice a day.

Pharmacodynamics is the study of how a medication affects the body. Drugs used in psychiatry generally bind to different receptors in different cells in the brain and regulate (increase or decrease) the action of specific neurotransmitters to bring out their effect. The agonist action of a drug stimulates a physiological action and the antagonist action blocks the receptor. The effects on receptors are responsible for both therapeutic as well as side effects.

Psychotropics help in restoring the normal functioning of the brain.

Choice of a psychotropic in clinical practice

Psychotropic medications can only be prescribed by a physician/psychiatrist. Choice and dosage of drugs are individualized for each patient and depend on the diagnosis, and past or family history of response to a drug. Usually, a drug is started at a low dose, which is gradually increased depending on improvement. Different patients may need different dosages of the drug. It is important to monitor treatment response and the emergence of side effects. Improvement takes place gradually. Sleep, appetite and agitated behavior are the first symptoms to improve followed by improvement in other symptoms. It is important to use the medication in an adequate recommended dosage for an adequate duration for the therapeutic effects to stabilize. In psychiatry, a drug generally needs to be taken for a minimum of 4-6 weeks in an adequate dosage to assess its efficacy and acceptability in an individual patient. The appearance of side effects while taking medication may also govern the change in dosage or medication.

Antipsychotics:

Antipsychotics are used to treat psychotic disorders, such as schizophrenia. These drugs may also be used to treat manic episodes in bipolar disorder and sometimes to augment the effect of antidepressants for treatment-resistant depression.

Antipsychotics are usually grouped into 'first generation antipsychotics (FGAs)' (or 'typical antipsychotics') that primarily act on the dopamine receptor system (thus also called dopamine receptor antagonists or DRAs) in the brain and 'second generation antipsychotics (SGAs)' (also called 'newer antipsychotics' or 'atypical antipsychotics') that act on both serotonin and dopamine receptor systems (thus also called serotonin dopamine antagonists or SDAs). Both groups have an equal effect in ameliorating symptoms but have different side effect profiles. Antipsychotics often need to be given for a long period, varying from 6-8 months for acute psychotic conditions to 2-3 years in first-episode schizophrenia, and sometimes even longer.

Some antipsychotic medications (fluphenazine, haloperidol, flupenthixol, risperidone, paliperidone, and olanzapine) are also available in the form of long-acting injection form that can be given fortnightly or at monthly intervals instead of daily oral dosages which helps in maintaining better adherence to the treatment. Commonly used oral antipsychotic medications are given in Box 1.

Antidepressants

Antidepressants are used to treat depression, generalized anxiety disorder, panic disorder, obsessive compulsive disorder and other similar ailments. They improve symptoms, such as sadness, hopelessness, low confidence, poor concentration, lack of energy and lack of interest in activities.

These drugs provide benefits through their action on the serotonin, norepinephrine and dopamine neurotransmitter systems. There is generally a delay of 2-3 weeks in the onset of the therapeutic effects of these drugs. These medications generally need to be given for a long period, varying from 6-9 months to 2-3 years.

Box 1. Commonly Used Oral Antipsychotic Medications

Name	Usual dose (mg/day)	Commonly available strength (mg)	Common side-effects
First Generation Antipsychotics (FGAs)			
Haloperidol	5-15	0.5, 1.5, 5, 10,	Tremor, rigidity, slowness of body movements, menstrual irregularities, abnormal spontaneous body movements (on long-term use)
Second Generation Antipsychotics (SGAs)			
Olanzapine	5-20	2.5, 5, 7.5, 10, 15, 20	Increased appetite, weight gain, somnolence
Quetiapine	150-600	25, 50, 100, 200, 300, 400	
Risperidone	2-8	0.5, 1, 2, 3, 4	Menstrual irregularities, weight gain, tremors, rigidity, slowness of body movements
Clozapine*	50-400	25, 50, 100, 200	Drowsiness, weight gain, nausea, increased heart rate, drooling of saliva, constipation, seizure (at very high dose), agranulocytosis (in <1% of cases, but require regular monitoring of blood cell counts)
Aripiprazole	10-30	2, 5, 10, 15, 20, 30	Headache, anxiety, nausea, restlessness

* Clozapine is used in cases of treatment resistant schizophrenia.

Sudden stoppage of many of these medicines may cause discontinuation or withdrawal syndrome. Hence, to avoid this problem, the dosages of these medicines are gradually reduced and stopped over a period of 2-3 months, when the treatment is complete. Commonly used antidepressant medications are given in Box 2.

Anxiolytics or Antianxiety Medicines:

Anxiolytics are used to treat anxiety states, such as generalized anxiety disorder or panic disorder. These agents may also help reduce agitation and treat insomnia. Some antidepressants, especially SSRIs, also have anti-anxiety effects. SSRIs are used in the treatment of anxiety disorders when the medications need to be given for a long period. Benzodiazepines have both anti-anxiety and hypnotic effects, i.e., sleep-inducing effects, and are also used for the treatment of anxiety and insomnia. But benzodiazepines are not used for more than 4-5 weeks due to the risk of dependence.

Another common class of drugs used to treat anxiety states is beta-blockers which act by blocking the β (*beta*) receptors of the autonomic nervous system thus reducing the autonomic symptoms of anxiety, like tremors, palpitations and tremors.

Box 2. Commonly Used Antidepressant Medications

Name	Usual dose (mg/day)	Commonly available strength (mg)	Common side-effects
Selective Serotonin Reuptake Inhibitors (SSRIs)			
Escitalopram	10-20	5, 10, 20	Nausea/vomiting, gastric distress, anxiety (during initial weeks), sexual dysfunction, dry mouth, may interfere in sleep (fluoxetine) or cause sleepiness (paroxetine)
Fluoxetine	20-80	20, 40, 60	
Sertraline	50-200	50, 100	
Paroxetine	12.5-50	10, 20 (normal release) 12.5, 25 (as slow-release preparation)	
Serotonin Norepinephrine Reuptake Inhibitors (SNRIs)			
Venlafaxine	75-225	37.5, 75, 150	Nausea, gastric distress, sexual dysfunction, dry mouth, increased blood pressure (at high doses)
Tricyclic Antidepressants (TCAs)			
Amitriptyline	75-225	10, 25, 75	Dry mouth, drowsiness, constipation, tremors, postural hypotension
Imipramine	75-225	25, 75	
Others			
Mirtazapine	15-45	7.5, 15	Drowsiness, increased appetite, dry mouth, weight gain
Bupropion	150-450	150, 300	Headache, insomnia, dry mouth, nausea, tremors, restlessness, seizure (at high doses)

Medications for Insomnia:

Hypnotics are the drugs used to manage sleep disturbances. As sleep disturbances are mostly a symptom of some mental disorders, the treatment of insomnia is continued till the effect of the medication for the treatment of the associated mental disorder is not observed, and afterward, the hypnotic drugs are slowly reduced and stopped. Both benzodiazepines and zolpidem (5-10 mg) can be used as hypnotics. However, these should not be used for more than a few days to weeks, as there is a risk of developing dependence. The cause of insomnia needs to be treated and principles of sleep hygiene should be followed. This is discussed in detail later in the chapter on sleep disorders.

Melatonin is another medication used for sleep disturbance. Melatonin is a hormone produced mainly at night and is associated with sleep regulation. It is used mainly for jet lags and sleep disturbances related to shifting work. It can sometimes cause fatigue, irritation, dizziness or headache, and has been associated with reduced fertility on long-term use.

Box 3. Commonly Used Anxiolytic Medications

Name	Dose (mg/day)	Commonly available strength (mg)	Common side-effects
Benzodiazepines (BZD)			Dizziness, forgetfulness, impaired motor skills, disorientation, blurred vision
Alprazolam	0.25-1	0.25, 0.5, 1, 1.5	
Clonazepam	0.25-2	0.25, 0.5, 1, 2	
Lorazepam	1-4	1, 2	
Diazepam	5-10	2, 5, 10	
Beta-Blockers (β blockers)			
Propranolol	20-80	10, 20, 40	Decreased heart rate, reduced blood pressure (not to be taken by patients with bronchial asthma)

Mood-stabilizers:

Mood stabilizers are used to treat bipolar disorder and have both therapeutic as well as prophylactic effects. Bipolar disorder is an episodic illness, characterized by episodes of mania and depression with intervening episode-free periods. Commonly used mood stabilizers include lithium carbonate, sodium valproate, carbamazepine and oxcarbazepine. Box 4 lists the usual doses, blood levels and common side effects of the mood stabilizers.

Certain precautions need to be observed when taking lithium. Dose of lithium is strictly regulated by monitoring blood levels. Its therapeutic blood levels are 0.6-1.2 mmol/L. Lithium has a narrow therapeutic range and can be neurotoxic as well as cardiotoxic, if the blood levels increase beyond 2 mmol/L. An important caution when taking lithium is to take plenty of liquids in any form. If fluid loss or dehydration occurs due to any reason like fever, vomiting, loose motions or excessive sweating, it may result in a rapid rise in the levels of lithium in the blood that may lead to lithium toxicity. Therefore, when starting lithium,

the patients, as well as their family members, need to be informed about such precautions. In case of occurrence of fever, loose motions or vomiting due to any cause, lithium should be stopped temporarily.

Lithium and carbamazepine also exhibit drug interactions with many drugs. Therefore, if a person is taking any other medicine, he/she should inform the doctor about it.

Psychostimulants:

Psychostimulants or stimulant drugs are used for the treatment of attention deficit hyperactivity disorder (ADHD). These include methylphenidate and atomoxetine. (Box 5)

Medications for Dementia:

Cognitive enhancers are used to treat various forms of dementia or neurocognitive disorders. Mild to moderate stages of dementia are treated by cholinesterase inhibitors and moderate to severe stages of the disease are treated by N-methyl-D-aspartate (NMDA) blockers. (Box 6)

Box 4.   Commonly Used Mood Stabilizing Medications

Name	Dose (mg/day) (Serum levels)	Commonly available strength (mg)	Common side-effects
Lithium	900-1200 (0.4-1.2 mmol/l)	300, 400, 450	Nausea, vomiting, tremors, increased urinary frequency, increased thirst, weight gain, nausea, hypothyroidism
Valproate	750-1500 (50-100 mg/l)	200, 250, 300, 500, 750, 1000	Gastric distress, nausea, drowsiness, tremors, weight gain, hair loss (**Not to be given during pregnancy; to be avoided in child-bearing age**)
Carbamazepine	400-800 (4-12 mg/l)	100, 200, 400	Nausea, gastric disturbances, drowsiness, double vision, low serum sodium levels (at high doses or after long-term use)
Oxcarbazepine	600-1200 mg	300, 450, 600	Dizziness, drowsiness, nausea, headache

Box 5.   Commonly Used Stimulant Medications

Name	Dose (mg/day)	Commonly available strength (mg)	Common side-effects
Atomoxetine	1.2mg/kg/day	10, 18, 25	Abdominal discomfort, anxiety, irritability/dysphoria, insomnia, increased heart rate, reduced appetite
Methylphenidate	20-60	5, 10, 18, 20, 36	

Box 6.   Medications to Treat Dementia

Name	Dose (mg/day)	Drug strength	Common side-effects
Cholinesterase Inhibitors			
Donepezil	5-10	5, 10, 23	Diarrhea, nausea, vomiting
Rivastigmine	3-12	1.5, 3, 4.5, 6	Reduced hunger, dizziness, nausea, vomiting, diarrhea, headache
NMDA Blockers			
Memantine	5-20	5, 10	Dizziness, headache, constipation, increased sleep

Medications for Substance Use Disorders:

Treatment of substance use disorders, like alcohol or opioid (smack/heroin) dependence, is done by specific medications in phases. For example, detoxification from alcohol is treated with benzodiazepines, while long-term treatment is done by anti-craving medications (acamprosate and naltrexone) or deterrents (disulfiram).

Opioid dependence is treated initially by opioid agonists like buprenorphine, and long-term treatment may require opioid agonists or antagonists. Currently, there is no specific medication available for cannabis dependence. Drugs used for maintenance treatment of opioid dependence are scheduled drugs and not available on prescription, and are directly dispensed in the de-addiction clinics or hospitals. (Box 7)

Nicotine gum is used for the treatment of nicotine dependence (smoking, smokeless tobacco, *gutka, khaini,* etc.). Bupropion, an antidepressant, also reduces the craving for tobacco. Varenicline is another drug used to reduce the craving for nicotine.

Other medications:

There are certain other medications that are used to treat some specific conditions, such as sexual disorders, (sildenafil, tadalafil), or to manage the extrapyramidal side effects of the antipsychotics (trihexyphenidyl and biperiden). (Box 8)

It is important to know certain important points for medicines used in psychiatry. These are elucidated in Figure 1.

Physical Methods of Treatment

Analyses of the brains of healthy individuals and those with mental or neurological disorders have brought critical insights into the underlying problem of mental ill-health. A human brain is composed of millions of neurons that are interconnected with each other over various regions of the brain and generate consciousness, thoughts, feelings, behavior, etc. The neurons communicate with each other using electirc current in form of ions traveling from one neuron to another, similar to the current flowing through the electrical wires

Box 7. Medications for Substance Use Disorders

Name	Dose (mg/day)	Drug strength (mg/ml)	Use	Common side-effects
Buprenorphine	8-16	0.2, 0.4, 2	Opioid addiction	Sedation, nausea, vomiting, constipation, headache, sweating, sleep disturbances
Methadone	15-40	15	Opioid addiction	
Disulfiram	125-500	250, 500	Alcohol addiction	Drowsiness, tiredness, headache, acne, metallic/garlic-like taste
Acamprosate	1332-1998	333	Alcohol addiction	Diarrhea, abdominal pain, vomiting
Naltrexone	50-150	50	Opioid/Alcohol addiction	Nausea, headache, tiredness, reduced hunger

Box 8. Other Medications for Specific Conditions

Name	Dose (mg/day)	Commonly available strength (mg)	Use	Common side-effects
Phosphodiesterase-5 Inhibitors				
Sildenafil	50-100	50, 100	Erectile dysfunction	Headache, flushing, abdominal pain, muscular pain
Tadalafil	10-20	5, 10, 20		
Anticholinergic Agents				
Trihexyphenidyl	2-4	2	Rigidity, tremors, slowness of body (extrapyramidal side effects of antipsychotics)	Dry mouth, nausea, vomiting, constipation, light-headedness, urinary retention
Procyclidine	2.5-5	2.5, 5		

General Rules of Psychiatric Treatment

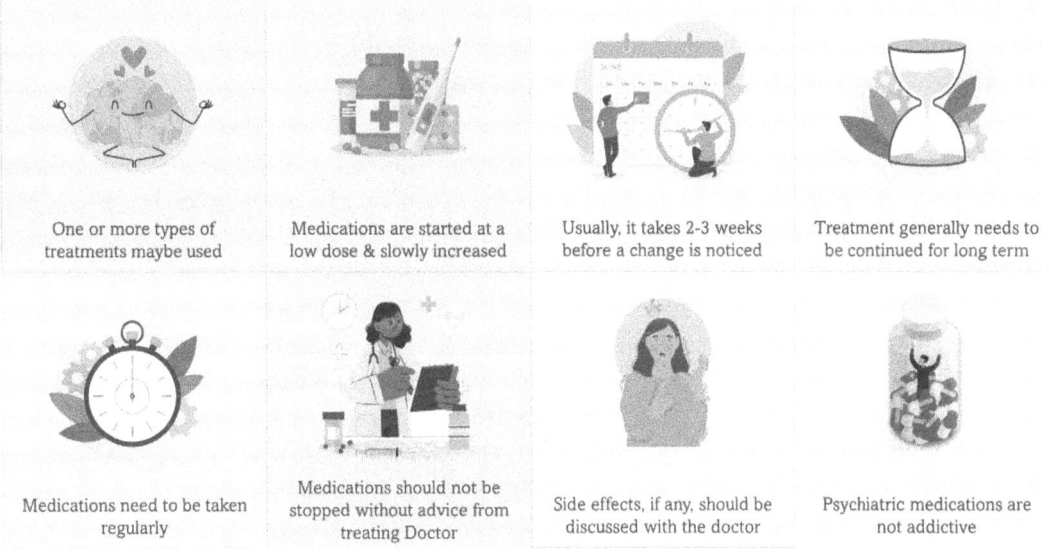

One or more types of treatments maybe used

Medications are started at a low dose & slowly increased

Usually, it takes 2-3 weeks before a change is noticed

Treatment generally needs to be continued for long term

Medications need to be taken regularly

Medications should not be stopped without advice from treating Doctor

Side effects, if any, should be discussed with the doctor

Psychiatric medications are not addictive

Figure 1. *Guidelines for Psychiatric Treatment*

in the household. It has been suggested that when certain brain neurons do not function well, the dysfunction manifests itself in the form of a mental disorder. There are certian physical methods of treatment, which directly act at neurons.

Commonly available and recommended physical methods of treatment include electro-convulsive therapy (ECT) and repetitive transcranial magnetic stimulation (rTMS).

Electro-convulsive therapy (ECT) is one of the oldest physical methods of treatment for mental disorders, which is in use for more than 80 years. ECT is the treatment of choice for psychotic disorder with catatonic symptoms and very severe depression.

ECT modifies neuronal current directly through electrical stimulation and is one of the earliest used effective treatments for treating mental disorders. It is performed under anesthesia and is called **modified ECT** and requires a setup comprising all life-saving instruments.

A pre-anesthetic check-up is usually done by an anesthetist to assess the individual undergoing modified ECT before providing anesthesia. The check-up requires evaluation of bodily functions through various blood tests, electrocardiogram (ECG) and chest X-ray. A dental and ophthalmological examination is also done during check-up to look for any loose tooth or raised intracranial pressure.

The duration of providing ECT is less than 8 seconds but the entire process of providing anesthesia takes around 15-20 minutes. Once the ECT is given, the individual is kept under observation for at least 30 minutes till the individual is fully awake.

Usually, it is given 2-3 times a week, delivering a total of about 5 to 12 sessions of modified ECT to treat depressive or psychotic symptoms.

rTMS has been introduced in psychiatry in the last 20 years. It modifies current in neurons through magnetic stimulation. A magnetic coil is placed over the head at a specific region without touching the head. rTMS does not require anesthesia and therefore no pre-anesthetic check-up is required. There is no pain during the procedure and the individual is completely awake during the procedure. The treatment duration for an individual session rTMS session is about 30 minutes for a single session and 10 to 20 such sessions distributed over 2-4 weeks need to be given. It has been found effective in the treatment of depressive disorder and obsessive-compulsive disorder.

Conclusion

Different kinds of mental ill-health conditions require varied approaches to management. Working together, patient, family members and the mental health professional can decide which treatment may be the best, taking into consideration the symptoms and their severity, personal preferences, side effects and other factors. As the treatment takes some time to generate an effect, the patients and their family members should maintain patience for the effects to appear.

KEY POINTS

➢ A large number and variety of medications are available for the treatment of different mental illnesses

➢ Most psychotropic medications are started at a low dose, which is gradually increased to reach the therapeutic dose

➢ It may take 1-2 weeks for the beneficial effect of a drug to begin and another 3-4 weeks for the beneficial effect to stabilize.

➢ Usually, sleep, appetite and agitation are first to respond to treatment followed by improvement in other symptoms

REFERENCES

1. World Health Organization (WHO). https://www.who.int/health-topics/mental-health

2. National Institute of Health and Care Excellence. https://www.nice.org.uk/guidance

3. American Psychiatric Association. https://www.psychiatry.org/patients-families

4. Royal College of Psychiatrists of the UK https://www.rcpsych.ac.uk/mental-health/treatments-and-wellbeing

CHAPTER 22

Psychotherapy and Counseling

Rachna Bhargava and Lini Philip

Introduction

Psychological interventions are an important mode of treatment for psychosocial and mental health problems. Psychotherapy and counseling are the two specific psychological interventions, which are conducted by professionally trained experts. These differ from a simple advice and guidance, given by friends or the family who may provide reassurance and advice. Due to lack of expertise in skills for specific techniques, friends/family cannot replace a trained counselor or a psychotherapist. In addition, they may also have difficulty in maintaining objectivity while providing help.

There are many types of psychotherapy and counseling. This chapter briefly introduces various kinds of psychological treatments that are useful in different mental health conditions.

What is Psychotherapy and How Does it Differ from Counseling?

Psychotherapy is a form of treatment by psychological means for problems of emotional nature conducted by a trained person with the goal of removing, modifying or alleviating existing symptoms, targeting disturbed patterns of behavior and promoting positive personality growth and development (adapted from The Technique of Psychotherapy by Lewis Wolberg, 4th Edition, 1977).

Counseling is an intervention in which a trained person listens to someone who has a problem and gives him/her advice on how to deal with it. Counseling can be done for multiple issues, related to interpersonal problems, family issues, career counseling, etc.

Though both psychotherapy and counseling aim at helping a person and are conducted by a professionally trained person, the two are distinct in terms of goals and duration. The issues that are taken up in psychotherapy are complex in nature and hence require a greater number of sessions than for counseling. The goals in psychotherapy can be variable, like obtaining insight, changing maladaptive thought patterns, resolving intrapsychic conflicts, management of negative emotional states, etc. At times, mental illness may result in other psychological issues which are also taken up in psychotherapy. Counseling is seen to be more appropriate for school/college settings and in other community settings, whereas psychotherapy is usually practiced in a clinical setting.

Why Does One Need Psychotherapy or Counseling?

Many psychological issues may emerge due to either one's inability to cope with life demands or interpersonal conflicts. The problems may vary from academic stress, work pressure, domestic violence, low mood and anxiety to more severe ones, like trauma or chronic severe mental illness. Stressful life events, like abuse, neglect, bullying, loss of loved ones, divorce and serious illness, can be very disturbing for any individual and the person may need support for coping with them.

There are individual variations in the ability to deal with stressors. These stressors can lead to lowered work productivity, missed classes, poor relationships and low mood for many individuals. Thus, the experience of chronic stress in one's life can have deleterious effects on both physical health and psychological well-being. For example, a person may be frustrated in an unrewarding job for years or may be continuing in a conflicting marriage for decades.

Apart from these stressors, some individuals may also suffer from mental illness. These disorders, too, create an enormous financial, emotional and social burden for the individual. In these conditions, psychotherapy and counseling sessions provide an effective mode of resolving issues. In some conditions, like interpersonal conflict, behavioral problems, mild anxiety and related issues, seeking psychological treatment may be sufficient for dealing with these problems effectively.

Counseling and psychotherapy are beneficial for all age groups and all population subgroups, including women, minorities and individuals with disabilities. Depending upon factors like age and mental health issues, counseling and psychotherapy may be conducted in individual or group format. For example, an individual with depression will benefit greatly from individual psychotherapy sessions, focusing on his/her negative emotional state and maladaptive thought patterns, while an individual with substance use disorder may benefit more from group therapy sessions focusing on enhancing his/her motivation and understanding reasons for relapse. In group psychotherapy, the group usually comprises 6-8 individuals with similar issues. The therapist moderates the discussion and helps the individuals to share their experiences. This sharing helps the other individuals to gain direction. Box 1 summarizes indications for psychotherapy.

Individual mental illnesses, like depression, anxiety, obsessive compulsive disorder, etc. respond

| Box 1. | Indications of Psychotherapy |

- Mental illness
- Intense negative emotions like anger/sadness
- Interpersonal issues /Relationship difficulties/conflicts with significant others
- Maladaptive pattern of behaviour
- Use of any psychoactive substance
- Chronic medical illness
- Having suicidal thoughts/ideas
- Difficulty in learning/academic difficulties
- Difficulty in coping with different life situationsimalcing decisions
- Sexual dysfunction

very well to psychotherapy. For those who do not have any deep-rooted issues, counseling is still useful if the issues are not being resolved on their own by them. For example, dealing with academic problems, coping with unhappy relationships, making difficult choices in life, etc.

Process of Psychotherapy and Counseling Sessions

Counseling and psychotherapy sessions are usually held once or twice a week depending upon the nature of the problem, feasibility of the person to come for sessions and availability of slots with the concerned therapist. A typical session may range from 60-90 minutes, focusing initially on the assessment of the person's problems and mutually agreeing on the goals for therapy/counsellimg. Formal psychological assessments are integral to psychological intervention as it helps the therapist to identify issues and plan goals and sessions.

Within a session, the therapist and the counselor make efforts to build a trusting relationship with the person and focus on providing a safe and confidential space to discuss his/her problems freely without hesitation. Counseling may take 10-12 sessions to help a person resolve his/her problems, while psychotherapy sessions may take 6 months to a year to help people make changes in their thoughts, behaviors and emotions. Effective sessions also require commitment from the client to work towards making difficult changes in his/her life. Regular attendance in sessions is expected from them. Finally, the sessions are terminated when all the goals are achieved and the person feels confident to deal with his/her life challenges and is able to think effectively.

Types of Psychotherapies

There are many different approaches used in conducting counseling/psychotherapy, depending on the kind of problem. Each approach follows different principles and goals and uses a set of techniques to achieve the goals in a series of sessions. There is a focus on changing maladaptive thoughts, feelings or behaviors using psychological techniques rather than changing the underlying biology of the brain. Some of the common psychotherapeutic techniques are described below:

A. Psychoanalytic Psychotherapy

It is one of the earliest approaches to psychological problems and involves understanding the unconscious motives and conflicts of an individual. According to this approach, the problems of an individual lay hidden in the unconscious mind, of which the person is not aware of. Hence, the psychotherapist encourages the client to talk about himself/herself freely and interprets to help the client resolve conflict. Sigmund Freud, the founder of 'Psychoanalysis', emphasized on the role of early childhood experiences, needs and sexual urges in genesis of conflicts and psychopathology. Hypnosis and dream analysis are some of the common techniques used psychoanalytic psychotherapy.

B. Behavior Therapy

Behavior therapy aims at identifying the maladpative behaviors and their genesis, and then attempts to modify these using specific techniques. Instead of asking about any past events, thoughts, motives or emotions, the behavior therapist generally asks about the current problems that are disturbing the person. It is based on the principle that all behaviors are primarily learned, and hence, can be unlearned or modified. There are various ways in which the behavior is learned: it can be acquired through association (**classical conditioning**) or through positive/negative outcomes or consequences (**operant conditioning**).

Classical Conditioning: If a neutral stimulus or object gets repeatedly paired with a stimulus which naturally elicits a negative response (like pain or fear), the neutral stimulus also starts eliciting this negative response. This process is called classical conditioning and is often in the background of development of phobias. The process of classical conditioning may be better understood with the help of an example. If a child goes for vaccination for the first time, he/she may experience pain after the shot and may start crying. Later on, the child may experience distress even at the sight of a needle, doctor or hospital. Needles, doctors and hospitals that initially did not evoke any response in the child may now become a source of fear for the child. This is how people learn to fear different objects or situations that, in themselves, are not fearful (e.g. fear of closed spaces, heights, dogs, lifts, injections, clowns, dentists, etc.).

In a classic study done in the 1920s, John Watson, the father of behavior therapy, conducted an experiment with a young child called Little Albert. This nine-month-old child was not fearful of objects, like rabbits, rats, masks, etc. It is well known that all children respond to loud noises by expressing some fearful response like crying. During the experiment, when Little Albert was playing with the white rat, Watson made a loud noise, which made the child fearful and he started crying. After pairing the white rat with loud noise repeatedly, the child began to cry just after seeing the rat. The child became fearful of other white objects like Santa Claus masks or white fur coats subsequently. Thus, little Albert generalized his fear of white furry rats to other white objects (a process called **generalization**).

Operant or Instrumental Conditioning: Behavior also gets modified based on the consequences of one's behavior, which is the basic premise of **operant conditioning.** In other words, the behaviors, that are retained or forgotten in the future depend upon the positive or negative response one gets for that particular behavior. Factors that increase the probability of increasing a specific behavior are called **reinforcements.** People will tend to engage in those behaviors more often for which they receive rewards, like praise, money, high marks etc. **(positive reinforcement).**

A behavior would also increase if it allows a person to escape from negative consequences, like a student studying to avoid getting bad marks or an employee working efficiently to avoid being criticized by the manager **(negative reinforcement).**

A particular behavior can also be decreased by giving **punishment.** For example, being scolded by parents for fighting with siblings or a child losing TV privileges after not eating vegetables or parents taking away car keys for misbehavior, etc. If parents/teachers are consistent and prompt in their actions, the child is highly likely to change his/her behavior. Reward and punishment would vary with context and one needs to identify them to ensure positive results. Additionally, the reward should not be otherwise made available to the individual, lest it would not be an incentive to modify behavior.

For teaching more complex behaviors to young children, like using a spoon to feed themselves, principles of **shaping** (i.e., reinforcing every small step taken by the child towards the desired behavior) and principles of **chaining** (by breaking the task into smaller steps, teaching those steps and reinforcing the targeted behavior) are used. For example, a counselor working with a socially withdrawn adolescent boy may want to teach social skills by reinforcing him initially when he makes eye contact with another person, followed by reinforcing him when he smiles and talks in a normal tone and then reinforcing him when he nods and interacts with two-three people around.

Since an individual's behavior is determined by the environmental responses, therapists and counselors need to spend a lot of time analyzing the chain of events around them. What happens before and after a behavior can be understood by using a behavioral analysis method called Antecedent Behavior Consequence Analysis or commonly known as **ABC analysis.** Consider an example (Box 2). As depicted in the Box, the child's disruptive behavior is likely to occur again since mother has reinforced his behavior by leaving her work and playing with him. Here, modifying the consequences by not leaving work when child

Box 2. ABC Model of Behavior Modification

Antecedent	Behavior	Consequence
Mother is working	Child throws a tantrum and demands to be played with	Mother leaves her work and plays with the child

throws a tantrum is a way of helping parents deal with the child's disruptive behavior.

Some commonly used techniques in behavior therapy are described below:

Token Economy. This technique is usually used in hospital and school settings, and uses tokens in the first step as a reward for good behavior. These tokens are later exchanged for other big rewards, like special food, holiday, free time, etc.

Modeling: Individuals learn by observing another person. In daily life too, one may have observed that children try to imitate their favorite star in terms of style of walking or dressing and so forth.

Contingency Management: This involves changing a particular behavior by rewarding or punishing that behavior. For example, a child may be given a piece of chocolate or allowed to watch TV for 15 minutes after dinner if he/she makes his/her own bed every day (It may be noted that chocolate would act as a reward only if the child is really fond of it and does not get it otherwise).

Systematic Desensitization: The individual is taught relaxation techniques, and while being in the state of relaxation, the therapist helps to imagine fearful situations in a hierarchical manner till the fear of a particular situation or object decreases. The least feared situation is visualized in mind and the individual learns to deal with it before going to the next feared situation.

Exposure: This technique involves exposing the individual (in vitro) to objects/situations that he/she fears the most and is prevented from avoiding the same. Coping skills are taught simultaneously to help the person deal with his fears.

Time out: It is defined as loss of positive reinforcement for a brief period of time after a child shows problematic behavior. For example, a young child is made to sit in another room for 10 minutes for poking another student in class. Time-outs should be brief and safe for the child.

Activity Scheduling: This technique involves charting a list of daily activities, that a person needs to participate in. Scheduling everyday activities help bring routine and predictability in one's life.

C. Cognitive Behavior Therapy

Our behaviors are often linked to our thinking processes. Alternatively, actions are determined by underlying thoughts. Hence, the 'cognitive' component is perceived as essential in dealing with individual's behavior. Cognitive behavior therapy (commonly known as CBT), initially developed for helping patients with depression by Aaron Beck, has been used for modifying maladaptive thinking processes related to various mental health issues. For example, individuals with depression typically have three forms of negative thought patterns - negative thoughts about themselves, about the world and about the future (known as the *cognitive triad*).

In CBT, besides using behavioral techniques (discussed earlier), the underlying cognitive errors are addressed to modify thoughts, behaviors and emotions. The negative thoughts due to mental illness or other stressors are associated with negative emotions, like anxiety, sadness, fear, etc., and eventually, impact behaviors. For example, if someone has experienced a relationship break-up and thereafter thinks that nobody will ever love him/her again, then he/she is less likely to go out and meet new people again. Over time, isolation and loneliness may eventually lead to depression. When an individual is under stress, he/she may view the surrounding situation as being challenging and his/her thinking might become distorted. Thoughts like 'I'm not smart enough', 'Nobody really loves me' or 'I can't do anything right' may stem from negative experiences in one's life.

In most mental health problems, the thoughts are maladaptive because these are extreme and inaccurate, and often lead to dysfunction. These distorted thoughts (cognitive errors) may interfere in routine activities like not being able to work or go to school, etc. Even maladaptive behaviors, like substance use, may be maintained due to distorted thoughts like 'one more drink won't hurt me'. CBT addresses the distortions and initiates the individual into adaptive behavior, like engaging in work and carrying out responsible tasks at home (activity scheduling). The distortions are challenged, tested and discussed in sessions with the patient.

Some common examples of cognitive distortions are:

All-or-None Thinking: Involves thinking that something has to be exactly as we want it to be or it is a failure. For example, a student who says, 'Unless I get an A grade in the exam, I have failed', is engaging in an all-or-none thinking, where grades like B would be seen as failure, and therefore, the student would experience sadness.

Mind-Reading: Involves thinking that we know what the other person is thinking about us. For example, a person may conclude that his presentation is terrible because he saw one person yawning in the audience or a student might think that he is a bad student because his teacher did not reply to his email.

Catastrophizing: This type of thinking involves exaggerating one's mistakes and expecting the worst-case scenario. For example, a student might think that failing one exam in school would mean that he will never be able to succeed in life.

Filtering: Focusing on the negative events and ignoring the positive events. For example, an employee might receive a good review from the manager but may focus on one negative remark made by a team member, thereby ignoring the good review about himself.

CBT sessions are structured and take around 12-16 weeks for completion. Generally, sessions are taken up once a week. The therapist helps the individual to learn about the inaccurate ways of thinking and how these have developed. However, severe and chronic problems may require more sessions. A hallmark of CBT sessions is the **homework assignments** given to the patients, in which they write down their thoughts between sessions and test their cognitive changes in home setting. One way of recording one's thoughts at home is by maintaining a **dysfunctional thought record**, which involves writing down one's distorted (automatic) thoughts in different situations. It is important to remember that thoughts, by themselves, do not cause any psychological disturbance; rather it is the interaction between thoughts, behaviors, emotions and genetic and environmental situations that causes mental health problems.

D. Family Therapy

Family is an important social unit for all individuals and exerts great influence on each of its members. Families act as support systems, protecting people from developing illnesses and making them resilient to deal with everyday challenges. However, they may also maintain mental illness sometimes. For example, understanding parents who support an adolescent navigate through a difficult relationship by listening to him/her, allowing him/her to ventilate and providing him/her with emotional support may prevent the adolescent from developing depression. However, parents who criticize, scold frequently or do not show emotional warmth may put the child at risk of developing adjustment issues in later life.

Some of the mental illnesses are relapsing in nature and, at times, the patient may not be able to regain his/her functioning level as per his/her educational and occupational profile. Cognitive decline and negative symptoms (lack of motivation, lethargy, inability to show emotions, etc.), associated with severe mental illnesses like schizophrenia may also lead to emotional exhaustion among caregivers. There is also an increased financial burden of taking the member for treatment regularly, paying bills, buying medications, etc. In such cases, taking care of persons with chronic mental illness can take a toll on the entire family (also known as caregiver burden), as discussed in chapters 3 and 24. Counseling sessions play an important role here in helping caregivers deal with multiple issues.

Different approaches have been used in conducting family-based interventions based on individual problems. Family therapies are different from individual therapies, in that multiple individuals from a family attend the therapy session with a common goal. The goal may range from improving communication among the family members to learning how to deal with a loved one's diagnosis. **Problem-solving** is a useful technique for helping families in dealing with individuals with mental illness and helping them in making long-term adjustments in their life. If there are specific marital issues between spouses that need to be resolved, then **couples therapy** is preferred.

A crucial aspect of family-based interventions is to work on the communication patterns of the family members. Sometimes communication may be characterized by interruptions, speaking for others and contradictory verbal and non-verbal messages. Critical comments towards patients' illness or high expectations from the patient (also known as **expressed emotions**) are known to occur frequently among families with severe mental illness. Few counseling sessions with family members may help them become aware of the impact of their behavior patterns as maintenance factors besides gaining a better understanding of the course and symptoms of the illness. The sessions may also address issues like marriage, career, long-term care, etc. (The topic is further discussed in the Chapter 23.)

Conclusion

Psychosocial issues are very common in psychiatric illnesses, and hence, psychological treatments are essential. Psychotherapy and counseling help people make changes in their thoughts, emotions and behaviors by making use of different techniques based on different scientific principles. In cases of children and adolescents, psychotherapy sessions with the parents help hone their parenting styles and improve interpersonal relationships. Choice of the type of psychotherapy depends upon the therapist's ease and orientation along with individual characteristics and mental health issues, which guide the counseling/psychotherapy sessions. An essential requirement for a practicing psychotherapist or a counselor in India is that he/she should be a certified professional by the Rehabilitation Council of India.

KEY POINTS

➢ Psychotherapy and counseling are two forms of psychological treatments that are focused on improving mental, behavioral and social functioning.

➢ Psychotherapy/counseling may be particularly useful in conditions that are psychological in nature and psychosocial in origin.

➢ Psychotherapy is the primary mode of intervention for mental health problems, like anxiety, depression, obsessive compulsive disorder, and adjustment disorders.

➢ There are different approaches used in psychotherapy and counseling. Each approach has its own goals and techniques based on its underlying theory.

➢ Psychotherapy and counseling use similar approaches but are distinct in their use in terms of goals, duration and purpose of sessions.

➢ Psychotherapists and counselors are licensed professionals who are specifically trained in helping individuals overcome psychological issues.

REFERENCES

1. Cognitive Behavior Therapy. https://www.rcpsych.ac.uk/mental-health/treatments-and-wellbeing/cognitive-behavioral-therapy-(cbt) last accessed on 18th Feb 2022

2. Psychotherapies and Psychological Treatments. https://www.rcpsych.ac.uk/mental-health/treatments-and-wellbeing/psychotherapies last accessed on 18th Feb 2022

CHAPTER 23

Family and Mental Health

GS Kaloiya

Introduction

Family is the first institution for socialization and one of the most important social groups in the life of an individual. Family is also an influential factor and predictor of mental health, especially among children. Effects of a familial atmosphere can be positive as well as negative on its members' mental health. A healthy family takes care of the needs of its members, whereas needs remain unmet in an unhealthy and dysfunctional family. This chapter discusses the role of the family in promoting mental health, caregiver's burden and family interventions.

Role of Family in Mental Health Promotion and Prevention of Mental Ill Health

Family plays a valuable role in promoting mental health by adopting preventive measures and participating in the treatment process. Family acts as a support system and helps fulfill the psychological and biological needs of a person with mental illness during treatment and in post-recovery stages and also helps in preventing relapse. Similarly, the family also plays a pivotal role in the prevention of mental illness by providing psychological and emotional support, warmth and healthy parenting by acting as a role model and inculcating healthy coping styles.

Various ways in which the family helps in mental health promotion and prevention of mental ill-health are discussed below:

Psychological and emotional support: Psychological and emotional support helps in coping with stressful situations and promotes the well-being of an individual. Family can serve as a cornerstone for the psychological and emotional support it provides to its members. It helps in reducing perceived helplessness, loneliness, anxiety, depression and isolation among its members.

Healthy parenting style: Healthy parenting style contributes to the mental health of children. Some of the healthy practices followed by parents that help in preventing any mental illness among children are: providing quality teaching and training, giving suitable advice when needed, helping children with their problems, teaching discipline, avoiding communication gaps, fulfilling their basic needs, expressing warmth and affection, giving them love and respect, focused listening to their viewpoints and teaching them to socialize in their environment.

Healthy coping styles: Healthy environment at home is required for developing healthy coping skills to cope with everyday stress and anxiety. One learns these coping strategies early in childhood by observing one's parents and significant others.

Coping strategies can be of several types. Some of these are discussed below:

- *Appraisal-focused (adaptive cognitive):* This involves thinking about a stressful situation from a different perspective to deal with the stress in a better manner.

- *Problem-focused:* This strategy involves analyzing the situation in terms of benefits and costs involved in choosing a particular option, obtaining more information about the problems, asking others for their help, etc.

For instance, if a person feels confused about choosing a particular career option, he/she may write down what are his/her broad areas of interest, what prospects each option holds, what will be the benefit in each career along with the disadvantages of each course. Further, he/she may talk to experts in that job so that more information is obtained that will help him/her make better choices.

- *Emotion-focused:* When problems cannot be solved, one learns to accept them and manage one's own emotional reaction towards the situation.

Emotional warmth: Emotional warmth includes love, affection and acceptance. These needs are primarily fulfilled by the family.

Open communication: Open communication is about expressing one's views and ideas within a family without hesitation and fear. Open communication is healthy for relationships and increases the active participation of each member within the conversation.

Self-esteem: Self-esteem refers to how one thinks about himself/herself, especially about one's abilities to solve his/her own problems.

Subjective sense of self-sufficiency: Much of our understanding of ourselves comes from our interaction with our family members. Praise, approval and validation from family lead to an increased ability of an individual to become autonomous and independent along with increased feelings of self-worth.

Positive regard: Supporting and showing acceptance towards a member of a family, regardless of his/her behavior, is known as positive regard.

Help-seeking behavior: Help-seeking behavior involves asking others, especially family members for help in times of distress. This involves asking for guidance or treatment options in case of an illness and general support for oneself.

Physical and social activities: Engaging in sports, community work or religious activities promotes social integration of family and individual with society.

Parenting styles: There are various types of parenting styles, among which the authoritative style leads to a better outcome for children. Authoritative parents express their warmth towards children rather than being overly harsh or lenient. They also demonstrate discipline with good reasoning behind it.

Within a dysfunctional family, mental health problems are very common. There could be many reasons for dysfunction, for instance, having a poor role model in the family, substance use in the family, history of abuse and violence, disturbed parent-child relationship, poverty, etc. Issues like increased conflicts, poor scholastic performance, psychiatric illnesses, severe medical conditions and behavioral issues among children and other family members are often seen in dysfunctional families. Similarly, chronic and severe mental health issues in an individual can lead to dysfunction in a family because of increased emotional, financial and social strain.

Table 1 summarizes some of the family characteristics associated with mental health problems amongst children.

Table 1. *Factors Associated with Mental Health Problems Among Children in a Family*

Factors	Explanation
Poor role model	Children spend most of their time with family and learn many behaviors through observations and imitations. They see their parents as their role models and try to imitate their behaviors. If a good role model is missing in the family, the children are more likely to learn the maladaptive behavior.
Substance use and mental illness	Presence of substance use or mental illness in the family causes undue stress and burden for other family members.
Marital discord and violence	Marital discord and violence in the family lead to neglect of the children and increase the risk of mental illness.
Child abuse	Physical, emotional and sexual abuse in childhood and adolescence is linked with a range of mental health problems, such as depression, substance use, post-traumatic stress disorder, eating disorders, etc.

Role of Family in Treatment and Recovery from Mental Illness

For individuals who suffer from mental illness, support and care from family members are essential. Family members provide valuable input to the consultation team in obtaining more information about the person, ensuring that he/she is regularly taking medicines and is coming for treatment. Helping them understand the prominent symptoms of illness and attributing them to biological causes can increase their understanding of the illness and decrease their emotional exhaustion over time. Family members can act as a moderator of effective therapy in the following aspects:

Emotional support: Emotional support can be provided by listening to what the patient is saying and nodding, and expressing warmth towards him/her. Doing this increases positive communication with the patient and he/she will feel heard and supported.

Seeking treatment: Family members are usually the first ones to observe any behavioral or emotional changes in the patient. They can identify such changes and seek treatment for the patient immediately. With a warm relationship and open communication, they can persuade the patient to seek treatment.

Supervising treatment: In some of the chronic psychiatric illnesses, where the patient does not have insight, supervising the treatment is very essential. Due to certain symptoms, the patient may refuse to take treatment, and hence, family members have to supervise it. For example, a person with paranoid schizophrenia may refuse to take medications. Here, family members can discuss various options with the doctors and ensure that medications are given timely to the patient.

Persuading the patient to remain in treatment and follow-ups: Symptoms of the illness generally subside after the initiation of the treatment because of which patients may refuse to adhere to the treatment. Family members are educated about the relapsing nature of illness and the long duration of observation, treatment and follow-up needed for the illness. The family can then persuade the patient to continue treatment and follow up.

Financial support for treatment: The family provides financial support for meeting the treatment costs of their ill family member. Treatment puts a financial burden on the whole family. This burden is not directly visible and includes hidden expenses related to the treatment, such as various tests, medicines, transportation expenses and loss of wages due to visits to the hospital.

Overcoming stigma: Due to stigma, family members and the patient may get reduced social support and have difficulty in maintaining social relationships, and continuing or finding a job. Family members, by participating in the treatment, can improve their knowledge about mental illness and its treatment and can overcome the stigma.

Managing their expressed emotions: Due to the chronic nature of the mental illness, family members get overburdened and exhausted. Some of the family members develop negative expressed emotions (over-involvement, critical comments and hostility). These expressed emotions increase the distress levels among family members and are seen as one of the causes of relapse in patients. However, positive expressed emotions (warmth and positive remarks) help in better recovery from the illness.

Role of family in post-recovery stages: It is evident that the family provides a support system to the patient in the early phases of the illness. However, in the post-recovery stages, there is a need for further support. The family often steps up to create a conducive environment to fulfill the needs of the patient. The family provides help to the patient by:

• Providing emotional support
• Supervising the treatment to reduce the possibility of relapse
• Engaging the patient in certain vocational activities in case of chronic illnesses
• Supporting the patient to lead his/her life as it was before the illness
• Supporting the patient in case of relapse or recurrence of the symptoms
• Motivating the patient for seeking help from various sources in case of any need

Figure 1 summarises the role of the family in treatment and recovery from mental illness.

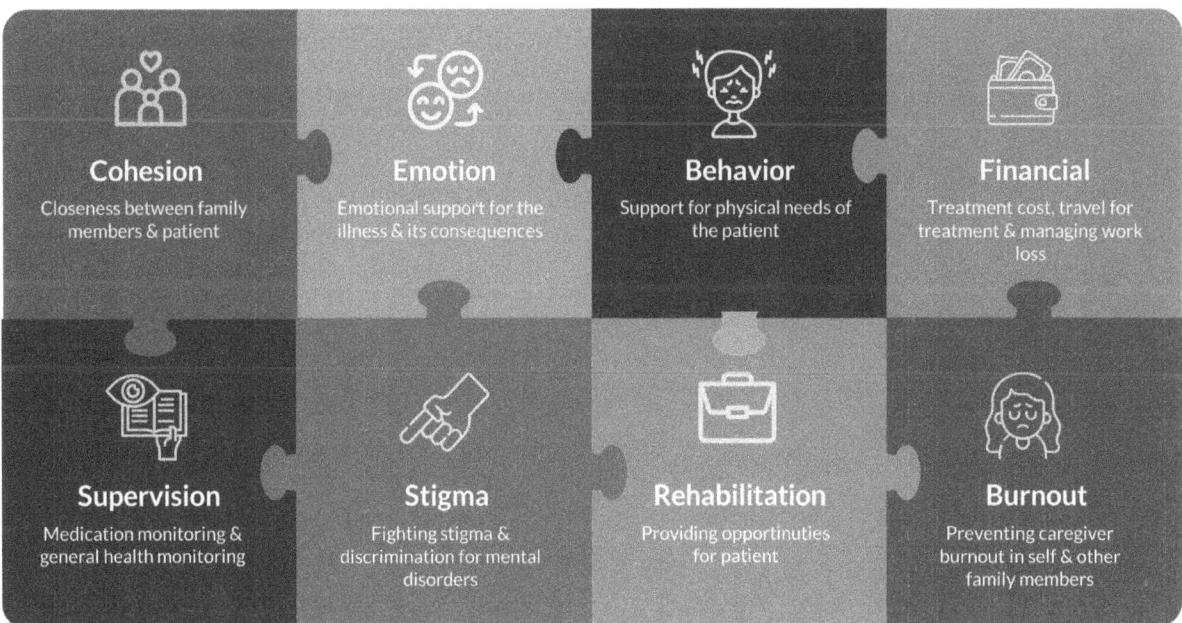

Figure 1. *Role of Family in Treatment and Recovery from Mental Illness*

Caregivers' Experience and Burden

The diagnosis of a mental illness in a family member has a negative impact on the quality of life of his/her caregivers. For instance, it can lead to a feeling of guilt and shame, affect social life and may be associated with feelings of loneliness and isolation, stigmatization, physical and mental strain and economic burden. This is also called the 'caregiver burden'. Caregivers are constantly worried about the patient's well-being, cure and availability of adequate treatment. This increases their anxiety and stress, which further contributes to the burden. However, it is important to note that the caregiving experience can also lead to positive feelings in family members by increasing their satisfaction in the caregiving role and may also increase their self-esteem due to praise and respect given to them in society.

While providing care to the patient, the role of *primary caregiver* is played by a responsible family member who is likely to spend most of the time with the patient and help in his/her treatment. Caregiver burden can be objective and/or subjective in nature. The impact of caregiver burden on family members is summarized in Table 2.

Why is it Important to Include Families in Patient Care?

There is a paucity of mental health professionals in India. Family members can serve as an important support in mental health care. Family members are generally the first ones to detect any abnormality in mood, behavior or any other psychological disturbance in their patient due to their proximity. Therefore, it is important to involve family members in treatment to get a full narrative of the patient's illness, assessment process and management, including therapy/counseling.

Involving family in treatment is associated with higher recovery rates and serves to provide effective physical and emotional support to the patient as well as other family members and primary caregivers. Such an approach is associated with a decline in feelings of helplessness and hopelessness among primary caregivers. It also helps in improving adherence to treatment and reduces the chances of relapse. This also improves the quality of patient care and increases patient satisfaction.

Family therapies have been found to be effective in reducing the anxiety and stress levels among family members as well as the patients.

Table 2. *Impact of Caregiver Burden on Family Members*

Impacts of Caregiver burden	Examples
Physical Impact	• Tiredness due to prolonged working hours • Lifestyle-related health issues (hypertension, diabetes, obesity, etc.)
Psychological impact	• Stress • Feeling of isolation or loneliness • Hopelessness and frustration • Irritation and anger outbursts • Feeling of guilt
Social impact	• Effect on interpersonal relationships • Stigmatization due to illness • Reduction of social support
Financial impact	• Income loss due to absenteeism or work loss • Increased expenses on treatment and traveling for seeking treatment

These are also known to manage the expressed emotions among family members and develop a healthy coping environment at home. Though a multi-modal system is generally followed in clinical practice, nevertheless, the inclusion of family therapy and psycho-education increases empathy and satisfaction among family members and helps them to develop better communication strategies.

When is Family Therapy Required?

Generally, family therapy is sought for finding solutions to the problems that are causing dysfunction within a family. However, there could be covert problems that are not in the forefront at the initial assessment and are often identified during the process of treatment. Some of the common situations, where family therapy is indicated are listed below:

- Conflicts between parents and children
- Adjustment and communication problems
- Marital discord
- Maladaptive parenting styles

Box 1. Goals of Family Therapy

- To explore the roots of psychopathology among relationships and its impact on family members
- To mobilize functional resources and internal strength of family
- To help strengthen the adaptive coping and problem-solving behavior among family members
- To restructure the maladaptive interactional styles so that their communication can be improved
- To assess and decrease the expressed emotions

- Presence of expressed emotions
- Chronic psychiatric problems and psychosocial issues
- Terminal and life-threatening illness

Box 1 summarizes the goals of family therapy.

There are many kinds of family therapy. Table 3 describes the steps of family therapy in general.

Table 3. *Steps of Family Therapy*

Steps	Description
Intake Session	• An intake session is scheduled and consists of about 20-30 minutes in which the therapist tries to understand the nature of the problem, the family's understanding of the illness/issues and the level of motivation. • The nature of therapy and the terms of the informal contract between therapist and family members are explained.

Family Assessment	• The assessment aims to delineate different aspects of the family functioning and communication gaps between members.
	• This phase usually includes the following steps:
	  o Drawing of 3-generation genogram to understand the dynamics of the family
	  o Exploration of roles played by the members and their functions (life cycle of the family)
	  o Problem-solving and coping styles in response to past events and stressors posing challenges. This is carried out to understand the cohesiveness and adaptability of family
	  o Generation of structural maps to understand familial systems

Steps	Description
Intervention Phase	• Assessment in some cases leads to resolution of the problem in patients but may further need treatment in the majority of the cases. • Before initiating the treatment phase, it is necessary to define an outline of the plan of action by which the family and the therapist work towards goals. • Goals can be long-term or short-term, depending on the type of issue and its resolution. • It is a general practice that once the patient starts making small changes, a snowball effect comes into action and more such changes start occurring in an amplified fashion. This is usually done by negotiating between the goals of family members and the patient. For instance, when a teenager demands freedom and family members want obedience, then a therapist finds a mid-way by helping them negotiate with each other so that the needs and wishes of both the family members and the teenager can be satisfied.

Disengaging	• When the treatment process enters this phase, the frequency of sessions is gradually reduced. This is typically done by increasing the interval between sessions. This process reduces the level of dependency on the therapist.
	• Questions pertaining to the process of change are posed in front of the family so that they can develop an understanding of the nature of the illness and the process to be followed for its resolution.
	• Relapse management planning is an integral component of this phase, as it helps the family members to visualize and predict their future actions and responses towards relapse(s).
	• Termination of the therapy or disengagement is a complex process. There are certain strategies that may be employed to make this process easier:
	   o Scheduling a follow-up with longer intervals
	   o Keeping touch via telephone on an urgent basis

Conclusion

Family is placed in the *innermost circle of social circles*, and plays an important role in the process of socialization, learning healthy coping styles, and adopting healthy and socially desired behavioral outcomes. Family plays an important role in recovery from mental illness, and also in post-recovery stages by providing psychological and emotional support, supervising the treatment, persuading the patient to remain in treatment and follow-ups, financial support and overcoming the stigma related to mental illness. Family can also help in the prevention of relapse of a mental illness following recovery. Family therapies are an important mode of treatment for a range of mental disorders.

KEY POINTS

➤ Psychological support, healthy parenting and coping styles, emotional warmth, open communication and positive regard play an important role in preventing mental health problems in a family.

➤ Poor role-modeling, substance use within the family, mental health problems in a member and disturbed parent-child relationships can lead to a dysfunctional family.

➤ Family can help in the healing and recovery of the patient with mental health issues.

➢ Caregivers are likely to experience physical, psychological, social and financial burdens as part of the caregiving process. Some may experience it as personal satisfaction, gain and experience.

➢ Family therapies are associated with higher recovery rates and help provide effective physical, emotional and support to the patient as well as his/her family members.

REFERENCES

1. Carr A. Family Therapy: Concepts, Process and Practice (3rd ed.). Wiley-Blackwell: 2012.

2. Chadda RK. Caring for the family caregivers of persons with mental illness. Indian Journal of Psychiatry 2014: 56(3), 221–227.

3. Jencius M. Experiential family therapy. In J. Carlson, & S. Dermer (Eds.), The Sage Encyclopedia of Marriage, Family, and Couples Counseling (Vol. 2, pp. 578-581). SAGE Publications: 2017.

4. Varghese M, Kirpekat V & Loganathan S. Family interventions: basic principles and techniques. Indian Journal of Psychiatry 2020: 62(Suppl 2), S192–S200.

CHAPTER 24

Long Term Care for Chronic Mental Illness

Amrita Roy and T Sivakumar

Introduction

Chronic mental illness (CMI) refers to conditions with severe and persistent symptoms, such as schizophrenia, bipolar affective disorder and other non-affective psychoses. The National Mental Health Survey of India, 2015-16, estimates the lifetime prevalence of severe mental disorders to be 0.8%.

Need for Long-Term Care

CMI may interfere with a person's ability to perform in various life domains, such as interpersonal, family, work, and social ones. Persons with CMI often have frequent exacerbations of symptoms or relapse, resulting in restriction of their functional capacities in the long run. Persons with CMI are at a higher risk of poverty. The emotional and behavioral functioning of persons with CMI can be impaired to an extent where it interferes grossly with their capability to remain in the community without supportive services for a long term. As a result, they have more complex health needs and may often require substantial care from family members and mental health professionals (MHPs).

Families, being the mainstay of caregiving for persons with CMI, often face physical and mental health consequences (stress, burnout, emotional exhaustion and feeling low or angry), leading to caregiver burden in the long run. The role of caregiving can also disrupt the family functioning and daily activities of family members.

Barriers to Long-Term Care

The provision of long-term care for persons with CMI is one of the critical challenges for mental healthcare systems for various reasons:

- Several barriers in the development of mental healthcare services at policy, budget, infrastructure and service delivery levels
- Lack of synchronization between mental healthcare services and services provided by the social sector
- Scarcity of essential mental healthcare services in rural areas; usually available at the district level. Specialized mental health services are concentrated in urban areas
- Increased prevalence of nuclear families. Urbanization has contributed to a change in traditional family ties and self-help mechanisms, hampering families to ensure informal care for a person with CMI
- Lack of supported housing facilities. There is a lack of residential/housing arrangements for persons with aged parents or no guardian or homeless. Many wandering homeless mentally ill persons never receive the required care.

Figure 1 summarizes the barriers to long-term care for persons with mental illness.

Long-Term Care Services

The long-term outcomes of CMI may include long-term institutionalization, repeated hospitalization

Barriers to Long Term Care

Lack at proper policy, program, act and Implementation

Lack of budget, infrastructure, and service delivery levels

Lack of synchronization between mental healthcare services and the social sector

Scarcity of essential mental healthcare services in rural areas

Urbanization hampering families to ensure informal care to person with CMI

Lack of supported housing facilities

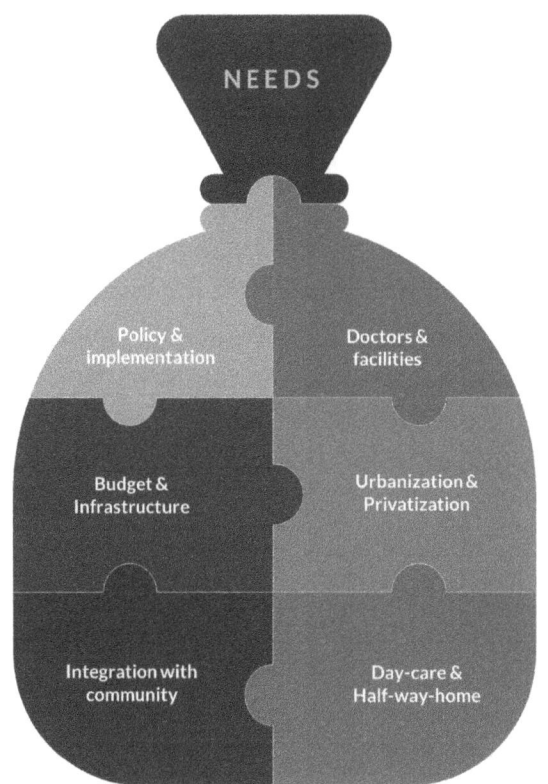

Figure 1. *Barriers to Long-Term Care for Persons with Mental Illness*

due to relapse, homelessness, death due to suicide and loss of follow-up. The goal of long-term care services must be to enable persons with CMI to eliminate or compensate for functional deficits, overcome environmental and interpersonal barriers and restore their ability for independent living and effective life management. Comprehensive long-term care of persons with CMI must include clinical, rehabilitation and welfare services:

1. **Clinical services**

   Inpatient mental health services: Inpatient mental healthcare services are primarily provided by general hospital psychiatry units of general hospitals or medical colleges, private organizations and several central and state government-run tertiary mental healthcare institutes.

   Follow-up outpatient services: There is a shortage of MHPs in India. Their availability

is concentrated at multi-specialty hospitals and tertiary care centers usually located in urban areas. However, ongoing efforts are being taken to integrate mental healthcare with primary healthcare services, increase the mental healthcare workforce and decrease the rural-urban divide under the 'District Mental Health Program'. Caregivers can visit nearby district hospitals for follow-up care. The augmented use of digital health services is a positive trend that has also boosted tele-mental health services, including consultations, medication reviews and therapies. Caregivers with access to smartphones and internet services can opt for online follow-up services. Caregivers can also select e-hospital services offered under 'Ayushman Bharat Digital Mission' (https://ehospital.gov.in/ehospitalsso/).

Pharmacy with needed medication: Families often report trouble getting relevant medications at nearby pharmacies. Thanks to online pharmacy platforms, medications can be ordered and delivered at doorsteps. Families can opt for online consultation/e-prescription for medication reviews. The Department of Pharmaceuticals, Government of India (GoI), runs more than eight thousand *Janaushadi Kendras* that provide affordable generic medicines under the 'Pradhan Mantri Bhartiya Janaushadhi Pariyojana.' The *Janaushadi Kendras* can be located on their website (http://janaushadhi.gov.in/StoreDetails.aspx). The Mental Health Care Act (MHCA), 2017, mandates all government-run or funded centers to provide essential medicines free of cost.

Physical health: Persons with CMI may have other physical health issues. Appropriate referrals must be made by MHPs whenever needed. Additionally, some might also suffer from medication's side effects that impact their physical health, such as metabolic syndrome. Physical health needs often get overlooked during hospitalization and follow-ups. Enhancing physical health is essential for overall well-being. Information about medication's side effects, necessary lifestyle modification and thorough physical assessments are a few of the simple tasks that MHPs can accomplish during outpatient visits.

2. **Rehabilitation services**
   a) **Rehabilitation needs of persons with CMI:**

Basic needs: Basic needs include shelter, food, clothing and safety. The family members of a person with CMI usually meet these needs. However, many persons with CMI may be abandoned, and hence, homeless. Homeless

persons with CMI usually remain in hospitals or shelter homes (such as shelters for women, old-age homes and beggars' colonies) or are sometimes spotted on railway stations/bus stops/roads. The MHCA 2017 mandates the provision of sheltered and supported accommodation and halfway homes apart from the hospital and community-based rehabilitation establishments.

Residential rehabilitation facilities: India's residential rehabilitation facilities include halfway homes and long-stay facilities. Halfway homes are utilized for short stay durations ranging from weeks to months. They are commonly used to facilitate the transition from inpatient to community care. Long-stay facilities are used for longer durations ranging from months to years. Comprehensive rehabilitation interventions are offered in the rehabilitation facilities to promote functioning and facilitate community integration. These residential facilities are usually located in cities. The Department of Empowerment of Persons with Disabilities (DEPwD), GoI, has formulated the revised 'Deendayal Disabled Rehabilitation Scheme' to provide halfway homes in community settings to facilitate psychosocial rehabilitation, vocational training and community reintegration.

Non-residential rehabilitation facilities: Various non-residential facilities include daycare centers, vocational training centers and sheltered workshops. Daycare centers offer productive engagement, socialization, recreation and various skills training services. Vocational training centers and sheltered workshops involve specific skills training or paid work activities. The 'NGO DARPAN portal' (https://ngodarpan.gov.in/) provides a repository of information about voluntary organizations and Non-Governmental Organizations (NGOs), sector- and state-wise. The portal has details of more than 20,000 organizations working for Persons with Disabilities (PwD), including the mental health area, listed under the 'differently abled' category. Like residential rehabilitation facilities, most non-residential services are also confined to urban areas. Families from rural areas can visit the nearby 'district disability rehabilitation center', which provides comprehensive rehabilitation services for PwD.

Social needs: Persons with CMI inadvertently face stigma, resulting in social exclusion risk. Mental health awareness, disability-inclusive policies and peer support services can be helpful in the long run. However, in current contexts, participation in rehabilitation programs might address a few social needs, such as making and meeting friends, learning social skills, interacting with various people and participating in various recreational and leisure activities.

Financial needs: Financial needs can range from earning an income to money management (bank account, transactions, savings, etc.). Persons with CMI commonly face work discrimination and unemployment. Thus, most of them are unable to earn a livelihood. In such cases, they are financially dependent on family income, including the treatment costs. Thus, caregivers/persons with CMI can look for alternative paid work activities, which offer an income, rather than remaining unemployed. For money management, caregivers must encourage the person with CMI to handle finances, including ATM withdrawal, updating the passbook and using different payment mechanisms (cards, online, etc.) under supervision initially and then empower them gradually to do so independently.

Educational and vocational needs: Poor functioning can impair one's ability to find, sustain or return to educational and vocational training courses or work. Thus, persons with CMI may need support from MHPs in finding suitable courses, ensuring reasonable accommodation at the institution/workplace, and continued support for overcoming challenges faced in education/training/work. Many rehabilitation facilities offer pre-vocational and vocational skills training services and opportunities for work in various sheltered and supported settings.

Assistance in daily living and instrumental activities: Many people with CMI cannot perform daily living (such as brushing, bathing, grooming, cleaning, etc.) and instrumental activities (such as medication management, personal communication, preparing meals, etc.) independently. Persons with CMI may be gradually encouraged and trained to perform these activities independently.

Having a daily routine: An absence of meaningful daily routine (productive activities) is a common challenge faced by persons with CMI. A caregiver can take the help of an MHP to prepare an activity schedule. An activity schedule (a plan of activities) can help keep the person engaged productively at home. The activities must be selected based on the person's interests and capabilities. The activities can combine creative, physical, informational and recreational activities. Caregivers can engage them in all possible household and outdoor work instead of allowing them to remain idle.

b) Addressing the needs of family caregivers:

Informational needs: Families need information about the nature and management of illness, medications and their side effects, ways to cope with problems related to the illness, handling symptom exacerbations and relapses and resources to gather the required information. The books 'Mental Illness and Caregiving' and 'Mental Disorders and You' provide a comprehensive overview for caregivers.

Managing crises: Caregivers may face various difficult-to-handle situations where persons with CMI display symptom exacerbations, erratic behaviors, physical or verbal aggression, suicidal ideations, etc. Caregivers can prepare a safety plan with the help of an MHP/doctor that includes a list of warning signs, ways of coping and managing that have worked in the past, what can be done to calm self and the person and who else can help in a crisis, and a list of contact numbers that can be contacted in an emergency.

Overcoming other challenges: Having a normal work-life balance is a common challenge that caregivers face. Caregivers often have to manage other household and work responsibilities in addition to the caregiving role. Other challenges that caregivers face are difficulty handling the illness and its unpredictability, struggles in relationships and communication (isolation, lack of social support, etc.) and fears about the future. Caregivers also face personal health issues related to the stress of caregiving and aging.

Respite from caregiving role: The caregiving role leaves very little time for self. To perform the caregiving role effectively, one needs to balance own physical, emotional, social and spiritual needs. Brief periods of time-out and assessment of self-need help look at one's situation, consider options and make decisions that allow one to take care of oneself within the context of caregiving responsibilities.

Social support: In simplest terms, social support means having somebody (family member, friends, organizations, etc.) to bank on, seek assistance or get supportive resources (emotional, physical, financial, informational, etc.). Recognition of their caregiving efforts is often the basic social support needed for a family caregiver. They also commonly need support in navigating the care system and planning for future care needs of persons with CMI. Social support helps one deal with stressors better. Rehabilitation organizations/ MHPs work to improve the social support for the caregivers by providing necessary psychosocial and informational interventions, such as organizing caregiver education programs, conducting family meetings and workshops and formulating caregiver support groups.

Financial planning services: Persons with CMI are likely to be financially dependent upon their families. Families frequently encounter the challenge of planning the person's financial security. Taking help from a financial advisor/certified financial planner can help make informed decisions about out-of-pocket expenses in the present and future care situations and help take control and manage finances better. Caregivers can choose to form a 'trust' [a legal arrangement where one or more individuals (the trustees) control money or assets (the trust property), which they must use for the benefit of one or more individuals (the beneficiaries)] and appoint a 'legal guardian' [discussed later under guardianship] if the person is not capable of handling finances.

Handling caregiver burden: The family caregivers bear a substantial burden due to the responsibility of caregiving. The caregivers are likely to have higher stress and negative expressed emotions, such as worry, anger, shame, grief and guilt. Family conflict, criticism and lack of acknowledgment by other family members further promulgate subjective burden and caregiver distress. Caregivers' mental health is equally important. Thus, caregivers must be equipped to cope with stressful situations and manage personal health. They should not hesitate to seek help to prevent or handle caregiver burnout. MHPs need to identify the early signs of caregiver burden, introduce appropriate interventions to reduce the burden and help develop healthy coping strategies. Box 1 enlists some of the measures that can be employed to prevent and handle caregiver burden.

Caregiver support groups/associations/ advocacy forums: The focus of these caregivers' groups is to provide mutual support to families that share similar situations. Caregivers can be part of various caregivers' associations, such as 'Association for MENtally Disabled (AMEND)' in Bengaluru, 'Aasha' in Chennai, 'Action for Mental Illness (ACMI)' in Bengaluru, 'Family AllianCE on Mental Illness (FACEMI)' – a pan-India organization, 'Marghadeepthi' in Guwahati, 'Nodal Association for the Mentally Ill (NAMI) India' in Mumbai, 'Sambandh' in Delhi, 'Schizophrenia Awareness Association (SAA)' in Pune, 'Subitcham' in Madurai and 'Turning Point' in Kolkata. Participation in support groups facilitates awareness and peer learning for the caregivers. They offer an emotionally supportive atmosphere and provide opportunities to learn from others' experiences and share feelings without any fear of stigma. Connecting with other families in similar circumstances leads to improved coping skills and social support and reduced perception of burden and distress.

Box 1.   Measures to Prevent and Handle Caregiver Burden

- Practice yoga or meditation
- Inculcate positive emotions like compassion and hope
- Indulge in any activity of choice or creative work, like preparing handicraft items, painting, tailoring, baking, etc.
- Develop new hobbies such as reading books, gardening and writing a diary
- Participate in spiritual practices
- Interact with other caregivers
- Join caregiver support groups
- Take a balanced diet and stay hydrated
- Take adequate sleep and rest
- Perform regular physical activities, such as walking, climbing stairs, in-home exercises, etc.
- Meet friends and relatives
- Take time-outs for self to watch a movie or TV or go out

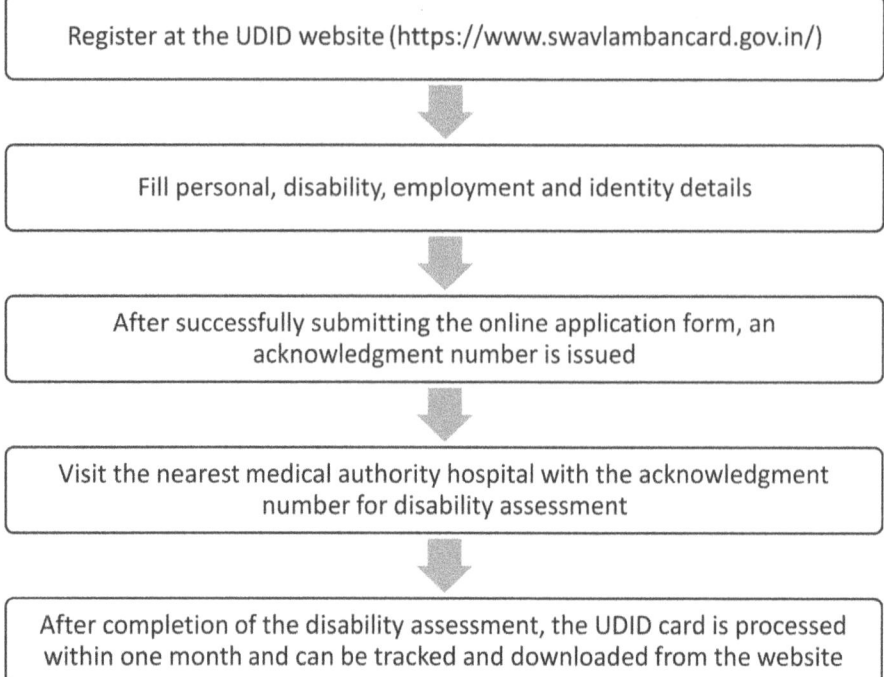

Figure 2. *Processing Unique Disability ID (UDID) Card*

'What after me' issues: As the caregivers continue to age, their health may worsen, and hence, they are forced to look for and rely on others for care and support. Several sessions may be needed to make the person with CMI understand, adjust and accept the idea of others being involved in their treatment, planning care, decision-making, daily and instrumental activities, and residential support. A well-planned and timely conversation with siblings/relatives about the person's care and support needs can help prepare for future transitions and care coordination.

3. **Welfare services**

Unique Disability ID (UDID) card: The Department of Empowerment for Persons with Disabilities (DEPwD), Government of India (GoI), has developed an initiative called UDID card for PwD. UDID is a digitally generated disability certificate that can be processed by following the steps depicted in

Figure 2. UDID card is a prerequisite to avail various welfare benefits.

Welfare benefits: GoI and various state governments offer many welfare benefits for persons with benchmark disabilities (person with >40% disability), including disability pension, unemployment allowance, travel benefits (concessional bus pass and train concession), reservation in employment and educational institutes, and income tax deduction. Families with good income can benefit from the income tax concessions (Box 2), whereas low-income families can benefit from a disability pension. These welfare benefits vary state-wise. The details of state-level disability benefits can be gathered from the nearby district welfare office/social welfare office, usually annexed with the district collector/district magistrate office. Caregivers can seek help from MHPs if they are eligible and wish to avail themselves of any welfare benefits.

Box 2. Income Tax Concessions

- ✓ Under section 80U of Income Tax Act 1961, a PwD can avail a deduction of ₹75,000 (for ≥ 40% disability) or ₹1,25,000 (for ≥ 80 % disability).
- ✓ Under section 80DD of Income Tax Act 1961, caregivers can avail a deduction of ₹75,000 (for ≥ 40% disability in dependent PwD) or ₹1,25,000 (for ≥ 80 % disability in dependent PwD).
- ✓ Anyone (either the PwD or the caregiver) can avail income tax concessions under section 80U/ 80DD.

Guardianship: To safeguard the rights of PwD, section 14 of the Rights of Persons with Disabilities Act (RPWDA), 2016, has made provision for guardianship. Any person (parents/siblings/relative) can be nominated as the legal guardian, who can make legally binding decisions in specific life domains for PwD. The family caregiver can approach a district court or any designated legal authority as notified by the state government to obtain guardianship.

Free legal aid services: Section 27 of MHCA 2017 and section 12 of RPWDA 2016 promote the right to access legal aid and justice. Section 12 of the 'Legal Services Authorities Act, 1987' entitles all persons with mental illness to seek free legal aid from the legal services authority of their respective states. An application can be given to the State Legal Services Authority for seeking free legal aid services. An online application can be submitted and tracked at the National Legal Services Authority website (https://nalsa.gov.in/lsams/). Families with android smartphones can opt for the 'Nyaya Bandhu app' – a legal services app, where lawyers and applicants have to register and make their profile free of charge. Depending upon the applicants' grievances and the lawyer's expertise, the applicant and lawyer will be matched by the app.

Insurance: The public health insurance scheme 'Ayushman Bharat - Pradhan Mantri Jan Arogya Yojana' covers the cost of mental healthcare treatment in government facilities. The insurance policies for mental healthcare are meager compared to coverage of other types of healthcare. Private insurance companies that have introduced policies to cover selected aspects of mental healthcare (such as outpatient treatment, hospitalization, counseling, consultation, etc.) include 'Max Bupa Go Active', 'Max Bupa Health Premia', 'Manipal Cigna Pro-Health Insurance', 'HDFC Ergo Health Suraksha', 'ICICI Lombard Health Shield' and 'Digit Health Plus Policy'.

Skills training services: Improving vocational/ skills training and employment opportunities for persons with CMI are critical for enhancing their quality of life and their families. The DEPwD, GoI, has developed a national action plan for the skill development of PwD by a network of skill training providers (NGOs and private and public sector training institutions). Free vocational training is provided to any unemployed Indian citizen aged 18 to 35 under the 'Pradhan Mantri Kaushal Vikas Yojana (PMKVY)' initiative. The PMKVY website (https://www.pmkvyofficial.org/) provides the details of centers and vocational courses. Though these courses are not designed exclusively for persons with CMI, they are open to all and can be utilized by them as well.

Services for government employees: Government employees having a dependent

LONG TERM CARE SERVICES

Clinical Services	Rehabilitation Needs	Needs of Caregiver	Welfare Services
• Inpatient mental health services • Follow-up outpatient services • Pharmacy with needed medication • Physical health check services	• Basic needs of living • Residential rehabilitation facilities • Non-residential rehabilitation facilities • Social engagement • Financial independence • Educational and vocational skills • Assistance in daily living and instrumental activities • Daily routine & monitoring	• Information regarding illness • Managing crises • Overcoming other challenges • Respite from caregiving role • Social support • Financial planning • Handling caregiver burden • Caregiver support groups/ associations/ advocacy forums • 'What after me' issues	• Unique Disability ID (UDID) card • Welfare benefits • Guardianship • Free legal aid services • Insurance • Skills training services • Services for government employees

Figure 3. *Long-Term Care Services*

person with a permanent disability are entitled to exemptions from routine transfer/rotational transfer subject to administrative constraints. Government employees can transfer their pension in the following sequence: Spouse → Permanently disabled children → Dependent parents → Permanently disabled siblings. The condition should be a permanent disability (a temporary disability certificate will not be considered valid) and the person should not be capable of earning a livelihood.

Figure 3 lists various long-term care services available for persons with mental illness.

Long-Term Care at Home

Persons with CMI need continued support in one or the other life domains. This has led to the exploration of alternatives to providing long-term care besides institutionalization. Presently, there is a broad consensus on the need to move towards community- and home-based care due to its cost-effectiveness, better accessibility and outcomes, increased met needs and user satisfaction. However, the current community-based mental healthcare services are not well developed, underutilized and do not adequately address the person's long-term care needs. Many alterations from policy to service delivery level are warranted to provide accessible, comprehensive, effective and high-quality rehabilitation services to people with CMI at home and community levels.

Task sharing and task shifting to non-mental health professionals (primary healthcare doctors, accredited social health workers, etc.) and non-health professionals, such as caregivers, lay health workers and peers (persons with lived experience of mental illness) are viable substitutions to address the considerable needs of persons with CMI at home and community level. Peer support providers and community volunteers can become crucial sources to assist in the recovery process of persons with CMI. Peer support services remain an underutilized resource in the mental healthcare field. Systemic changes and peer movement are necessary to catalyze the growth of peer support services.

Family caregivers typically function as the 'informal caregivers', who provide long-term home-based care to persons with CMI, without due recognition, support and economic gain. Apart from the pension given to the person, the caregivers must also be provided with monthly assistance, as they are often unable to take up employment due to the caregiving role. The Government of Kerala runs the '*Aswasakiranam*' scheme to assist the caregivers (family members or relatives) of PwD (including mental illness) with ₹600 monthly aid. Other states can adopt similar initiatives to support home-based care of persons with CMI.

Supported accommodation is essential to resolve long-term care issues for homeless mentally ill and recovered long-stay inpatients. Congregate or scatter housing with supportive services can be considered wherein a group of 4-5 persons with CMI can stay together in rented accommodation in ordinary rural or urban neighborhoods with on-site health staff support. The 'home-again' initiative (reintegrates people with mental illnesses by accommodating them in rented and shared homes in the community) by a Chennai-based NGO – 'Banyan' – is a pragmatic and sustainable model to replicate.

Conclusion

Persons with CMI may have severe and persistent symptoms that might interfere with their ability to perform in various life domains, such as interpersonal, family, work and social domains. As a result, they have more complex health needs and often require long-term care. Comprehensive long-term care of persons with CMI must include clinical, rehabilitation and welfare services. There is a need to address various barriers to ensure community- and home-based long-term care for persons with CMI.

KEY POINTS

➤ Persons with CMI might have impaired functioning in various life domains, such as personal, family, social and work, thus requiring long-term care from family members and MHPs.

➤ Various long-term services include clinical, rehabilitation and welfare services.

➤ The family caregivers bear a substantial burden due to the caregiving role, and hence, might need support in overcoming the caregiver burden and other associated challenges.

➤ Participation in caregiver support groups may successfully address the social and informational needs of the caregivers.

REFERENCES

1. Aswasakiranam, Kerala Social Security Mission, Government of Kerala [Internet]. Socialsecuritymission. gov.in. [cited 17 January 2022]. Available from: http://www.socialsecuritymission.gov.in/scheme_info.php?id=NQ==

2. Ministry of Law and Justice. The Mental Healthcare Act. New Delhi: Government of India; 2017.

3. Ministry of Law and Justice. Rights of Persons with Disabilities Act. New Delhi: Government of India; 2016.

4. Ministry of Law and Justice. Legal Services Authorities Act. New Delhi: Government of India; 1987.

5. Nyaya Bandhu (pro bono legal services), Department of Justice, Ministry of Law and Justice, Government of India [Internet]. Probono-doj.in. [cited 17 January 2022]. Available from: https://www.probono-doj.in/home/index

6. Pradhan Mantri Jan Arogya Yojana (PM-JAY), National Health Authority, Ministry of Health and Family Welfare, Government of India [Internet]. Pmjay.gov.in. [cited 17 January 2022]. Available from: https://pmjay.gov.in/

7. Singhai K, Sivakumar T, Angothu H, Jayarajan D. (2021). Review of person health insurance policies for mental health conditions. *Indian J Priv Psychiatry*, *15* (1), 3-9.

8. Unique Disability ID, Department of Empowerment of Persons with Disabilities, Ministry of Social Justice & Empowerment, Government of India [Internet]. Swavlambancard.gov.in. [cited 17 January 2022]. Available from: https://www.swavlambancard.gov.in/

CHAPTER 25

Coercion in Mental Health Care - What Might the Future Hold?

Andrew Molodynski, Louise Penzenstadler and Yasser Khazaal

Introduction

While you are reading this book, many millions of people all around the world will be working with health care professionals to get help for their mental health, regardless of location, religion, creed, gender, age or any other characteristic. Two of the great developments over recent years have been the increasing willingness of people to seek help and the reduced stigma about having mental health problems. These, combined with improved community services in many countries and regions and the closure of large and often oppressive institutions, have led to a much more collaborative and positive approach in general.

However, many people with severe mental health problems, such as psychosis or severe mood disorders, still receive treatment and support without their agreement or consent. This chapter will give an overview of this aspect of mental health care, its history, and how it may develop in this new era of enhanced technology. This chapter is deliberately designed to be accessible to all readers. For more detail, you may visit the website of the World Association of Social Psychiatry coercion group (www.coercioninpsychiatry.com).

The most commonly used term by those involved in clinical care and research regarding treatment against an individual's will is *coercion*. Coercion is commonly defined as 'The use of force or the threat of force to make somebody do something they otherwise would not'.

Legal definitions can be very complicated indeed, but the above captures the essential point that a person is compelled to have treatment that they would not otherwise agree to. There are very strong feelings about coercion, as one might imagine, in people who are subject to involuntary treatment and among those who provide it, as well as among lawyers and human rights activists. The debate has become broader and more open over the recent decades as mental health care has steadily emerged from the shadows. This has been both welcome and necessary. Books by Burns, Szmukler and Szasz demonstrate widely varying views amongst psychiatrists (Burns 2013; Szmukler 2008; Szasz 2009) and there are plenty of other examples from the wider clinical, academic and legal communities! The views of those who have experienced involuntary treatment are fortunately much more widely available today than they previously were thanks to the internet and growing support networks.

There is no doubt that the huge changes in what we can achieve with technology are already changing this debate and pushing the boundaries of current thought on what is proportionate and what is not, if indeed such a distinction can be made.

Figure 1 summarizes the concept of coercion in mental illness.

History

Mental health services have always varied between and within countries; however, certain generalizations can reasonably be made. In High Income Group (HIG) countries, there has been a

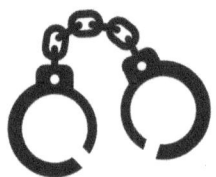

Concept of coercion in mental illnesses

Coercion, or the use of pressure, is common in mental health care

Coercion, a global phenomena, can happen either in institutions or in the community

Rapid advances in digital technology and monitoring need to be carefully evaluated for their potential harms

Figure 1. *Coercion in Mental Illness*

progressive move of services and, therefore, people from large institutions into the community, in the last half of the last century and the first decades of this one. This has been almost universally regarded as a positive change, allowing people more chance of a family and personal life with fewer restrictions on their freedoms. However, it has led some to question the living conditions and lack of care and support that many with mental illness receive in these wealthy societies. The story is different in many Low- and Middle-Income Countries (LAMICs). These countries do not generally possess the large asylums of HIGs, so there has not really been a progressive deinstitutionalization. Indeed, in some places, the only mental health care that is available is still within fairly basic facilities, often with very poor conditions and little regard for individual human rights (WHO 2018). At the same time, there are some really new and ground-breaking initiatives in less wealthy countries that are improving peoples' lives in significant ways.

It is not fair to say that there is a clear distinction between the haves and the have-nots. Some wealthy countries, notably Japan and Saudi Arabia, still have very high levels of stigma about mental illness and still have much coercive care as a result. There

is no country or region that can say it does not have coercive care of some sort for the mentally ill; for example, in the UK, new records are now regularly set (almost annually!) for the number of people forced to accept treatment for mental health problems against their will. In the USA, it is reported that there are more people with severe mental illness in prison than there are in hospitals (Fazel 2012), surely not what was intended by the architects of deinstitutionalization.

Recognizing and Measuring Coercion

Some coercion is easy to recognize. If people are chained to trees or are locked in hospitals and given forced medication, then it is easy to agree that coercion is occurring. Frequently though, this concept is less clear. What about the deeply caring family who cannot afford health care and who resort to giving their only son medicine for his psychosis secretly so he doesn't get taken away and 'kept' somewhere where they cannot see him? Or the family whose mother has dementia and they lock her door at night to stop her wandering in the street? Or the mother that looks after her son's money because he is addicted to drugs and would use it all on his addiction and become unwell and unable to look after himself? Can we say we would act otherwise or that these things are inherently wrong? I remember a discussion many years ago with a family who offered to bring their very psychotic family member to the hospital after tying them up and putting them in a car. As a young psychiatrist, I was horrified by the suggestion, but as we talked about the difference between that and the police coming in uniform, as strangers, and using handcuffs to do the same, it became clear that there were a lot of similarities. This highlighted to me the crucial importance of culture and family experience in such matters and the need to listen to (and more importantly to hear) different perspectives.

Examples of clear coercion, such as involuntary admission, the use of legislation in the community to insist on medication, the use of seclusion and the use of restrictive devices (straps, caged beds, etc.) can be counted and compared. Other forms of coercion almost certainly cannot be quantified in this way but we know from large-scale research in a number of countries that they are commonly reported. We know that coercion may also manifest in different forms around the world, but that it is ubiquitous (Molodynski et al 2016).

These less formal and unregistered types of coercion are hard to measure, but people have tried and continue to do so. Some useful tools do exist for the interested reader and have allowed comparisons to be made between different countries and services. Prominent examples are the coercion ladder, the Experiences of Coercion Scale, etc. On a bigger level, looking at systems, the World Health Organization has developed the very useful Quality Rights Toolkit for both inpatient and community mental health services. This ultimately aims to reduce coercive practices by identifying and measuring them.

Key Global Themes in Coercion

As mentioned earlier, there is no simple divide between those countries with wealth and those without. However, there are issues that are more relevant in different settings, based both on the economy and upon prevailing social practices and attitudes. Perhaps, the most important example of the latter is the differences between cultures that predominantly enshrine the rights of the individual and those that hold the rights of the community paramount, so-called collectivist cultures.

In wealthy countries that have deinstitutionalized, the use of force in mental health care is generally governed by the law of one sort or another. Such laws typically provide safeguards and rights of appeal, but despite this, there have been disgraceful breaches of the rights of individuals or groups, such as the sustained ill-treatment and abuse of a group of patients with learning disabilities at a private hospital in England some years ago that was exposed on a television program. Outside hospitals, there has been a substantial increase in the use of legal powers to compel the acceptance of treatment and support for the mentally ill in a way that would be unthinkable for people with other health concerns. The reasons for this are unclear, but relate, at least in part, to natural risk aversion, the role of the media and high profile (but rare) tragedies where people with mental health problems have committed terrible acts of violence. The increasing use of such powers is especially troubling as there is no evidence that they actually make any positive difference to the person or those around them or indeed prevent the tragedies alluded to above. Alongside such powers, we also know that the harder to define pressures, often referred to as 'leverage' or 'informal coercion', frequently occur. These can include financial management, housing provision, contact with children being made contingent upon accepting

Informed Coercion

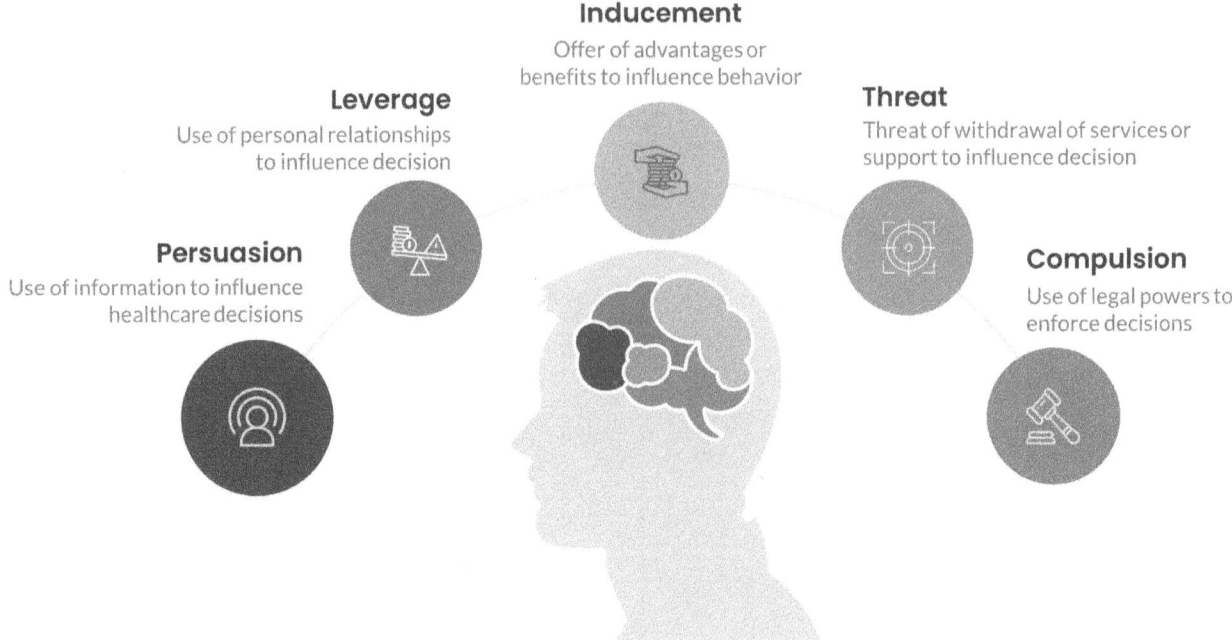

Figure 2. *Examples of Informed Coercion*

treatment (Szmukler and Appelbaum 2008), etc., as illustrated in Figure 2.

In less well-off countries, the role of state-funded and organized community mental health services is often much smaller, making the role of the family and community much more central. These are of course generalizations, but they do allow us to draw some worthwhile contrasts. Where economic and political factors dictate that mental health services are either absent or grossly inadequate (nowhere in the world can they be said to truly meet the demand), probably the most coercive factor is the absence of care. This can leave families with desperate choices between 'sending away' their loved one to a facility of some sort or trying to make the best of things at home. Facilities may be run by the state, a non-governmental organization or a traditional/faith healer. In any of these facilities, the loved one may

be far from home and subjected to harsh and/or degrading conditions.

Fighting coercion and discrimination against individuals with mental health issues are key aims of the Convention on the Rights of Persons with Disabilities. Coercive measures are often but not always used when a patient is in a crisis situation and is unable to decide which treatment would be helpful. A number of efforts are being made worldwide in order to help patients express their own will and preferences about health-related decisions in order to anticipate situations in which coercive measures may be needed. Guidance and concrete strategies to help caregivers ensure that patients can make their own healthcare-related decisions can be found in the training manual provided by WHO Quality Rights (World Health Organization, 2019).

The Effect of Technology

It will be clear from the preceding sections that most of what is thought and written about coercion involves interpersonal relationships, family relationships and established mental health services, whether that means institutions or community staff and services. Internet-based technology (as opposed to technological devices generally) has now begun to change things at a rapid pace, particularly in the last 5-10 years with advances in 'smart' technology and vastly increased access to the internet globally. This has made many things possible that simply were not possible 10 years ago. This has both positive and negative effects on coercion in mental health care. On the one hand, wherever one is in the world (almost), it is now possible to access crucial information easily and cheaply about mental health problems, services, and crucially, the beneficial and problematic effects of treatments. This liberates people from only being able to know what they are told by those around them and vastly increases their autonomy and capacity in decision-making. On the other hand, technology brings 'opportunities' for greater monitoring, surveillance and communications that can shame and reinforce stigma. The latter has been pointed to in many countries as a key problem with social media that leads to increased mental health problems, especially in the young. Monitoring, often self-monitoring, and the measurement of activity and biological parameters have been hailed as great breakthroughs in overall health care - mental health care is no exception. One only has to look at the Apple Store or Google Play to see just how popular these are, with commonly available apps measuring diet, activity, sleep, mood and many other things.

There is, however, a less positive and more coercive side of such things - their use to monitor individuals in the community with health problems to determine levels of compliance with treatment plans and changes in activity that may or may not be relevant to their health status but that generally ought to be a private matter. We are now seeing the first-time use of 'technology-augmented treatments' with well-documented trials of medications containing tiny transmitters that confirm that they are swallowed and are linked to transponders that measure the person's activity until they are excreted out to be replaced by those in the next dose. While these may indeed increase our understanding of mental illness and help some individuals make progress, one cannot help but wonder where it may lead. By measuring movement, such programs also have the capability to monitor the location and certainly will give a clear picture of activity to third parties, something that many would not welcome. In addition, the person's social media and personal contacts can be examined alongside their internet and social media usage. The term 'digital phenotyping' has been applied to such activities.

As in other branches of medicine, such as reproductive health and genetics, the ethical debate has not been able to keep up with the rapid advances in what we are able to do. While there is considerable reassurance in the case of technologically-assisted medications and their use in research being subject to stringent ethical oversight (as long as proper procedures are abided by), a plethora of apps that use smartphone technology to monitor the whereabouts and the amount and the type of activity (including online activity) are largely unregulated and only limited by the imagination of those who develop them. The fact that some of the academic discourse around the so-called digital phenotyping is enthusiastic about the prospects of using such profiling to predict, or at least attempt to predict, the development or recurrence of mental health problems must be of concern. While some rightly point out that it could enable early intervention by the individual or others, it clearly raises a host of issues around the collection and use of personal information and the potential outcomes, especially in an area where we know our powers of prediction are low and where legislation is not comprehensive.

While, in theory, one must consent to an app being downloaded onto a personal device, these decisions can be influenced like any other by coercive forces. A health care provider might make the use of such technology a requirement for insurance programs or, at the very least, strongly promote it in a way that minimizes potential harm and privacy issues. We have seen numerous examples of such behavior in the digital realm over recent years. So, it is okay to be cautious, while not setting aside the enormous potential benefits for some that technology may bring.

In order to benefit from the potential of such technologies without unwittingly taking on the associated risks, a number of safeguards are needed, such as the involvement of end-users and people with mental disorders, during the conception, design and assessment of such technological tools and better management of the imbalance between innovation and regulation.

Conclusion

Coercion has been a part of human relationships in one form or another since they came into existence and in mental health services since they were first developed. It is unfair to say that all coercion is inherently 'bad', as a lot of coercion is borne out of love and for lack of better alternatives; it can be the least bad option at times. This seems most true in cases where families in low-income group countries have little alternative other than to 'look after' or 'contain' a family member with severe mental illness in the absence of either treatment or support. Conversely, we know all too well that there are egregious breaches of the human rights of the mentally ill all around the world, whether that be in highly financed and sophisticated health care systems or in communities. Some of the worst excesses happen inside institutions, away from prying eyes, but many occur in plain sight in our communities, amongst us.

It is crucial that all who provide care and support to people with mental illness remain aware of these issues and the danger of being coercive, either intentionally or by omission or unintentional action. We must also recognize and monitor the developing technology and remain vigilant about the problems it may bring with respect to the privacy and sensitive data that could allow them to be 'phenotyped' without full knowledge. Things are changing fast, hopefully with great benefit to people with mental health problems from greater openness, communication and scrutiny of services. These positive changes must be counterbalanced against the risks described above in order to minimize and mitigate them.

KEY POINTS

➢ Coercion, or the use of pressure, is very common in mental health care.

➢ Coercion can happen either in institutions or in the community.

➢ Rapid advances in digital technology and monitoring need to be carefully evaluated for their potential harms as well as their undoubted benefits.

REFERENCES

1. Burns T. Our Necessary Shadow: The Nature and Meaning of Psychiatry. Penguin UK; 2013.

2. Fazel S, Seewald K. Severe mental illness in 33 588 prisoners worldwide: systematic review and meta-regression analysis. The British Journal of Psychiatry 2012, 200: 364-373.

3. Molodynski A, Rugkåsa J, Burns T, editors. Coercion in Community Mental Health Care: International Perspectives. Oxford University Press; 2016. Oxford, UK.

4. Molodynski A. 'Regional themes' in Molodynski A, Rugkasa J, Burns T (ed). Coercion in Community Mental Health Care- International Perspectives. Oxford University Press 2016. Oxford, UK.

5. Szasz T. Coercion as cure: A Critical History of Psychiatry. Transaction Publishers; 2009.

6. Szmukler G. Men in White Coats: Treatment under Coercion. Oxford University Press; 2018.

7. Szmukler G, Appelbaum PS. Treatment pressures, leverage, coercion, and compulsion in mental health care. Journal of Mental Health 2008; 17:233-44.

8. World Health Organization. Mental Health, Human Rights and Standards of Care. Assessment of the Quality of Institutional Care for Adults with Psychosocial And Intellectual Disabilities, in the WHO European Region. Geneva: World Health Organization, 2018.

9. World Health Organization. Mental Health, Disability and Human Rights. WHO Quality Rights Core Training - For All Services and All People. Course guide. Geneva: World Health Organization, 2019.

CHAPTER 26

Therapeutic Community: An Overview

Naveen Anand, Prioma Das, Sayani Samanta and Aniruddha Basu

Introduction

As long as history can be traced, there has always been a formation of a cohesive group of individuals with a common interest for excellence in any field. The Gurukuls of the Vedic ages put together the knowledge seekers with the gurus, the learned ones, in a homely environment. The institution, in its own right, was effective in the fulfillment of its goal of knowledge dissemination. Across the globe, there have been many such residential programs running with a varied range of goals and objectives, not just limited to education. The common entity across such residential programs was the outcome that viewed the individual to have been a changed one in its entirety. Either instinctually formed or inspired by the already existing ones, forming a group, creating a conducive niche for themselves to achieve the common endpoint, along with others, enabling and empowering individuals taking part in it, has been a consistent model for the individual excellence. This model has been applied to persons with severe mental illnesses, delinquent behaviors, addictions, etc. with positive outcomes, and is called the **therapeutic community (TC)**. The approach has been used most commonly for substance use disorders.

TCs are a self-help approach that provides a drug-free residential setting. The main goal is to rehabilitate drug users socially and through abstinence, while it is social integration in case of severe mental illnesses (SMI). A hierarchical model is used in TC, which mainly focuses on peers in different stages of treatment that increases the level of personal and social responsibilities. At the start of a TC program, the participant needs to be abstinent from alcohol and drugs. In SMI, patients who have passed through the acute phase of treatment are included.

In the TC treatment model, all the participants are taught to perform team activities under the guidance of staff members. The community members act as role models for each other by promoting a self-help approach. This works in two ways. Firstly, the residents actively participate in group therapy to identify the often-unconscious motives, unresolved conflicts and maladaptive self-protective behaviors, which result from previous traumatic or abusive formative experiences. Secondly, the involvement of residents in specific activities in the community and the nurturing of an interdependent, cohesive, pro-social environment is beneficial to the individual and other community members.

In essence, TC is a psychosocial method and program of treatment, where troubled people regularly attend a structured social community group to understand, lessen and overcome their personal, psychosocial and other emotional problems.

Background History

The modern-day concept of TC was first developed by Maxwell Jones in 1953. His book titled 'Social Psychiatry' was first published in England, which was changed to 'Therapeutic Community' when published in the United States later on. The concept drew inspiration from the self-help groups like Alcoholics Anonymous (AA) and Synanon.

AA was founded by two recovering alcoholics, Bill Wilson and Dr. Bob Smith; in 1935. There are 12 steps and 12 traditions used in AA that help any individual in the recovery process. The main goal of attending AA meetings was maintaining abstinence. AA prioritized spirituality but its basic concept was 'self-help'. The meetings in the AA group were mainly focused on stories of maintaining sobriety and understanding the issues of staying sober.

TCs were mostly developed during the World War II to provide treatment for the traumatized military personnel suffering from acute dissociative, neurotic and hysterical disorders. Previously, the psychiatric hospitals used to follow an authoritarian, oppressive and dependency-inducing culture that ultimately aggravated the self-damaging behaviors, as the treatment was going on within an anti-therapeutic environment. So, in reverse, a more humane, tolerant and empowering environment was decided to be provided, which was more flexible, structured and interactive and was more effective in reducing the patient's distress. It was soon realized by the psychiatrists that interactive group discussion had a positive impact on the patients' morale, understanding and self-esteem.

On the other front, in the year 1958, Synanon, a drug rehabilitation program evolved. The important elements of contemporary TCs, like the concepts, program model and basic practices, were used in the Synanon program. The most noticeable change was the non-residential setting of AA shifted to the intensive 24-hour residential community, which included the entire daily activities, therapeutic groups, relationships, recreations as well as community meetings. The Synanon collected funds from public and private sectors and provided treatment through a hierarchal structure.

Synanon provided a treatment option for users of narcotics and other illicit drugs who were not benefitted from the conventional medical and mental health systems. The Synanon Program and, later on, the TCs, evolved to focus on psychological and lifestyle changes. The main aim of the new treatment model was to help individuals to raise self-awareness and develop personal honesty, self-disclosure and commitment to self-change. Thus, TC brought in a revolutionary change in the treatment of addictions and psychological issues.

Principles of Therapeutic Community

The concept of 'community as a method' is the core of the practice of TC. It is the purposive use of peer community to facilitate social and psychological change in individuals.

Box 1 lists the principal themes of the TCs.

'Permissiveness' encourages the expression and enactment of disturbed feelings and relationships of an individual so that they can be examined by the peers and trained staff of the TCs alike. It allows the individuals for catharsis, self-disclosure and the assumption of self-responsibility.

'Communalism' promotes communication with each other, sharing responsibilities, emphasizing on the abandonment of fixed social roles and attitudes, and enabling the capacity to build new relationships. The democratic principle allows equal participation, self-management and altruism to flourish amongst the residents and contributes meaningfully to the treatment of others. Every

---

Box 1. Principal Themes of Therapeutic Communities

- Permissiveness
- Communalism
- Democratic decision-making
- Reality confrontation

resident in the TC is continually confronted with their own image as perceived by other residents and staff. This reality confrontation promotes a sense of self-awareness and the development of identity and self-concept and learning through interpersonal actions.

While the above concept is based on Rapoport's observation at Henderson Hospital in the 1950s; Haigh (1999) wrote about principles or universal qualities of therapeutic culture in TCs based on object relations theory, self-psychology and group analysis, and called it the quintessence of a therapeutic environment. This model is able to bring improvements in all members of the TC by bringing a feeling of belonging, safety, openness, group participation and empowerment, all of which contribute to their improvement. (Box 2)

The Generic TC Model

The generic TC model emphasizes on bringing out the person from their addiction and aims to inculcate the right living practice through a specific program that differs from an institution-based program. However, the existing models for severe mental illnesses (SMI) are not standardized. People with SMI, like schizophrenia, are often included in TC with a different perspective of 'recovery'. It aims to help improve the quality of life, autonomy and social integration. The TC activities include a range of psychological therapies and psychosocial

> **Box 2. Quintessence of a Therapeutic Environment**
>
> - Attachment - Culture of belonging
> - Containment - Culture of safety
> - Communication - Culture of openness
> - Involvement - Culture of participation and citizenship
> - Agency - Culture of empowerment

> **Box 3. Therapeutic Communities are Useful in**
>
> - Children and adolescents
>   - ✓ With delinquent behaviors
>   - ✓ Emotionally deprived and abused
> - Substance use disorders
> - Long standing psychosis
> - Learning disabilities
> - Personality disorders

activities alongside the TC activities. Box 3 lists various situations related to mental and substance use disorders, where the concept of TC has been used.

The clients in residential settings of TCs stay away from external influences, 24 hours a day for several months, and indulge in TC-oriented programs. This separateness helps clients to detach from old networks and relate to drug-free peers in the TC. The TC setting offers an environment that promotes a sense of commonality and engages the clients in collective activities. These include at least one meal prepared, served and dined together, seminars and meetings, team job function, organizing recreational and leisure periods, holding and organizing ceremonies and rituals like birthdays, etc.

Within a TC, recovered members, recovered professionals and trained professionals are all part of the community and have equal participation as any other residents. They facilitate the smooth functioning of the TCs as rational authorities and guides in the self-help community method. Clients who demonstrate expected behaviors and reflect the values of TC are viewed as role models. Multiple role models ensure the spread of social learning effects. The treatment protocol in the community and the activities are organized in stages, reflecting the developmental view of the change process.

With the TC's self-help approach, residents are responsible for the daily management of the whole facility. Every person in the community is assigned work for the day, which helps individuals develop a sense of affiliation and provides an opportunity for skill development, self-evaluation and responsibility.

A peer encounter group operates within the TCs as the major therapeutic group under professional directions. The purpose is to create individual awareness of specific attitudes and behavioral patterns that need a change. An adequate opportunity for emotional expressions and constructive management of emotions for individual and interpersonal growth is encouraged.

The rigorous schedule of TC is meant to internalize the teachings of TC within the residents. The duration of treatment is decided on the basis of growth, an individual achieves at each stage of treatment. After the termination of primary treatment, sustenance of an individual's recovery in the form of healthy lifestyle requires the assistance of family support services, vocational education and individual or group psychotherapy.

Each day in TC is ruled by a specific routine, comprising specific therapeutic and educational activities with a fixed time frame and format. Routine activities are followed through strict order of activities to eliminate unhealthy lifestyles leading to negative thinking and boredom, ultimately leading to relapse. Structured community activities make an individual self-disciplined to manage time, foster self-planning skills, challenge self to meet goals and become accountable like senior residents.

The TC model works phase-wise to observe the development of the client through the therapeutic and educational activities s/he chooses or gets assigned. The incremental learning witnessed phase-wise, helps an individual to move towards recovery. The self-help community method engages an individual in daily activities of the residents, for example, dusting, cleaning, preparation of meals, maintenance, security, purchasing, schedule preparation and monitoring, conducting seminars and meetings, etc. Thus, it helps juniors and new residents to become more absorbed in the activities. Further, it helps in gaining management skills, self-growth and discipline, reflecting TC's effectiveness. The scope and depth of resident job functions rely on the program setting (e.g., institutional versus free-standing facilities) and his/her resources (level of psychological functioning supported by life and social skills). Box 4 summarizes the stages a person goes through in a TC.

TC's goal of recovery is far from the concept of recovery from a medical model of treating mental illnesses and substance use disorders with pharmacological therapies. While it is often sufficient to have control over psychotic experiences and behaviors for clinical practices, TCs aim at socio-occupational integration of the individuals back into mainstream society. TCs mediate recovery in individuals by inculcating a sense of belongingness and individual responsibility.

It is a human's innate drive to form and maintain, at least a few, good, lasting, significant

Box 4. Program Stages

Stage 1 – Induction	Assessment and orientation into the TC	0 – 2 months
Stage 2 - Primary treatment	Focus on social and psychological goals	2 – 12 months
Stage 3 – Re-entry	Preparation for healthy separation from TC	13-24 months

interpersonal relationships. For the achievement - 'to belong', there is a need for frequent pleasant interactions with others in the context of a stable enduring framework of mutual concerns. The suitable circumstances for such interactions are provided by the TCs. The belongingness affects self-esteem and the social acceptance affects self-regulation. The resultant attitudinal and behavioral changes help cope with suicidal thoughts, anxiety and depression through self-help. The activities in TCs are explicitly structured to promote mutual concern and shared responsibilities. The regular meetings, formal and informal activities and crisis support system enable each member to stand by the other in the TC, enabling positive supportive environments.

The promotion of responsible agency, as in any psychotherapeutic model, is ingrained in the structure and basic functioning of the TCs. The individual is given an opportunity to reflect on his/her own knowledge and skills acquired, and re-approach the stresses of life with new ideas for resolution. This enables positive behavioral change, attitudinal change and self-efficacy. The individual takes responsibility for his/her actions and omissions, making himself/herself as a responsible agent for change around him/her.

The proponents of TCs for various indications, such as addiction or personality disorders have reported an overall individual recovery, which otherwise has no good prognosis in long term with any other non-community-based treatment modalities. The uniqueness of the TCs and the adaptations with respect to socio-cultural differences, which, in fact, are the strength of TCs, renders it difficult to compare with other community-based treatments methodologically. The scientific community is yet to evaluate the TCs in a standardized modern approach to recommend them as an effective treatment modality. The

immeasurable social outcomes of TCs come at a cost of long duration of treatment protocols and a need for financial support from external agencies, like the state or charitable organizations. Owing to the long treatment protocols, dropout rates are often high and jeopardize the treatment outcomes in other dimensions too. Though the concept is voluntary engagement in the TCs program, the imposition of 'right living' impinges on one's right to live, and ethical dilemmas as to what and who judges right and wrongs always exist.

Figure 1 summarizes various processes that are in the background of bringing a change in the members of the TC.

Conclusion

Therapeutic communities (TCs) are a treatment modality for various indications in individuals who have significant psychosocial issues. These use community as a resource for mediating a change in the individual, within the context of a residential program. The treatment protocol is psychologically structured and guided by rules and standards, allows for stepwise learning and brings about the expected changes. The perspective is to view the problem in holistic and humanistic terms, and the goals are set in social and psychological domains.

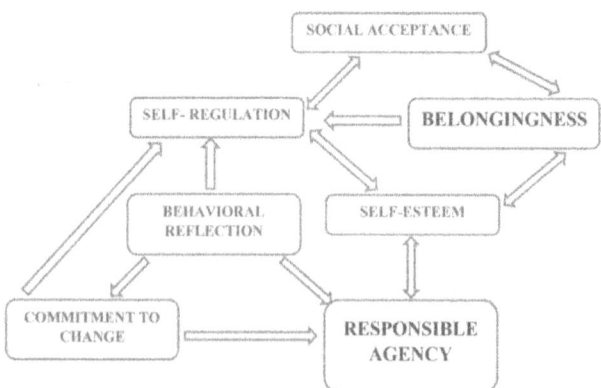

Figure 1. *Processes Underlying Changes in the Members Belonging to a Therapeutic Community*

KEY POINTS

➢ Therapeutic communities (TCs) use community as a method and the context in which the individuals change.

➢ TCs have well-defined protocols, with appropriate activities that induce expected changes.

➢ The problem is not the disease but the individual with the disease.

➢ The goal is to attain a socially integrated and empowered individual.

➢ The structure and functioning of the TCs provide individuals the opportunity for self-reflection, self-regulation, self-help and responsibility to change.

➢ The step-wise learning of skills culminates in a healthy separation from the TCs.

REFERENCES

1. Alcoholic Anonymous India. http://www.aagsoindia.org/ accessed on 17th Feb 2022.

2. European Monitoring Centre for Drugs and Drug Addiction. Therapeutic communities for treating addictions in Europe: evidence, current practices and future challenges; 2014.

3. Fountain House. Fighting to improve health, increase opportunity, and end social and economic isolation for people most impacted by mental illness. https://www.fountainhouse.org/ accessed on 17th Feb 2022.

4. Fountain House Lahore. http://www.fountainhouse.com.pk accessed on 17th Feb 2022.

5. De Leon G. The Therapeutic Community: theory, model, and method. New York: Springer Pub; 2000.

6. Society of Service of Narcotics Anonymous. https://naindia.in/ accessed on 17th Feb 2022.

CHAPTER 27

Disability and Rights of Persons with Mental Illness

Raman Deep and Dhandapani Nandakumar

Introduction

The last few decades have witnessed several developments in the field of disability with an emphasis on rights-based provisions. Disability is now understood not only from a medical perspective (i.e., originating in the individual's body or brain) but also from a social perspective (that is, arises from the interaction of an individual with society). The concept of disability includes the social context within which disabled individuals live and emphasizes on societal barriers that may cause or contribute to disability.

We shall begin with an overview of concepts related to disability, followed by a discussion on the rights and legal provisions for persons with disabilities, especially in relation to mental illness.

Concept and Definition

The World Health Organization (WHO) defined disability as '*disturbance in or inability to perform social roles that would be normally expected of an individual in the habitual milieu, arising in association with a physical or mental disorder.*' People with impairment face disability largely because of the lack of services available to them in society. In addition, they face attitudinal and environmental barriers in their everyday lives, which aggravate the problem.

Impairment, disability and **handicap** are three related terms, often used with slightly different connotations and are defined as below:

Impairment: It reflects the disturbance at the level of the organs or body parts, and is focused on the *actual malformation or malfunction* in the body.

Disability: Simply put, it is the *functional limitation* due to impairment.

Handicap: Handicap reflects the disturbances in the individual's interaction with and adaptation to the surroundings. Simply put, it means the *experience of a disadvantage in fulfilling a social role.*

The concepts of these terms are further clarified in Figure 1.

Adapting and modifying the environment to assist and accommodate the persons with functional limitations helps prevent the transformation of disability to handicap (Box 1).

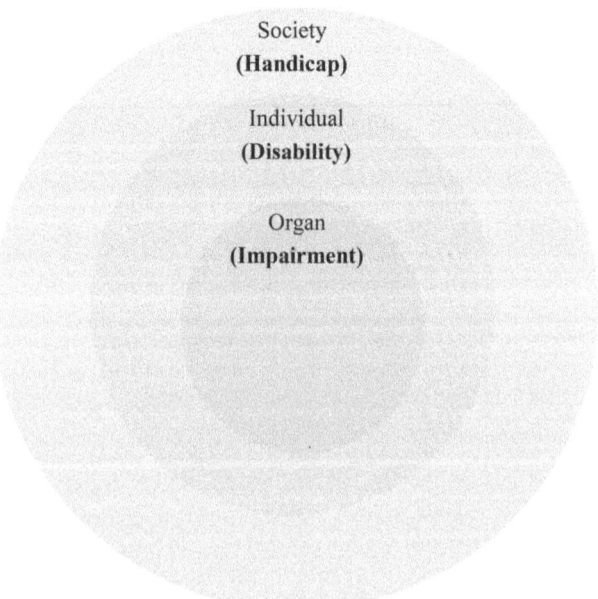

Society
(Handicap)

Individual
(Disability)

Organ
(Impairment)

Figure 1. *Impairment, Disability and Handicap*

Box 1.   Examples of Interventions to Reduce Functional and Role Limitations

	Physical condition (Trauma)	Interventions	Psychiatric disorder (Dyslexia)	Interventions
Impairment	Below knee amputation	Cosmetic limb	Inability to read or write	Provide special lighting or acoustics, space with minimal distractions
Disability	Inability to walk	Functional prosthetics, Wheelchair	Inability to learn (learning disability)	Multi-sensory teaching approach
Handicap	Disadvantages in performing the normal social roles in his or her environment	Policies conducive to special needs (e.g. wheelchair-friendly buses or buildings with ramp/elevator access)	Failures or poor grades in school, inability to secure college admission, limited career choices	Policies allowing the use of a 'scribe' and extra time during exams

Impact of Mental Disability

Severe mental disorders have a chronic and relapsing course with generally incomplete remissions, functional decline and reduced quality of life. Mental disability may have a tremendous impact at various levels, from an individual to the community.

Impact on individuals: It may be difficult to take care of daily activities, self-care, interpersonal relationships, social communication or finding a job or employment. The inability to carry out any work might lead to low self-esteem and low self-worth.

Impact on families: The family members may experience a considerable burden of care (physical, financial, social restrictions, etc.), which might manifest as psychological distress and ill-health. Further, the family members may also face stigma and discrimination.

Impact on community: Society also bears socio-economic consequences of mental illnesses in form of the inability of the person with mental illness to contribute, and by providing for treatment and care for the person with an illness.

Purpose of Disability Assessment

Assessment of disability can be done for various purposes, as listed below:

1. Ascertaining functional status of the patient, especially prior to psychosocial rehabilitation services
2. Facilitating adequate provisions, such as travel concession, disability pension, etc.
3. Litigation purposes in court, initiated by either party or by insurance agencies
4. Research and policy purposes

Approaches to Assess Disability

Previously, the methods used to measure disability included activity of daily living (ADL), which refers to basic personal care tasks of everyday life, such as grooming, maintaining personal hygiene, dressing, toileting, ambulating and eating. Lawton's Instrumental Activities of Daily Living (IADL) scale focused on eight tasks (using a telephone, shopping, preparing food, housekeeping, doing laundry, using transportation, responsibly taking medication and handling expenses), which are considered important for independent living. However, such methods do not incorporate the socio-occupational impairment, which is a limitation of this scale.

Another approach to quantify the burden of disease from a public health perspective is the use of Disability-Adjusted Life Year (DALY) (Figure 2). The DALY denotes the overall disease burden due to a particular illness and is often expressed as per 100,000 people. Essentially, it is the sum total of Years of Life Lost (1 YLL = 1 full year of healthy life lost due to premature death from a particular illness) and Years Lived with Disability (1 YLD = 1 full year of life lived with ill health or disability due to a particular illness). Such an approach is better suited to understand the impact at a global or population level rather than at an individual level.

From a research perspective, disability is assessed by means of multidimensional scales, such as the WHO Disability Assessment Schedule (WHO-DAS 2.0). Two Indian scales are also available to assess the functioning of mentally ill persons: Schedule for Assessment of Psychiatric Disability (SAPD) and SCARF Social Functioning Index (SSFI).

Assessment of the certifiable disability

Given below are the recommended tools, as per the Indian government's Gazette notifications, for certifying disability.

A. *Mental Illness:* The Indian Disability Evaluation and Assessment Scale (IDEAS) is used to assess mental disability for individuals with known mental illnesses. The scale assesses four items (self-care, interpersonal activities, communication and understanding and work) with an additional 'duration of illness' score. The global score is used to categorize disability into none (0%), mild (<40%), moderate (40-70%), severe (71-99%) and profound (100%).

B. *Intellectual disability* is assessed using Vineland Social Maturity Scale (VSMS) for adaptive functioning. VSMS is applied to the established diagnosis after testing the IQ. Reassessment is required for minors at 5 years, 10 years and 18 years of age.

C. *Specific Learning Disability* (SLD) is evaluated using the NIMHANS battery for SLD, after

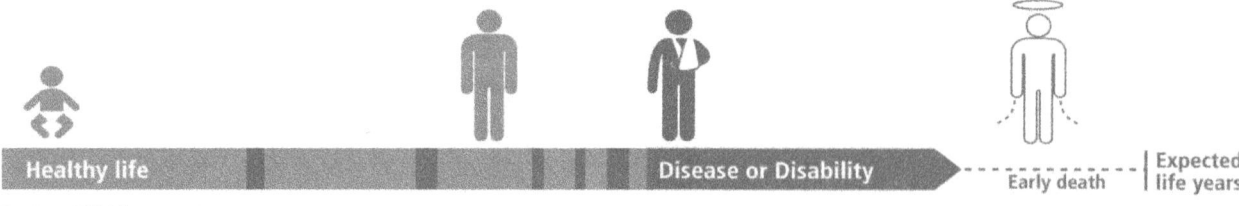

Source : Wiki Commons

**DALYs = Years of life lost due to premature mortality (YLL)
+ Years lived with disability (YLD)**

Figure 2. *Disability-Adjusted Life Years (DALYs)*

the physical examination (hearing and vision) and IQ testing (>85) yield normal results. The minimum age of assessment is 8 years, with reassessment required at 14 and 18 years of age.

D. *Autism spectrum disorder* is assessed using the Indian Scale for Assessment of Autism (ISAA) after diagnosis is already established by appropriate diagnostic instruments. The minimum age of assessment is 6 years, with reassessment required every 5 years till 18 years of age.

Policies and Laws for Persons with Disabilities in India

The Government of India brought out the *National Policy for Persons with Disabilities in 2006*. The policy deals with the physical, educational and economic rehabilitation of persons with disabilities. The Ministry of Social Justice and Empowerment (MSJE) is the nodal ministry to coordinate all matters related to policy implementation.

Laws on disability have evolved over time. To begin with, the Persons with Disabilities Act (PwD Act) was passed by the Indian government in 1995. It recognized a total of seven disabilities, including mental illness and mental retardation. It directed the government for several initiatives for prevention, promotion and rehabilitation. However, PwD Act was not comprehensive in terms of disability and rights coverage. For example, it reserved 3% of the government jobs for certain disabilities only, with the exclusion of mental illness. Further, it did not include developmental disabilities, such as autism, which was later addressed to some extent by the National Trust Act (2000). In the year 2006, a landmark international treaty was adopted by the United Nations. The Convention on the Rights of Persons with Disability (CRPD) emphasized the need for a paradigm shift from 'charity-based' to a 'rights-based' approach. India signed and ratified

the treaty in 2007. As a result, it was important to amend India's laws as per this international treaty. Consequently, the Rights of Persons with Disability (RPwD) Act came into existence in the year 2016 and replaced the earlier law. Many newer provisions came with the Act, including an expansion in the number of recognized disabilities to a total of 21.

At present, India has three laws that pertain to the subject of disabilities.

I. Rights of Persons with Disabilities (RPwD) Act, 2016 and RPwD Rules (2017)
II. National Trust Act for the Welfare of Persons with Autism, Cerebral Palsy, Mental Retardation and Multiple Disabilities, 1999 and associated Rules, 2000: This Act led to the constitution of a national body (National Trust) to enable and empower the persons with autism, cerebral palsy, mental retardation and multiple disabilities. It also extends support to registered organizations providing need-based services to families with disabilities. The Act also lays down the procedure for the appointment of guardianship and trustees for persons requiring such protection.
III. Rehabilitation Council of India Act, 1992: The act primarily deals with manpower development and research promotion in rehabilitation. It regulates and monitors the training of rehabilitation professionals and personnel in the country.

Recently, Mental Health Care Act (MHCA), 2017, was enacted for mental healthcare and treatment aspects. Chapter V of the Act has covered the rights of persons with mental illness, as stated below:

(a) Right to access mental healthcare
(b) Right to community living
(c) Right to protection from cruel, inhumane and degrading treatment

(d) Right to equality and non-discrimination

(e) Right to information

(f) Right to confidentiality

(g) Restriction on the release of information with respect to mental illness

(h) Right to access to medical records

(i) Right to personal contacts and communication

(j) Right to legal aid

(k) Right to make complaints about deficiencies in the provision of services

In addition, other provisions in mental healthcare, such as advanced directives and nominated representatives, also reflect the intent to protect the autonomy of persons with mental illness.

Rights-Based Provisions Under Current Legislation

The RPwD Act has a broad range of rights-based provisions to ensure dignity and to enhance the socioeconomic participation of persons with disability.

1. *Rights and entitlements:* These have been comprehensively covered in this legislation, including equality and non-discrimination; equal rights for women and children with disabilities, the right to community living; protection from cruel and inhuman treatment, protection from abuse, violence and exploitation; right to equal protection and safety in disasters or humanitarian conflict situations; right to home and family in case of children; reproductive rights; access to voting; and access to justice without discrimination due to disability, legal capacity and guardianship as per the degree of support required.

2. *Limited guardianship:* The Act has a provision for the grant of limited guardianship under which there is joint decision-making between the guardian and the persons with disabilities, thereby maximizing the autonomy of persons with disabilities to the extent possible.

3. *Legal capacity:* Persons with disabilities have the right to own or inherit property; to control their financial affairs; and to have access to bank loans, mortgages and other forms of financial credit.

4. *Inclusive education:* All educational institutions funded or recognized by the Government need to have inclusive education.

5. *Workplace establishments:* There are provisions to ensure non-discrimination at all establishments, including maintenance of records of employees with disabilities and facilities provided to them. A grievance redressal officer is to be appointed in all government establishments.

6. *Social security measures:* There are provisions to enhance social security (including *disability pension, caregiver allowance, unemployment allowance, insurance*, etc.), healthcare, rehabilitation and recreation.

7. *Enhanced accessibility of various services:* The Act has laid down the duties and responsibilities of appropriate government entities to take measures towards accessibility of services (such as access to transport, etc.) within a specified time frame. For example, all public buildings (be it government or private) are to be made accessible for all persons with disability within 5 years from the date of notification of the Act.

8. *Special provisions for persons with benchmark disability:* Any person with at least 40% of any of the specified disabilities certified by the medical authority or concerned notified authority is considered to have benchmark disability. Listed below are the special provisions as specified for individuals with benchmark disabilities.

   a. Every child between 6-18 years of age with a benchmark disability has the right to free education in a neighborhood school, or in a special school, of his or her choice

b. All government and government-aided institutions of higher education need to reserve at least 5% seats for persons with benchmark disabilities. Upper age relaxation of 5 years needs to be provided.

c. Every government establishment needs to reserve at least 4% of total vacancies in the cadre strength in each group of posts, of which 1% shall be reserved for autism, intellectual disability, specific learning disability, mental illness and a combination of multiple disabilities.

d. Provision of incentives to the employer in the private sector to ensure that at least 5% of their workforce is composed of persons with benchmark disability

e. Appropriate government and local authorities to make schemes in favor of persons with benchmark disabilities (with appropriate priority to women), to provide (a) 5% reservation in allotment of agricultural land and housing in all relevant schemes and development programs; (b) 5% reservation in all poverty alleviation and developmental schemes; and (c) 5% reservation in allotment of land on concessional rate for housing, shelter, business, recreation, etc.

9. *Special provisions for persons with high support needs:* Any person with a disability who is in potential need of high support may apply to the notified authority and request for assessment. Certifying for high support requires an assessment by a board for (a) the presence of benchmark disability along with (b) the need for high support and its nature. The concerned authority is required to take steps to provide support in accordance with the assessment report, subject to relevant schemes and orders of the appropriate government on this behalf.

10. *Grievance redressal:* The Office of Chief Commissioner of Persons with Disabilities and State Commissioners of Disabilities act as regulatory bodies and grievance redressal agencies and monitor the implementation of the RPwD Act, 2016. The same powers as vested in civil courts have been provided in matters of summoning the witness and documentary evidence.

Listed below are some of the other benefits under legislations other than the RPwD Act or by other ministries, which may be of use to patients with disability and their families:

- **Transfer of family pension:** Rule 50(9) of the Central Civil Services (Pension) Rules, 2021, states that the family pension shall be paid for life to the child of a deceased government servant/pensioner, who is suffering from any disorder or disability of mind, including the mentally retarded, which renders him or her unable to earn a living even after attaining the age of twenty-five years. A similar clause was there in the earlier CCS (Pension) Rules, 1972.

- **Income tax benefits:** Section 80U of the Income Tax Act, 1971, offers tax benefits for an individual suffering from a disability (that is, 40% or above), while Section 80DD offers tax benefits if an individual taxpayer's dependent family member(s) suffer(s) from a disability. A deduction of Rs. 75,000 is allowed for people with disabilities (40% and above) and Rs. 1,25,000 deduction is provisioned for people with severe disability (80% and above). No other documentation of expenses or bills is required apart from the disability certificate from a recognized medical authority. If the disability is temporary, the deduction can still be claimed for the time period or financial year during which the certificate is valid.

- **Railway concessions:** Railways provide 25% to 75% travel concessions (depending on the class of travel) for the persons with disability and one escort, on the production of the certificate in the prescribed format from a registered medical practitioner. Also, there is a *Divyangjan* quota (2 berths per 3-AC coach, 4 berths per sleeper coach) for booking tickets for a person with a disability (at lower berth) and his/her escort (at middle berth).

Offenses and Penalties for Rights Violation

Designated special courts handle the cases concerning the violation of rights of persons with disabilities. Penalties have been specified for various offenses pertaining to the RPwD Act.

  i. Any person who violates the RPwD Act or its rules will be punishable with a maximum fine of Rs. 10,000 for the first time and between Rs. 50,000 to 5 lakhs for repeat offenses.
 ii. Any person who deceives and fraudulently avails the benefit shall be punished with a maximum fine of Rs. 1 lakh or imprisonment for up to 2 years or both.
iii. Further, punishment has also been specified for the act of cruelty towards a person with a disability, which is 6 months to 5 years of imprisonment with or without a fine.

Role of Center versus State Governments

The Central Government plays a key role in policy and legislative matters. It has initiated social welfare schemes and measures through MSJE and is also committed to the CRPD at an international level. The Department of Empowerment of Persons with Disabilities (*Viklangjan Sashaktikaran Vibhag*) within MSJE is responsible for the coordination of all disability matters pertaining to the Central Government. Considerable inter-sector coordination is required across ministries and agencies.

The subject of disability is referred to in the State List as 'Relief of the Disabled and the unemployable' in the 7th Schedule of the Constitution. State governments run schemes for financial assistance, self-employment and social welfare of persons with disabilities, and educational assistance and scholarships for children with disabilities. The disability pension is provided at the state level (such as Rs. 2,500 in the state of Delhi) and varies from state to state. Overall, the subject of disability gets a varying degree of attention across different states.

There is also a provision for National and State funds for persons with disabilities. These funds support the schemes and benefits provided by the central as well as various state governments. More details on schemes are available at the official websites of the Department of Empowerment of Persons with Disabilities, UDID portal National Trust and respective state government websites

How to Apply for Disability Certificate

Any person with an illness that potentially causes disability can apply in a prescribed format to a certifying authority.

A dedicated online portal (https://swavlambancard.gov.in/pwd/application) is now made available under the UDID project for filing the application, the appointment for assessment and tracking of progress of the application.

On receipt of an application, the certifying authority shall assess the disability in accordance with the notified guidelines. The disability certificate is issued within one month of the date of receipt of the application. A permanent certificate of disability is issued in cases where there are no chances of variation in the degree of disability over time; else a temporary certificate is issued, which indicates a period of validity.

If an applicant is found to be ineligible for a disability certificate, the reasons for rejection are conveyed in a prescribed format. There is also a provision to approach the designated authority in case the applicant disagrees with the assessment.

UDID Project: An Initiative Towards National Database

The Unique Disability ID (UDID) project is an initiative by the Department of Empowerment, MSJE, to build an end-to-end encrypted, integrated system for the issuance of unique ID and disability certificates carrying the personal identification and disability details. It leads to the creation of a national database for persons with disabilities, which shall encourage transparent delivery of government benefits.

The UDID project seeks to capture all the information in one place, thereby avoiding multiple documentations, single universal identification (UDID card), leading to streamlining and ease of tracking benefits at different levels (village, block, district, state and national).

Barriers and Concerns Pertaining to Disability Provisions

In spite of ongoing efforts and advocacy, several barriers still remain, which are listed below.

- Lack of awareness is one of the main challenges. Only a small proportion of those with severe mental disabilities are aware of the various benefits and provisions provided by the government.

- The stigma associated with a mental disability may deter a person to seek disability certification. There may be apprehension about the label of disability and its potential implications, despite legal protection.

- Many psychiatric diagnoses continue to remain underrepresented at the level of certification despite a disability.

- More research and refinement are needed for the assessment tools currently used for disability assessment.

- Fraudulent information to avail certificate, especially for educational or job benefits, is another area of concern.

- Implementation of schemes varies from state to state.

Conclusion

Chronic or severe mental disorders are a significant cause of disability and affect the quality of life. Recent times have witnessed a paradigm shift from a charity-based approach to a human rights-based approach toward persons with disabilities. The legal provisions and welfare measures for persons with disabilities aim to provide better opportunities and enhance their social participation, in addition to ensuring their rights and dignity. There is a need to spread awareness regarding such provisions among persons and families who are impacted due to mental disability.

KEY POINTS

➤ Disability should be understood from a medical as well as a social perspective.

➤ There is a paradigm shift from a charity-based approach to a human rights-based approach.

➤ The dignity and rights of persons with disabilities are well protected by current legislation.

➤ Social welfare measures and benefits aim to provide equal opportunities and effective participation.

➤ Barriers such as stigma, lack of awareness and delay in implementation need to be addressed.

REFERENCES

1. World Report on Disability 2011. World Health Organization, Geneva; 2011. https://www.ncbi.nlm.nih.gov/books/NBK304079/

2. International Classification of Functioning, Disability and Health. World Health Organization, Geneva; 2001. https://www.who.int/classifications/icf/en/

3. Department of Empowerment of Persons with Disabilities, Ministry of Social Justice and Empowerment, Govt of India. https://disabilityaffairs.gov.in/content/page/acts.php

4. Rights of Persons with Disabilities Act, 2016, Government of India. https://legislative.gov.in/sites/default/files/A2016-49_1.pdf

5. The National Trust, Ministry of Social Justice and Empowerment, Govt of India. https://www.thenationaltrust.gov.in/

6. Unique disability ID (UDID), Department of Empowerment of Persons with Disabilities, Ministry of Social Justice and Empowerment, Govt of India https://www.swavlambancard.gov.in/schemes/

CHAPTER 28

Learnings in Mental Health from Ancient India

RK Chadda

Introduction

Ancient Indian treatises, including Vedas, Upanishads, Bhagwat Gita and epics like Ramayana and Mahabharata, are a great source of knowledge in a wide range of areas, including mental health. Ayurveda, the ancient system of medicine, also recognized mental health and included maladies for mental illnesses. Some of the principles of mental health as described in the ancient texts have got applicability even in the current period. Yoga and meditation being practiced today have history tracing back to ancient India. This chapter focuses on the learnings and principles from the ancient Indian treatise that have applicability in mental health promotion in the current times.

Learnings from Vedas and Upanishads

Vedas are four sacred Hindu texts, including *Rig Veda, Yajur Veda, Sama Veda* and *Atharva Veda*, which are a great source of knowledge encompassing different fields. *Yajur Veda* and *Atharva Veda* describe the mind as the inner flame of knowledge and the basis of consciousness (Figure 1). *Rig Veda*, the oldest of the Vedas, gives descriptions of various prayers and methods to strengthen willpower and promote mental happiness, and how to empower the mind and build up intelligence. *Rig Veda* and *Yajur Veda* also suggest that certain *mantras* can help in developing noble thoughts that can prevent development of depression. *Rig Veda* discusses about the speed of mind, methods and

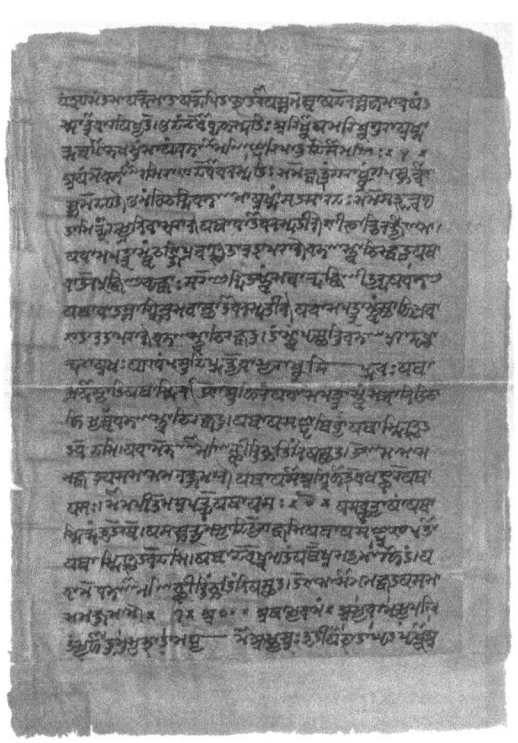

The Atharva Veda

A page from the Atharva Veda Samhita, the most ancient version of the text known.

The picture is courtesy of Prof. William Dwight Whitney (1827-1894), American linguist and lexicographer known for his work on Sanskrit grammar and Vedic philology.

Copyright: Public domain, through Wikimedia commons.

prayers for mental happiness and for increasing intelligence. There is an emphasis in Vedas on positive mental health and preservation of will power, consciousness and regulation of emotions. There are descriptions of emotional states, like grief, envy, pleasure, hostility, attachment and laziness, and their resolution. Vedas suggest culturally determined observances, like religious rituals, and dietary restrictions, like fasting to treat or resolve guilt emanating from *karmic* deeds (of previous life). Religious fasting is still considered a way of life in most parts of India, though the practice has become relatively uncommon in the younger generations.

Upanishads, which are a kind of synopsis of Vedas and are relatively of recent origin, give descriptions of consciousness, memory, thought and perception, which are all functions of the mind. There are also descriptions of the concept of *prakriti* (personality), dreaming state, waking state, deep sleep and *samadhi* (a state of intense concentration achieved during meditation) in the *Upanishads*. It is not that everything described in Vedas is applicable or perceived as correct in current understanding. However, certain principles have definite applicability in the current period.

Learnings from Ayurveda, the Ancient Indian System of Medicine

Ayurveda literally means the science of life and its origin dates back to the 6th century BCE. Sushruta and Charaka have been two famous physicians of Ayurveda in the ancient Indian history, who also wrote famous treatise on medicine, called *Sushruta Samhita* and *Charaka Samhita*, respectively. The former primarily deals with medical diagnosis and treatment and the latter refers to surgical practices. There is an emphasis on holistic health in Ayurveda, as also stated in the WHO's definition of health. Ayurveda also

stresses upon maintaining a balance between the three body humors; wind (vata), bile (pitta) and phlegm (cough). For optimal health, a person must have clarity of mind, senses, and soul, and be blessed with tranquility. Right conduct can help in preserving physical and mental health. Mind, the essence of life, is responsible for cognition. It directs the senses, controls the self, reasons and deliberates. Type of food also influences health, including mental health. Food could be *satvik* (sweet, based on natural products, vegetables and fruits, giving strength, health and equanimity), *rajasic* (saltish or sour food that stimulates thirst and may make the person restless) or *tamasic* (onion, garlic, meat, over-ripe or under-ripe vegetables or fruits, making an individual dull or aggressive). Parallel to it, three types of personality or *trigunas* have also been described: the intellectual '*satvika*', the emotional '*rajasik*' and the lustful '*tamasik*'. Food contributes to the development of personality characteristics and maintains a balance between different body humors.

Ayurveda describes four types of mental illnesses, those caused by exclusive involvement of emotions or exclusive involvement of the three body humors, disorders of body-mind involvement like *unmada* (psychosis), alcoholism and disorders with mind-body involvement. Treatments recommended in Ayurveda include medications (herbals), psychotherapy (mind control therapy), psycho-shock therapy, magico-religious practices and dietary modifications. One main difference between Ayurveda and modern medicine is the focus on separation of soul and body in the former and the body-mind dichotomy in the latter.

Learnings from the Bhagwat Gita

Bhagwat Gita or Gita is a concise guide to Hindu philosophy. Though, originally a religious text, it has much wider applications to different aspects of life's secular dimension. The text is based on a

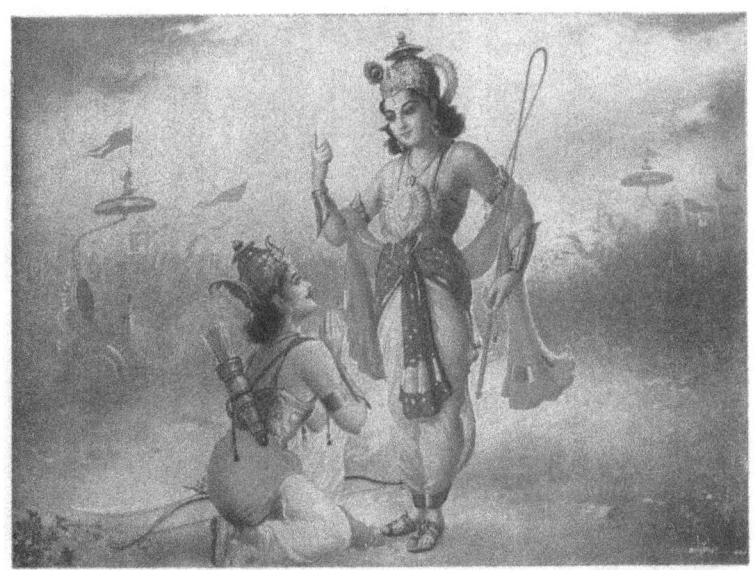

The Bhagwat Gita

An illustration of Lord Krishna reciting the Gita to Arjuna at the war of Mahabharata.

The picture is courtesy of Mahavir Prasad Mishra, author of the Sanskrit work - "महामुनि का संग्रह".

Copyright: Public domain, through Wikimedia commons.

conversation between Lord Krishna and Arjuna, the warrior prince, in the battlefield of Kurukshetra in the famous Indian epic Mahabharata, having happened around 5000 years ago. In the conversation, Lord Krishna explains to Arjuna his duties as a warrior and prince on the battlefield in response to his confusion and moral dilemma in fighting against his family elders, the Gurus (teachers) and the cousins, who are on the enemy side. The text, spread over 18 chapters, elaborates on several philosophical tenets for everyday living. Gita is a self-contained practical guide to life. There are descriptions on gaining mastery over vacillating mind, how to come out of worldly attachments and how a person has to make a decision in the background of adversities.

Gita has been translated into many languages and its application has been well recognized all around the world beyond India and Hinduism. Dilip Jeste, an American psychiatrist of Indian origin and also a past president of the American Psychiatric Association, and his group have conducted a text analysis of Gita using the QSR NVivo software. The group has identified 10 domains of the Gita: knowledge of life, emotional regulation, control of desires, decisiveness, love of and faith in God, duty and work, self-contentedness, compassion and

sacrifice, insight/humility and yoga (integration). Gita teaches a person to be his/her own master.

Dr. Matcheri Keshavan (another American psychiatrist of Indian origin) stresses on three principles described in Gita, which can help in building up resilience. The first one is the path of knowledge (*Jnana Yoga*), which helps in shifting our focus from 'I' to 'we', bringing a concept of collectiveness in the person, especially relevant in periods of crisis like the pandemic. The second is the path of action or duty (*Karma Yoga*), applicable to everyone and encouraging to do one's duty. The third principle is the path of meditation (*Raja Yoga*), which can help in reducing stress and further developing resilience.

Learning from the Ramayana

Ramayana is probably one of the most popular epics from ancient India and is highly revered by the Hindus. There are many small stories embedded within this mega epic, which have relevance in providing the lead for resolving stressful situations in day-to-day life.

The personality of Rama (Lord Rama), the central character, offers an extreme example of maintaining solace in various situations. It is rare to see Rama in anger or distress except when Queen Sita is kidnapped by Ravana and when Lakshmana, his younger brother, falls unconscious during the war. Two examples from the epic are shared here that are relevant to mental health.

One important event in the Ramayana has a specific message for patients going through depression. This has been called the 'Hanuman complex' by Late Professor Narendra Wig, former Professor and Head, Department of Psychiatry, PGIMER, Chandigarh, and AIIMS, New Delhi. The anecdote is of immense use in boosting the morale of a patient who has lost confidence. The story goes like this: Hanuman, who was always considered very brave and wise, had forgotten about his extraordinary powers to fly and many other strengths due to a curse. He had been asked to go on a mission to search for Queen Sita, who had been kidnapped by Ravana and taken to Lanka. Hanuman could not realize his actual potential, till he was reminded by Jambvanta about his ability and power to fly. The concept has been used in psychotherapy and counseling, especially in depression, when the patient or client has lost confidence and finds himself/herself unable to meet the challenges of life. The person is explained that in the past too, he/she had been able to meet the same challenges successfully and has not lost his/her abilities. The responsibility to meet the challenges lies in him/her and he/she is fully capable of meeting the challenge.

Another event refers to how we tend to misjudge situations. While in exile, when Lakshmana comes to know about the Bharata coming from Ayodhya to meet Rama, Lakshmana and Sita, he gets angry and distressed, suspecting Bharata's intentions. At that time, Rama counsels him that he should not reach such presumptions without going into details. The crisis resolves when they meet Bharata. A lesson to be learned here is that one should not make impressions before fully analyzing the situation.

Yoga:

The word 'Yoga' means 'union'. It refers to uniting one's personal consciousness with the divine consciousness. Descriptions of Yoga can be found in *Rig Veda* and Upanishads. Basic aim of yoga in relation to mental health is growth, development and evolution of mind. Swami Vivekananda has described Yoga as 'a means of compressing one's evolution into a single life or a few months or even a few hours of one's bodily existence'. Sri Aurobindo refers to Yoga as 'a methodological effort towards self-perfection by the development of potentialities latent in the individual'. The ultimate goal of Yoga is to have control over one's body and desires and conquer the endless worldly demands.

Maharishi Patanjali, also called the father of Yoga, describes the eight-fold path of Yoga, also called 'Ashtanga Yoga' for all round development of personality. Ashtanga Yoga is also considered as a key to attain the ultimate spiritual goal of self-realization. The eight-fold path includes *Yama* (self-control), *Niyama* (observation of rules), *Pranayama* (regulation of breath), *Asana* (assuming certain postures), *Pratyahara* (restraint of senses), *Dhyana* (meditation), *Dharana* (steadying of mind) and *Samadhi* (contemplation of universal consciousness).

The goal in all systems of yoga is to achieve an altered state of consciousness, known as the cosmic consciousness, transcendental illumination or samadhi. Regular practice of yoga helps in personality growth, managing emotions and reducing psychological tension. Research has shown beneficial effects of yoga in anxiety disorders, depression, dissociation and psychosomatic disorders.

It is important to mention here that yoga should be learned from a trained instructor and one should not attempt to learn it by watching others or reading instructions.

Meditation

Meditation refers to a practice of focussing concentration on a specific object, image or breathing. The origin of meditation can also be traced to the Vedas of the ancient India. Meditation has also been a part of religious practice in Buddhism and Sikhism. In the modern period, transcendental meditation has been popularized by Maharishi Mahesh Yogi. There are many schools of meditation, like Vipassana meditation, Art of living and transcendental meditation. Regular practice of meditation helps improve concentration and awareness of self, reduce negative emotions, and control stress and anxiety. It also contributes to creativity and personality growth.

The basic principle of most schools of meditation includes controlled deep and slow breathing, focusing attention on breathing, concentrating on feeling and listening, as one inhales and exhales. It may also include focusing attention on different parts of the body and becoming aware of various sensations, feelings of warmth, cold, tension or relaxation. Some techniques of meditation may include recitation of some *Mantras*, which may be religious or secular. One could also engage in prayer depending on one's religious beliefs, which is also a method of increasing concentration and works on the same principle as meditation.

It may be better to learn mediation from a formal instructor and then practice it regularly.

Conclusion

There is a treasure of knowledge available from the ancient Indian wisdom that has relevance for mental health. Vedas, Ayurveda, the ancient Indian system of medicine, Indian epics like Ramayana and the Gita, include many important principles regarding how to keep oneself in good mental health and for crisis intervention. It is thus important to be aware of this ancient Indian source of knowledge so that it can be used beneficially.

KEY POINTS

➤ There is a lot to learn about the principles of mental health from the ancient Indian texts.

➤ Bhagwat Gita is an important source of knowledge with application in modern times.

➤ Yoga and meditation can help in stress management and developing resilience against stress and anxiety.

➤ Practices of Yoga and meditation should be learned from a trained instructor.

REFERENCES

1. Avasthi A, Grover S, Kate N. Indianization of psychiatry utilizing Indian mental concepts. Indian J Psychiatry. 2013;55(6):136.

2. Bhide SR, Kurhade C, Jagannathan A, Sushrutha S, Sudhir PM, Gangadhar BN. Feasibility of using counseling techniques from Ramayana for managing negative emotions: An anecdotal review and analysis. Indian J Psychol Med.2021;XX:1–5.

3. Jacob KS, Krishna GS. The Ramayana and psychotherapy. Indian J Psychiatry. 2003 Oct;45(4):200-4

4. Jeste D, Vahia I. Comparison of the conceptualization of wisdom in ancient Indian literature with modern views: Focus on the Bhagavad Gita. Psychiatry: Interpersonal and Biological Processes. 2008;71(3):197-209

5. Keshavan M. Building resilience in the COVID-19 era: Three paths in the Bhagavad Gita. Indian J Psychiatry. 2020;62(5):459–61.

CHAPTER 29

Spirituality and Mental Health

Anju Dhawan and Sumegha Mittal

Introduction

Spirituality has been known to be a protective factor in preventing mental disorders and in promoting mental health. Spirituality is defined as developing a connection with oneself (atman) and the universe or the transcendent. It explores an understanding of consciousness. It deals with questions like 'who I am' and 'what the purpose of my existence is'. Spirituality is an individual's inward journey that aids in a better understanding of oneself. It provides an insight that external circumstances and people only influence how we think, feel, perceive and understand, but do not determine it. Spiritual growth may be achieved through certain practices. Spirituality helps develop the values of love, compassion, generosity, contentment, forgiveness, acceptance, wisdom, truth and gratitude inside us.

Relationship between Spirituality and Religion

Spirituality is an umbrella term and includes the concept of religion. The relationship between religion and spirituality is complex. There are many similarities and many differences between these two concepts.

- In spirituality, the questions are 'who am I?' and 'how do I find the meaning of life?'.
- Religion refers to a set of beliefs, rituals and practices that are common among a group of people, and are experienced individually and/or socially.

In contrast to religion, spirituality is more difficult to define. Spirituality is considered more personal and individualistic, something people define for themselves. Spirituality is largely free of the rules, rituals and responsibilities associated with religion. For many individuals, religion is intertwined with spirituality. For others, the two are separate. There are large groups of people who have started identifying themselves as spiritual-but-not-religious, and deny any connection at all with religion, seeing it as more divisive and conflicting and understanding spirituality entirely in individualistic and secular terms.

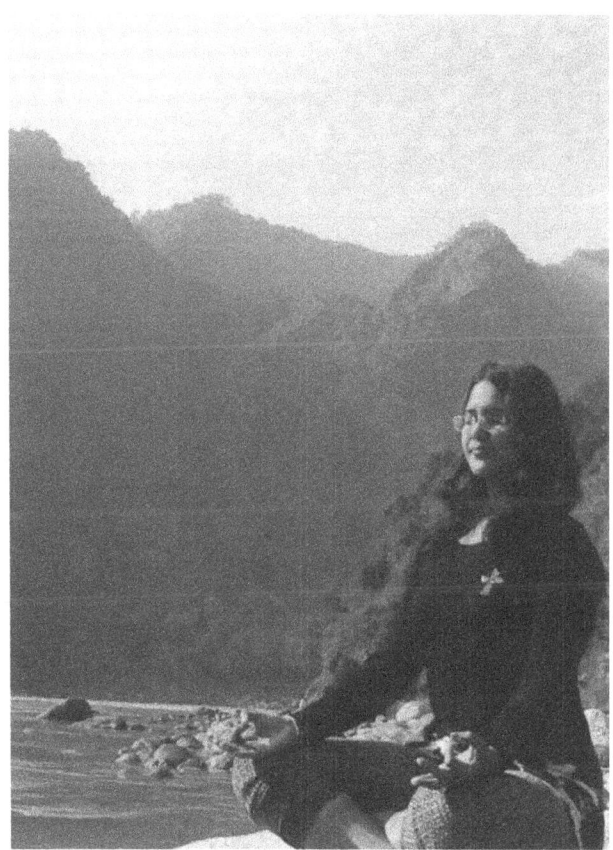

While spirituality is the core of all religious teachings, techniques such as yoga (including physical asanas, breathwork or pranayama and meditation) are also associated with spiritual growth as described in the yogic scriptures. Although meditation originated in Vedic scriptures and has been mentioned subsequently in Buddhist, Jain and other religious texts, the practice per se can be considered separate from any religious affiliation. Acceptance of these practices in the scientific western world and the introduction of the term 'mindfulness' has further increased their acceptability as a non-religious entity. Research conducted largely in the west, has supported the role of meditation in the promotion of mental health and the prevention of mental disorders.

Meditation has also been defined as the fourth state of consciousness with electrophysiological changes that are distinct from waking and sleeping states. Meditation is a state of deep rest but with full awareness, unlike sleep, which is rest without any awareness. During meditation, we sit with our eyes closed with the intention that for some time we have to do nothing. We drop our roles and desires temporarily and try to witness our thoughts and emotions. Thus, a mind in the present moment refers to meditation.

There are many types of meditation. Current literature pertains to mindfulness meditation and mantra-based meditation among others. **Mindfulness** is one of the most popular meditation techniques in the west. It has two main parts: attention and acceptance. The attention part involves directing your awareness to the physical sensations in the body, breath, thoughts and feelings you are experiencing. The acceptance part involves being a witness to your thoughts and feelings without any judgment. Instead of responding, resisting or reacting to those thoughts or feelings, your aim is to just observe and let them go. **Mantra-based meditation** requires attention on a mantra or sound to facilitate meditation. Other techniques of meditation are breath-based, such as **Sudarshan Kriya.**

Meditation helps experience the state of deep rest, inner silence, immense joy and happiness. Research has shown that meditation helps in managing emotions, reducing stress, improving concentration and confidence, facilitating clarity of mind, etc. Figure 1 summarizes the benefits of meditation.

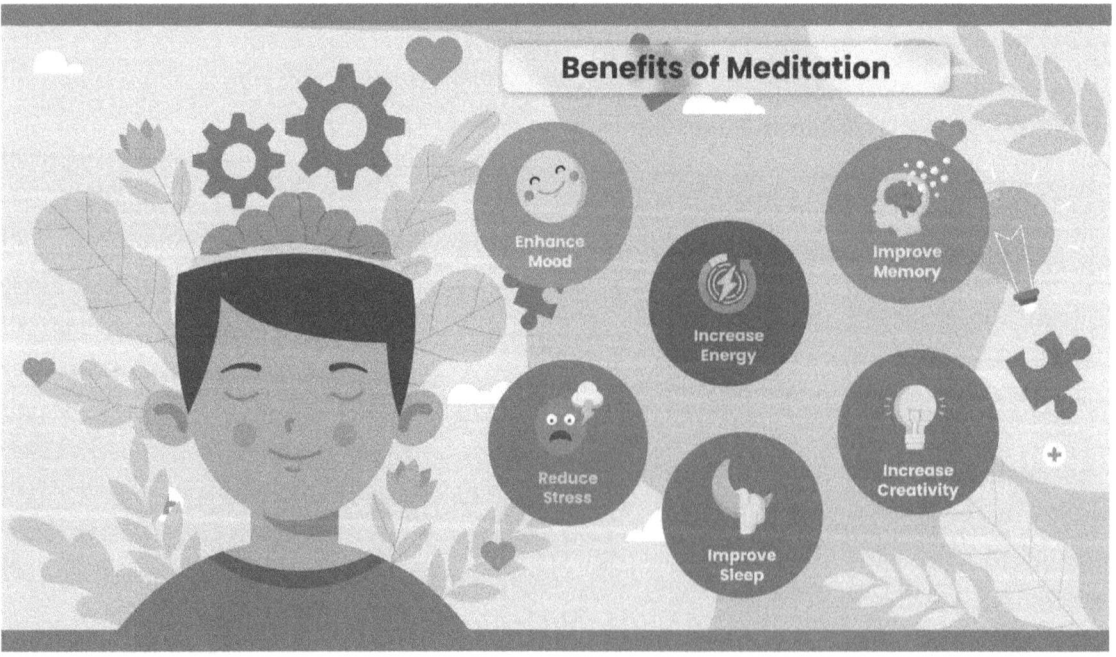

Figure 1. *Benefits of Meditation*

Spirituality and Mental Health

Both religion and spirituality have played a significant role in the lives of human beings. In times of stress, individuals look for internal or external sources of help and support.

Historically, mental health care was primarily provided in religious institutions by religious groups. Later, mental disorders were considered to have roots in religion or spirituality. Freud and Charcot considered spirituality and religion to be important causes of hysteria or neurosis. Again, in the early- to mid-twentieth century, a different perspective prevailed when spirituality and mental health problems were seen as separate. Recently, research has suggested that religion or spirituality (R/S) may play a protective and healing role in the face of emotional suffering.

Spiritual coping is a powerful coping strategy. During periods of stress, most people turn to their spiritual and religious beliefs to cope with the situation. Spiritual coping includes spiritual beliefs, prayers, meditation, breathing techniques and spiritual knowledge (reframing of stressors, spiritual support, spiritual connectedness, etc.) and is associated with better emotional health and overall psychological wellbeing. Unlike other coping methods, R/S is available at all times and in all circumstances. Looking inwards provides a sense of relief and betterment and gives a broader vision to resolve any problem. Spiritual beliefs also give meaning and purpose to existence and help see problems from a larger perspective instead of getting stuck in our small minds. Spirituality gives the wisdom that life has both good and bad phases and nothing stays forever, and teaches us to be equanimous in either of these situations. This helps accept suffering and gives strength and courage to go through adverse situations happily. Religious or spiritual affiliation provides a sense of belongingness and real or perceived social support. Spiritual coping is helpful not only for people facing day-to-day life issues or general medical illnesses but also for life-threatening illnesses like cancer. Even those

with psychiatric symptoms and disorders may rely heavily on their spiritual resources.

Mental health treatments incorporating mindfulness/meditation and user groups like Alcoholics Anonymous and Narcotics Anonymous involving principles and concepts of spirituality have become widely accepted. Professional psychiatric organizations, including the Royal College of Psychiatrists and the World Psychiatric Association, have recognized the importance of spirituality in psychiatric treatment and the need to include it as a part of the training of mental health professionals. Overall, there has been a growing academic recognition of the implications of R/S for mental health.

Scientific literature shows a remarkable increase in high-quality research publications in the past decade, providing insights and evidence-based information that suggests the role of spirituality in the promotion of mental health and quality of life. It has also been seen to play a key role in reducing stress, enhancing coping skills, improving sleep, and bringing a sense of well-being. A positive relationship has been associated with optimism, meaning and purpose of life, self-esteem and belongingness. R/S has been found to be inversely associated with mental disorders, such as depression, substance use, suicide and overall mortality.

Incorporating R/S into the treatment modality has been systematically found to be beneficial. Research on twelve-step therapy has also revealed its effectiveness in treating alcohol dependence. Although the number of studies is limited, some of them have shown higher patient satisfaction with spiritual or religious interventions.

Meditation and Mental Health

Mediation has recently gained a lot of attention owing to its effect on handling stress and negative emotions, facilitating the pursuit of happiness and well-being, and more recently, its integration into the management of psychiatric disorders.

There have been hundreds of scientific studies on the effects of meditation on healthy people which have found that meditation-based therapy is especially effective in reducing stress.

Research on changes in physiological parameters, both as state markers and as trait markers, has revealed activation of the parasympathetic system during and with continued practice of meditation. Meditation triggers the relaxation response with a reduction in heart rate, respiratory rate, systolic blood pressure, oxygen metabolism and skin resistance. A review of several studies shows that meditation is associated with increased heart rate variability and vagal activity. Heart rate variability (HRV) is associated with reduction in stress and negative mood states and improved resilience to stress and psychological flexibility. Regular practitioners of meditation are found to have increased vagal tone during practice as well as while at rest compared to non-practitioners. Studies that have compared brain structure or function in meditation as compared to controls have found differences in diverse and multiple regions of the brain between meditating and non-meditating groups.

Besides promoting mental health, the effect of meditation has also been studied in the treatment of anxiety and depression. Some studies, for example, have discovered that Meditation-Based Cognitive Therapy (MBCT) can aid in the reduction of depressive symptoms and the prevention of relapse in patients with depression. Some studies have also shown a reduction in anxiety of people with anxiety disorders. Studies on *Sudarshan kriya* have also found it to be effective for depression and post-traumatic stress disorder (PTSD).

Some real-life examples of the beneficial effects of meditation are given below:

Case Vignette 1

I am a 25-year-old college student doing my post-graduation in Delhi. Three years ago, I was facing an adjustment disorder due to an erratic ongoing relationship, which had affected my sleep quality, concentration and efficiency. I was introduced to spirituality by my friend. The continuous practice of meditation and breathing techniques helped me calm my mind immensely and has helped me regain the quality of sleep and concentration. It has made me more resilient in handling any ongoing stress by boosting my confidence levels and alleviating my fears.

Case Vignette 2

Initially, I used to think spirituality was just for Yogis clad in saffron clothes. However, after regular practice of meditation, I realized it has nothing to do with what you wear, where you live, which god you worship and which language you speak, but rather it is an experience that takes you within yourself where you feel how each and every creature in this universe is connected and is made of the same thing.

All boundaries get loosened up, and you feel immense love, peace, compassion, freedom and a sense of expansion inside you. In a sense, spirituality is a journey from the outside world to the beautiful world inside you.

Case Vignette 3

After many failed attempts to handle my emotions, when I discovered meditation and breathing techniques, I thought how can these simple techniques help me handle my emotions and improve my relationship? But after a few years of doing regular breathing and meditation, I know it helps me to be in the present moment, away from the guilt and regrets of the past and fear and anxiety of the future, thus keeping me fully aware, calm and content in the present moment.

Conclusion

The concepts of religion and spirituality are intertwined but distinct from each other. Spirituality has been seen to play a key role in the promotion of positive mental health and well-being, the reduction of stress and the improvement of coping abilities. Spiritual beliefs and non-beliefs can be integrated into clinical management, as has also been increasingly recognized by many psychiatric organizations.

KEY POINTS

➢ Spirituality promotes positive mental health, reduces stress and acts as a barrier to the development of certain mental disorders.

➢ Spiritual practices, such as meditation, can work as positive, preventive and intervention strategies for common mental disorders.

➢ Research has documented physiological, structural and functional changes in the brain with regular practice of meditation.

REFERENCES

1. Goyal M, Singh S, Sibinga EM, et al Meditation programs for psychological stress and well-being: a systematic review and meta-analysis. JAMA Intern Med. 2014 Mar;174(3):357-68.

2. Tang YY, Hölzel BK, Posner MI. The neuroscience of mindfulness meditation. Nat Rev Neurosci. 2015 Apr;16(4):213-25.

3. Koenig HG. Religion, spirituality, and health: the research and clinical implications. ISRN Psychiatry. 2012 Dec 16;2012:278730.

4. Moreira-Almeida A, Mosqueiro BP, Bhugra D, eds. Spirituality and Mental Health Across Cultures. Oxford, UK: Oxford University Press; 2021.

CHAPTER 30

Resilience and Mental Health

Priyanka Saha and Siddharth Sarkar

Introduction

Resilience refers to an individual's positive adaptation to the experience of adversity. The process of adapting would include facing events like trauma, tragedy, threats or stress. These adversities or difficult life circumstances can be of various types, including health issues, relationship problems, workplace difficulties and financial stressors. To simplify, we can say that resilience is the capacity of an individual to adapt to challenging situations while maintaining stable mental health.

Is resilience a personality trait? The answer is no. Resilience is something that anyone can take measures to develop or strengthen. When it comes to resilience in mental health, it is commonly considered as capacity for handling an adverse situation with good coping. Resilience usually pertains to 'bouncing back' from difficult circumstances, which can further help in personal growth, sometimes in a significant manner.

What is not resilience? Being resilient does not mean that a person is immune to distress or difficulties of life. Resilience involves thoughts, behaviors and actions, which anyone can learn and develop with time to deal effectively with situations and circumstances.

Many people experience similar setbacks in their life; however, their responses to such setbacks are different. Individuals who take such setbacks as a learning experience are more optimistic. Such individuals are less likely to become upset and depressed.

A few examples of resilience are described below:

- Response to the terrorist attack in America on September 11, 2001, where individuals took adequate efforts to rebuild their lives after the tragedy.
- Response of the world following an ongoing COVID pandemic and taking efforts to rebuild their families after profound grief.
- Someone loses a job, learns how to outweigh the negatives, learns from his/her mistakes and attempts to find another job.

The road to resilience is not easy and differs amongst different individuals and is likely to involve considerable explicit or implicit efforts to ward off emotional distress.

Models of Resilience

It has been suggested that, broadly, there are three classes of resilience models to explain how resilience influences and alters the path from risk factors to negative outcomes. These are the compensatory model, the protective model and the challenge model (Figure 1).

1. **Compensatory model**: This model refers to a situation when a resilience factor opposes a risk factor. It does not interact with the risk factor and has an independent and direct influence on the outcome. One example could be a resilience factor, like self-esteem, counteracting the risk factor of stress in

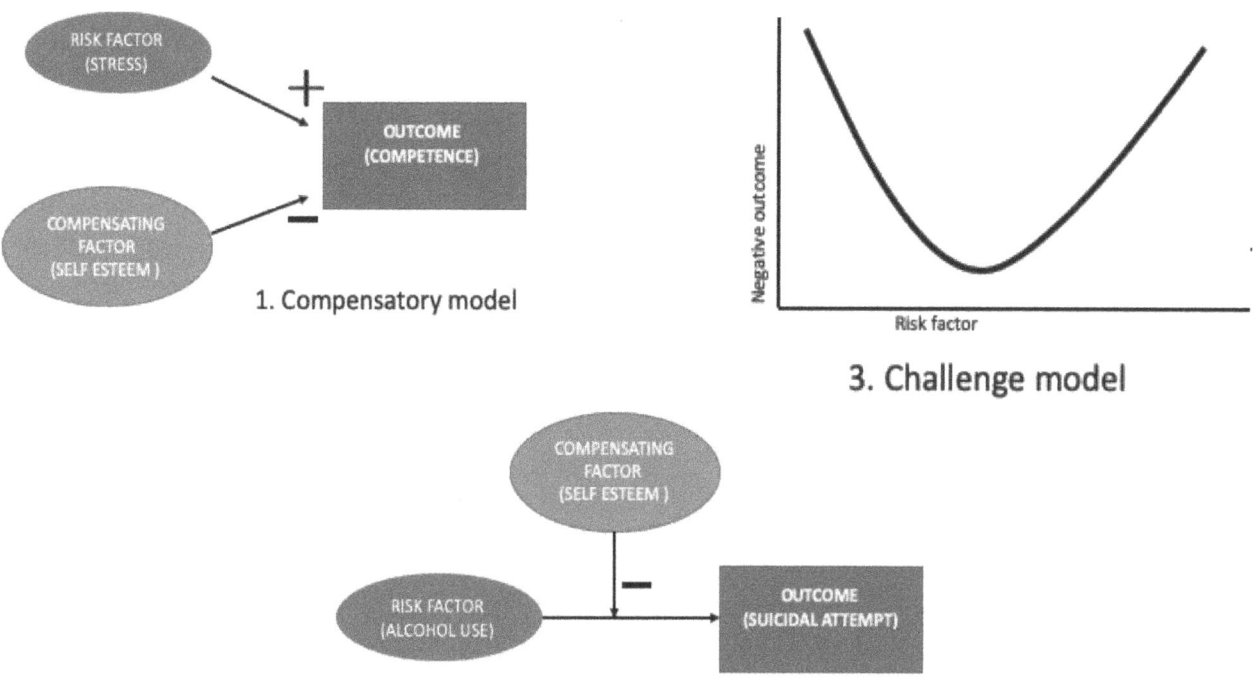

Figure 1. *Models of Resilience*

predicting the competence of a person. Resilience works in the opposite direction of the risk factor. Another example is daily heavy alcohol use that can worsen the outcome (hypertension, stroke, hepatitis, cirrhosis), but a compensatory factor of resilience would be moderating the alcohol use or stopping it, which will reduce the complications of alcohol use and increase self-worth and confidence.

2. **Protective model**: This model focuses on the moderating effects of resilience on negative outcome. Protective factors may enhance a promotive factor or neutralize a risk factor, and thus, lessen the negative outcomes. For example, parental separation may lead to depression in adulthood. However, the intelligence level of the child may moderate this relationship with a higher intelligence quotient being a protective factor. Some of the protective factors include problem-solving skills, caring and supporting relationships, sense of competency and meaningful life.

3. **Challenge model**: In this model, exposures to risk factors at both high and low levels lead to negative outcomes. However, moderate risk levels are not related to negative outcomes. Moderate levels of stress challenge an individual and enhance competence. Now if the person overcomes the challenge, it will prepare him/her for the next level of a difficult or challenging situation. For example, too much conflict in the home environment may have a deleterious effect on the well-being of an adolescent. Too little conflict in the family is likely to make him/her unable to resolve interpersonal conflicts as he/she enters into relationships and social discourse outside the family.

The models described above are one of the ways of understanding how resilience can be described. There may be many other ways of theoretically conceptualizing resilience, like the thriving model or the multi-system model of resilience. Each model has its own merits and characteristics.

Trajectories of Resilience

Resilience is often tested in times of traumatic events. Based upon the effect of resilience, the impact of severe traumatic events on mental health has been described in the form of four different trajectories. These are schematically depicted in Figure 2. Line A depicts an individual with good mental health prior to exposure to a traumatic event. The individual shows a temporary decline in mental health after the event without any recovery. Line B shows an individual with good mental health prior to the exposure. Following the exposure, there is a temporary decline in mental health but the individual further recovers quickly to the pre-exposure levels of mental health after a gap in which the individual has features consistent with mental illness. Line C depicts an individual with good mental health prior to exposure. Following the exposure, there is a relatively brief and temporary decline in mental health. This is followed by recovery and the mental health is found to be similar or somewhat better than before the exposure to a traumatic event. Line D depicts an individual with good mental health prior to the exposure. Following the traumatic exposure, the mental health is impaired but it recovers quickly to pre-exposure levels and mental health continues to increase, surpassing pre-exposure levels of mental health (this can be seen as post-traumatic growth). Thus, resilience factors may determine the development of mental disorders in some individuals, while at the same time, may be a facilitator for personal growth after experiencing a traumatic event. Therefore, it is very important to understand the factors that may help an individual successfully cope with adverse situations. In view of the diverse nature of adversities, resilience can further be considered as a protective factor.

Resilience and Mental Health

There are myriad factors that promote resilience. Characteristics of resilient people are mentioned in Box 1. Greater global improvement corresponds to greater improvement of resilience. Also, higher resilience has been found to be correlated with better quality of life.

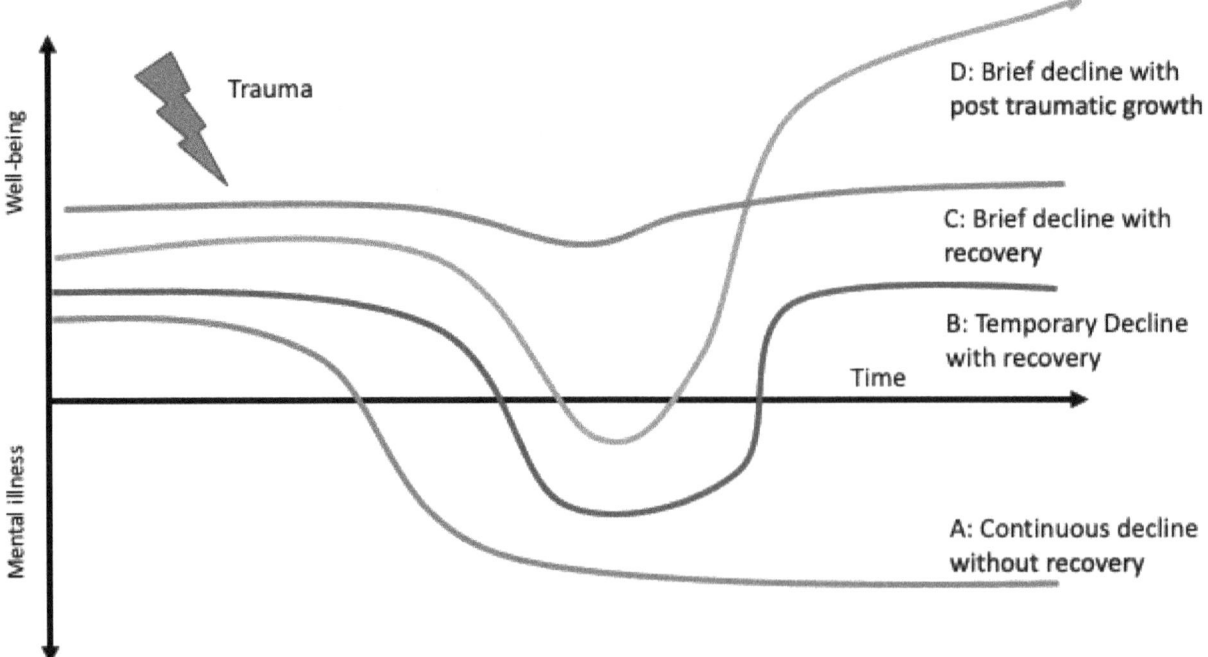

Figure 2. *Trajectories of Resilience After Severe Traumatic Event*

Box 1. Characteristics of Resilient Individuals *

- Viewing change as a challenge or an opportunity
- Having a close and secure attachment
- Recognition of one's limit to control
- Self-efficacy
- Taking support of others
- Commitment
- Having trust in others
- Having a goal-oriented vision
- Strengthening oneself during stress
- Having a realistic sense of control/having choices
- Having a good sense of humor
- Tolerance of negative affect
- Action-oriented approach
- Adaptability to change
- Patience
- Having optimistic approach

* Connor KM, Davidson JR. Development of a new resilience scale: The Connor-Davidson Resilience Scale (CD-RISC). Depression and Anxiety. 2003;18(2):76-82.

How to Build Resilience?

Resilience can be increased in many ways. Some of these include maintaining positive relationships, having a good support system, having a positive attitude towards life and having a good self-image. Resilience is a skill that can be enhanced with efforts.

Following are the means by which one can build resilience:

1. Identify the stressful situation.
2. Identify one's strength.
3. Build a positive view of oneself.
4. Avoid seeing crisis as an unbeatable problem.
5. Make meaningful connections with people.
6. Accept that change is a part of living.
7. Move towards the goals.
8. Look for opportunities for self-discovery.
9. Maintain hope.
10. Take care of self.

Another way to build resilience is the 4-factor approach. The elements of the 4-factor approach are shown in Figure 3. Following this 4-step process, one can train oneself to think differently. The more one engages in this process, the more resilient one can become and have mastery over self. Let's consider the following example to understand this approach. Suppose one had a breakup and feels dejected. The first step is simply talking about the event or listing it without magnifying it. For example, 'I got dumped, the relationship did not work out.' The second step is about taking ownership. Rather than blaming the other, one could acknowledge: 'All right, sometimes, relationships do not work out.' The third step dwells on re-evaluating and reframing the event in one's mind. 'Things could have been worse. We might have ended up hurting each other physically.' Reframing involves taking another perspective of the situation and trying to find something to be thankful for. Finally, the fourth step is about giving oneself some time to heal and adjust after the trauma. Engaging in this simple process can help one to become more resilient.

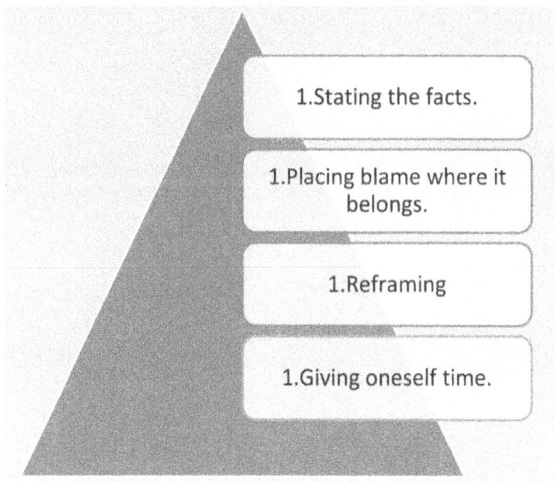

Figure 3. *The 4-Factor Approach*

Though genetic, personal or environmental factors have an effect on resilience, training can also help improve resilience. Training to improve resilience can be helpful in the following manner.

- It helps identify the stressful situation and embrace the problem.
- While communicating, it reduces the stress and brings up ideas to come forward with.
- It also helps in the refinement of executive skills, like planning, decision making, strategic thinking, self-reflection and information processing.
- Finally, it helps in taking responsibility, balance and acceptance.

Interface of Resilience and Mental Health

It has been seen that stress, trauma and early childhood adversity result in changes in the brain, which leads to vulnerability to the development of depression and other psychiatric disorders like post-traumatic stress disorder. Resilience can act as a protective factor against the development of these psychiatric disorders by modulating the impact of these adverse events on the individual and lessening the risk of development of a psychiatric disorder (as depicted in Figure 4).

Many individuals do not develop psychiatric illness despite facing stress or trauma or any adverse life situation, and they are considered resilient. Being resilient is being able to successfully adapt or cope with the challenges, which furthers the immunity to the effects of stress. Hence, understanding the factors that promote resilience is important.

Mental health professionals like psychiatrists, psychologists or psychiatric social workers play a special role in promoting and enhancing resilience when an individual is suffering from psychological pain. It may be better to communicate and express the distress or the pain that one is going through. Since resilience is an interactive concept, it can only be identified in terms of the response to some adversity. Resilience-oriented treatment should be provided in a manner that encourages patients to consider that they can 'act' to improve their situation, rather than feel that all benefits derive from what the clinician does. One needs to pay more attention to one's ongoing relationships and successful coping, which encompasses the social as well as the psychological dimension.

The following vignette provides an example of how resilience affects mental health.

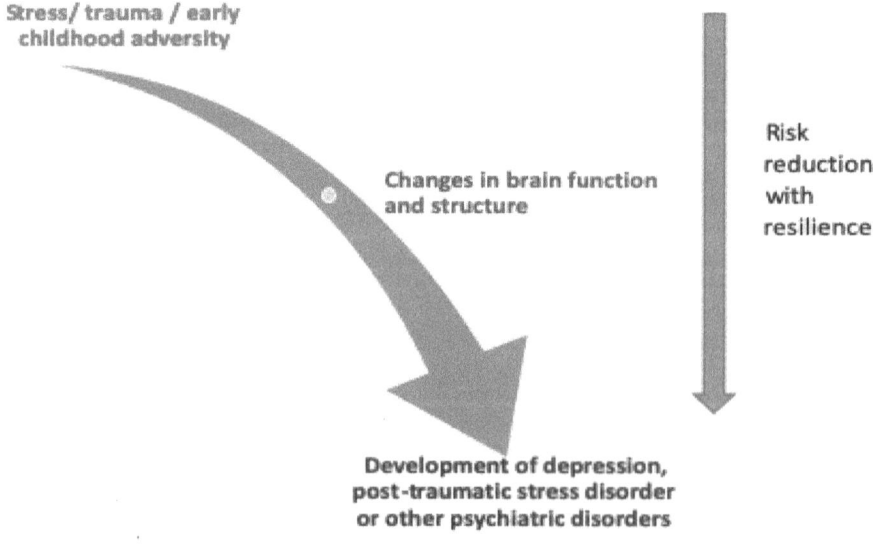

Figure 4. *Resilience Modulating the Vulnerability to Mental Illnesses*

Vignette: Two students A and B in class 10 have failed in physics exam. Student A and student B had the same exposure to stress (failure in the exam). Student A takes it in stride and keeps working hard and starts preparing himself to pass the next exam. He engages with others as well and seeks help from seniors to do better in the examinations. Student B keeps on cursing himself and starts crying and is unable to read further and his performance keeps on declining. A month later, student B is brought to the hospital by his family members in view of keeping himself aloof from everyone, not showing interest in any activities, decreased sleep and appetite and is further diagnosed to have mild depression. In this case scenario, we can assume student A has a higher resilience.

Resilience for Health Promotion

Resilience can be considered as a process or an end result. Development of resilience can start as early as childhood or during the transition or in adulthood. It is a skill that one learns during any kind of adverse situation and the learning usually can happen anywhere – home, school, peers or community. The response can be healthy or unhealthy. There lies the role of a mental health professional to identify and engage in the process and help the individual in having a positive view,

maintain hope and, at the same time, take adequate care of self.

Resilience has been often considered an important component of health promotion efforts. Resilience enhancing interventions can be part of a package of interventions to promote psychological health or can be a focus in itself. Training for improving resilience can be provided by a range of individuals, including parents, teachers, human resource managers and mental health professionals. Such interventions can be directed at communities, risk groups (like academically poorly performing adolescents) or those with behavioral or emotional problems.

Conclusion

Resilience is an important factor that determines the vulnerability to mental illnesses in the face of stress as well as the manner and promptness with which individuals deal with adversities. Resilience, as a concept, has many facets. Resilient individuals have been suggested to have certain characteristics. The resilience of individuals can be enhanced. In the mental health care setting, resilience needs to be worked upon, so that the mental health outcomes can improve and the individuals can experience a higher level of psychological well-being.

KEY POINTS

➢ Resilience refers to overall physical and psychological health, and has been defined as the ability to 'bounce back from adversity'.

➢ Resilient people look into their strengths and support systems to overcome challenges and work through problems.

➢ Resilience can help in protecting an individual from various mental health conditions, such as depression and anxiety.

➢ Resilience helps one not only in building balance but also in developing confidence and self-acceptance.

REFERENCES

1. 7 Steps to Manage Stress and Build Resilience. https://orwh.od.nih.gov/in-the-spotlight/all-articles/7-steps-manage-stress-and-build-resilience

2. Building your resilience. https://www.apa.org/topics/resilience

3. Vella SL, Pai NB. A theoretical review of psychological resilience: Defining resilience and resilience research over the decades. Arch Med Health Sci. 2019;7(2):233–39.

CHAPTER 31

Mental Health Promotion

Gagan Hans

Introduction

Mental health promotion is one of the core components of the larger field of health promotion and is an important strategy for both primary as well as secondary prevention in psychiatry. The World Health Organization (WHO) defines health promotion as the process of enabling people to increase control over their health and improve it. Mental health promotion refers to positive mental health, which is the desired outcome of health promotion interventions. There are a number of advantages of integrating promotion and prevention in the field of mental health.

Need for Mental Health Promotion

Mental illnesses are not uncommon and are seen across all societies and countries all over the world. According to the WHO, mental and behavioral disorders are responsible for around 12% of the global burden of disease. It has been estimated that 197.3 million people in India suffer from mental disorders, with a gross majority of this population having no or very limited access to mental health services. Mental illnesses result in significant morbidity in the affected population along with an additional economic burden to society.

Efforts made to increase awareness about the mental health conditions globally have been minimal and the people suffering from these conditions continue to face stigma due to a multitude of reasons. Various estimates over the last few decades have consistently shown that there is a wide gap between the number of people who require mental health care and the available mental health resources, particularly in less developed countries of the world. Mental illnesses result from a multitude of interdependent social, psychological and biological factors, all of which play an important role in determining the outcomes and have a significant association with factors like poverty, low income, low education, domestic violence, limited access to educational opportunities, substance abuse and human rights violations.

Scope of Mental Health Promotion

World Health Organization (WHO) defines health as '... a state of complete physical, mental and social well-being and not merely the absence of disease or infirmity.' This definition implies that physical, mental and social functioning are dependent on each other. People tend to describe health in terms of their current circumstances. For instance, some people equate it to freedom from disease, while others may define it in terms of autonomy and vitality. Elderly individuals may equate health to inner strength and the ability to cope, whereas the younger people may emphasize more on fitness, energy and strength.

There are three messages referring to the mental health in the WHO's definition of health:

• Mental health is one of the key components of health

- Mental health does not simply imply the absence of mental illness
- Mental health is intricately related to physical health and well being

Mental health has been defined by the WHO as '... a state of well-being in which the individual realizes his or her own abilities, can cope with the normal stresses of life, can work productively and fruitfully, and is able to make a contribution to his or her community.' Thus, an individual in the optimum state of mental health should not only be able to realize his/her abilities but also achieve full potential, thus contributing productively to the community. Hence, mental health is equally important for all members of society to ensure optimal productivity and well-being.

Mental health promotion is one of the core components of the larger field of 'health promotion', and is as important as developing treatment and support services for persons with mental illnesses and related disabilities. There is tremendous scope for improving the mental health of the communities, but most mental health professionals and health policymakers are often overwhelmed with the task of resolving the problems of people with illnesses. Also, rapidly changing socio-environmental conditions globally due to unprecedented events, such as the emergence of Covid-19, pose a great challenge to the mental health of the populations at a never-before-seen magnitude. Thus, until mental health promotion is given appropriate importance, the mental health crisis is only going to worsen. A major problem in this context is the reluctance of the society to talk about a mental health issue, which interferes with developing strategies for mental health promotion. Here, it is important to clarify that prevention of mental disorders and mental health promotion are two different, though overlapping concepts, and the target audience for mental health promotion is much wider.

Mental health plays a very important role in the determination of behavior in all stages of life. There is sufficient evidence supporting the association of mental illness with social factors, such as poverty, crime, substance abuse, low education and unemployment. These factors also drive other high-risk behaviors, such as road rage, unsafe sexual practices, domestic violence, civil violence and suicide, which are indicators of mental ill-health. Any strategy for mental health promotion needs to take into consideration all these facts.

Strategies for Mental Health Promotion:

Public Health Interventions: Public health interventions are the most viable intervention for improving the mental health of the population. These interventions have been shown to result in improved outcomes for several physical illnesses. For instance, some of the risk factors associated with cardiac illnesses can be managed by environmental changes, encouraging lifestyle modifications and introducing a tobacco control policy. There is evidence to support that mental health is significantly affected by policies related to housing, education and childcare, etc., thus making all these sectors a target for mental health promotion.

Shared Community Values: In various communities, throughout the world, there are well-established practices that help in promoting the mental health of the individuals, although this may not be identified as a direct outcome of these practices. Community leaders, policymakers and other significant people should play an active role in encouraging mental health promotion activities in the society and bringing relevant changes in health policy matters. It is important to emphasize here that although the basic principles of mental health promotion are universal, these need to be modified as per local requirements and resources. Understanding the local expression of the mental health issues and available resources is of utmost significance before strategies are planned for their improvement.

Upholding and Protecting Social, Economic, Political, Cultural and Human Rights: In any society in the world, protection of social, economic, political, cultural and human rights is a basic necessity without which just and fair systems of functioning cannot be established. These systems are required to support individuals and safeguard their mental health. Human rights enable people by granting them civil liberties, which are a legal binding on the government. Human rights also ensure the distribution of power uniformly in the society thus reducing social injustice. The constitutional values of equality before the law and no discrimination help ensure that the marginalized sections of the community are not exploited and their interests, including health-related needs, are adequately addressed. It is not possible for the institutions to solely ensure safeguarding the human rights of the citizens, as it encompasses social, economic, political, cultural and human rights dimensions, and thus requires participation from all community members.

Intersectoral Coordination: It has been well established that the mental health of the population can only be significantly improved by the joint efforts of various stakeholders. Any visible changes in the mental health of the society require definitive policies from the government as well as a coordinated effort from various stakeholders in the other fields as well, such as health, justice, education, housing, environment, and social welfare.

Prioritizing Mental Health: Issues related to mental health need to be prioritized particularly by the decision-makers in the government both

> ## Box 1. Strategies for Mental Health Promotion
>
> - Public health interventions
> - Shared community values
> - Upholding and protecting social, economic, political, cultural and human rights
> - Intersectoral coordination
> - Prioritizing mental health

at the national and the local levels because their actions impact mental health. International bodies also have a crucial role to play by ensuring that countries in different phases of development sensitize their population about the importance of mental health promotion.

Strategies for mental health promotion are summarized in Box 1.

Key Challenges in Mental Health Promotion:

Multiple Risk Factors for Health: There are multiple determinants of health that can either enhance or threaten the health status of a community or an individual. Some of these factors comprise an individual's choices, like smoking, daily exercise, eating preferences, etc. There are other factors that are beyond the control of the individual, such as access to education, housing quality, supportive relationships and level of social and civic participation. Both these sets of factors are not mutually exclusive from one another with one set of factors having a significant impact on the other set of factors. While it is desirable that an individual should adopt a healthy lifestyle, it is equally desirable that the set of uncontrollable factors should have no or minimal effect on an individual's capacity to live a healthy and respectable lifestyle. Thus, until concerted efforts are made to improve the socio-economic and environmental conditions to support the determinants of health in general and mental health in particular, improvement is unlikely to happen.

Mental Health of People with Mental Illnesses: The realization that mental health is greater than a mere absence of illness can be helpful for people living with mental illness and their caregivers. Persons with mental illnesses are usually struggling on multiple fronts simultaneously, such as maintenance of meaningful employment, relationships and social life. Mental health promotion in this subsection of society is particularly difficult because of the complexity of the challenge it poses. Thus, special consideration is required for people with mental illnesses so that they can build on their strengths to live well with their mental and other illnesses.

Improving Nutrition: Poor nutrition continues to be a key challenge in many underdeveloped regions of the world, especially among children. Scientific evidence suggests that improving nutrition in children from impoverished backgrounds improves development, cognition and educational outcomes among them. Food security for people from all socioeconomic backgrounds can help improve mental health and prevent many diseases. For example, the use of iodized salt globally has helped in protecting many million newborns from iodine deficiency, preventing mental and physical health problems.

Achievable Improvements in Housing Sector: Lack of access to good housing is an indicator of poverty having an impact on public health. Homelessness is a known risk factor for mental illness. Improvement in housing has been associated with an impact on mental and physical health in the long term, along with the perception of safety with a visible reduction in crime and good community participation.

Improving Access to Education: Low literacy rates continue to be one of the major challenges in many countries of the world, including India, especially among women. It directly limits an individual's ability to access economic entitlements. Improved literacy is directly linked to mental health promotion for several reasons, such as acquiring new skills, increased assertiveness in expressing one's rights, better employment and ease of availing economic opportunities.

Reducing the Use of Addictive Substances: Addictive substances, such as tobacco, alcohol and other such products, are a major contributor to mortality and morbidity among the users. Substance use is associated with several factors, such as poverty, low income, low education, domestic violence, limited access to educational opportunities and human rights violations. In addition, the use of addictive substances may worsen the outcome of mental illnesses. Thus, controlling the use of the addictive substances can help promote mental health not only of the users but also of the family members of substance users and the community in general.

Reducing Unemployment: Lack of employment can result in serious mental health problems. Recently, during the Covid-19 pandemic in India, the loss of immediate employment during lockdown for many migrants and daily wage workers in the private and unorganized sector led them to walk hundreds of kilometers to reach their native places. They experienced extreme anxiety and worry about their ability to sustain themselves during the prolonged period of lockdown, which had serious implications on their mental health. There is a significant association between high rates of unemployment and substance abuse, violence and human rights violations, which can have a considerable impact on the mental health of the population.

Empowerment of Women and Marginalized Sections of Society: Empowerment can be defined as the process by which the traditionally disadvantaged groups in a community can overcome the barriers that affect their growth and exercise all the rights due to them, with the aim to lead a perfect life in the best of health. Empowerment of the women and the marginalized sections of society continues to be a challenge in many regions of the world. Domestic violence is associated with a significant negative impact on the physical, emotional and mental well-being of the victims. The problem of domestic violence in traditional societies is associated with various evil practices, such as dowry, child marriage and normalization of violence against women. It is also associated with several other factors like low socioeconomic status, poverty, low income, low education, limited access to educational opportunities and alcohol and other substance abuse. The exposure of young children and adolescents to domestic violence is associated with a multitude of psychiatric difficulties in later life.

Effect of Covid-19 Pandemic on Mental Health: The emergence of the Covid-19 pandemic has been one of the worst humanitarian crises in decades, which is likely to have long-lasting adverse effects on mental health. The negative effects on mental health experienced by different subgroups of the population are likely to vary depending on their vulnerabilities. Poor socioeconomic status, loss of employment, limited access to essential supplies, special support needs, duration of lockdown, fear of infection, inadequate information, comorbid medical conditions and advanced age could all be possible determinants of these psychological sequels. Measures such as simple and clear information, minimum necessary period of lockdown, adequate supply of essentials, protection of employment and financial assistance to the poor can go a long way in minimizing these negative psychological effects. As waves after waves of the Covid-19 pandemic keep on resurging, it is imperative that programs

Box 2. Key Challenges to Mental Health Promotion

- Multiple risk factors for health and mental health
- High prevalence of mental ill-health
- Nutritional deficiencies
- Inadequate housing
- Lack of access to education
- Increasing use of addictive substances
- Unemployment
- Marginalized sections of the society
- Covid-19 pandemic in the current time

to strengthen mental health, especially of the vulnerable population, are implemented to reduce these negative consequences.

Key challenges to mental health promotion are summarized in Box 2.

Conclusion

An optimal state of mental health is essential for an individual to make a positive contribution to their community. Thus, mental health promotion is an essential component of overall health promotion and needs to be prioritized. Inability to recognize the importance of mental health promotion in the community can result in high social and economic costs. There is a need to develop and invest in sustainable programs for mental health promotion. Once introduced in the community, these can become self-sustainable in long run and continue to deliver positive results as well as to adapt to newer challenges with minimal intervention. Promoting mental health must take into consideration issues like poverty, substance abuse, violence, unemployment, gender discrimination and unhealthy lifestyle. Safe and secure housing, access to education and protection from human rights violations are also essential for mental health promotion.

KEY POINTS

➢ Mental health promotion needs to be a public health priority.

➢ Strategies of mental health promotion need to include various stakeholders from sectors like health, education, social welfare, labor agencies and community leaders.

➢ Targeting risk factors for mental ill-health, such as illiteracy, unemployment, homelessness, social insecurity, substance use, crime and violence, is crucial for mental health promotion.

REFERENCES

1. Barry MM, Clarke AM, Petersen I, Jenkins R. Implementing Mental Health Promotion. Springer Nature: Switzerland AG: 2019.

2. Kobau R, Seligman ME, Peterson C et al. Mental health promotion in public health: perspectives and strategies from positive psychology. Am J Public Health 2011; 101(8): e1 -e9.

3. WHO. Promoting Mental Health: Concepts, Emerging Evidence, Practice: a report of the World Health Organization, World Health Organization: Geneva, 2005.

CHAPTER 32

Preventing Mental Ill Health

Mamta Sood

Introduction

In the previous chapters, important facts about mental illnesses have been highlighted. Mental illnesses are common, are of many kinds, start early in life and affect all aspects of day-to-day functioning, thereby resulting in significant disability in individuals and a burden to the families and the society. Although evidence-based effective and affordable treatments are available, about 70-90% of the persons with mental illness, especially in low resource settings, do not receive any treatment. Prevention of mental illnesses has been proposed to be an important sustainable strategy to improve the treatment gap for mental health conditions.

Prevention is a public health approach that refers to intercepting the development of ill health and promotion of health. Preventive interventions help in decreasing the rates of developing an illness, preventing relapse or recurrence and limiting the associated complications and dysfunction. On the other hand, health promotion interventions directly aim at improving health.

Initially, preventive strategies were recommended for acute communicable (infectious) diseases on the premise that the causes of these diseases could be identified and by removing the cause, the occurrence of the disease could be prevented. For example, malaria is caused by malarial parasite that spreads to human beings by the bite of Anopheles mosquito – the vector for the parasite. Malaria can be prevented by taking antimalarial drugs or taking steps to prevent mosquito bites and breeding of mosquitoes. As the research advanced in this field, preventive strategies could be applied to chronic non-communicable diseases, like diabetes and hypertension. These diseases do not have a single cause but are the result of a combination of multiple complex genetic and lifestyle factors. Similar to these diseases, mental illnesses are caused by interactions of multiple factors. Therefore, in the last few decades, the concept of prevention has been applied to mental health.

In this chapter, we will discuss the concept of prevention in mental health, preventive efforts for mental illness and preventive strategies that can be adopted by persons with mental illnesses and their caregivers and persons without mental illness. The promotion of mental health has been discussed in a separate chapter.

Prevention in Mental Health

Preventive efforts in health have been divided into primary, secondary or tertiary prevention based on the population targeted and the expected outcome. Primary prevention targets the population with no current illness to prevent the onset of illness. Secondary prevention interventions target persons with a known illness to decrease its duration and prevent relapse. Tertiary prevention targets the consequences of illness to improve the functional outcome of the persons having the illness.

Prevention in mental health has been discussed in detail in the World Health Organization (2004) summary report titled "Prevention of Mental Disorders – Effective Interventions and

Policy Options" and aims at "*reducing incidence, prevalence and recurrence of mental disorders, the time spent with symptoms, or the risk condition for a mental illness, preventing or delaying recurrences, and also decreasing the impact of illness in the affected person, their families and the society*".

Primary prevention targets the healthy population to prevent the onset of mental illnesses. Mental health promotion, risk factor reduction and education are some of the areas that are the focus of intervention with an overall aim of alteration in the risk profile of the entire targeted population. The measurable outcome of primary prevention is a reduction in the onset of a new case (incidence) of a specific mental illness. Primary prevention interventions have been further divided as universal, selective and indicated. Universal interventions target the general population, selective interventions target the at-risk groups and the indicated interventions target the high-risk persons with minimal but detectable signs or symptoms of mental illnesses.

Secondary intervention targets the symptomatic population, particularly in the early stages of illness so that time spent in illness and chances of its recurrence are reduced. Improving access to treatment and early institution of effective treatment, both pharmacological and psychosocial, is the focus of secondary interventions. The measurable outcome of secondary prevention is reducing the number of existing cases (prevalence) of a specific mental illness. Reducing the duration of illness is also an important outcome.

Tertiary prevention targets persons with established mental illness to reduce functional deficits. Rehabilitation, reintegration into the community and enhancing social support are some of the interventions for tertiary prevention. Improving functionality and reducing disability in

affected persons and the cost of mental illness are important outcomes of tertiary prevention. Both secondary and tertiary preventions aim at reducing the overall burden of mental disorders.

Reduction of risk factors and enhancing protective factors related to individuals, families and social and environmental determinants of mental health are the targets of primary intervention. Risk factors increase the probability of onset, duration and severity of a mental illness, whereas protective factors improve an individual's resistance to developing these illnesses.

Risk and protective factors exist at macro and micro levels. At the macro-level, social, environmental and economic risk and protective factors play an important role in ensuring mental health. The risk factors are poverty, unsafe housing, war, limited education facilities or employment opportunities, poor job conditions, etc., while the protective factors include social support, social services, empowerment, etc. At the micro-level, risk and protective factors work on individuals, small groups like families, or social networks. Protective factors at the individual level include self-esteem, emotional resilience, positive thinking, problem-solving and stress management skills.

There is a need for international, national and local level policies for effective implementation of interventions to reduce risk factors and enhance protective factors for reducing the incidence of mental disorders. The macro-level risk factors can be improved by macro-policies that improve nutrition, housing and education, and decrease economic insecurity. Parenting and early interventions enhance protective factors, like resilience in children and adolescents. Taxation of alcohol products to target harmful use of alcohol and implementation of various measures in the workplace are some of the macro-level strategies intended for the adult population. Exercise, social support and community participation are helpful in improving the mental health of elderly people.

Table 1. *Prevention in Mental Health (Based on WHO, 2004)*

Type of Prevention	Population	Intervention	Outcome
Primary	Healthy population	Mental health promotion Risk factor reduction Education	Reduction in the number of new cases (incidence) of a specific mental illness
Secondary	Symptomatic population	Improving access to treatment Early treatment	Reduction in the number of existing cases (prevalence) of a specific mental illness Reduction in duration of illness
Tertiary	Persons with established mental illness	Rehabilitation Reintegration Social support	Improvement in functionality Reduction in disability

Prevention of Mental Illnesses

Preventive strategies have been used and researched in many mental illnesses based on the risk and protective factors involved in these conditions.

Common mental disorders: Depressive and anxiety disorders are among the most common mental illnesses.

Risk factors for onset and recurrence of depressive illness are parental depression, depressive thinking, inadequate parenting, child abuse and neglect, stressful life events and bullying. Protective factors include a sense of self-mastery, self-esteem, self-efficacy, stress resistance and social support. There is strong research evidence that effective preventive strategies for depression can be implemented for children and adolescents. Some of these strategies include strengthening cognitive, problem-solving and social skills of children and adolescents in schools, interventions for parents of aggressive children, strategies for decreasing child abuse and bullying, support for children of depressed parents or those who have experienced the death of a parent. Provision of social and economic support for persons exposed to wars, conflicts or natural disasters helps in preventing depression. It is important for elderly persons to remain physically healthy; regular physical exercise is one of the recommended strategies to prevent depression in them.

Similarly, for the development of anxiety disorders, common risk factors are traumatic events, anxious parents and perceiving oneself as having poor self-efficacy, self-control and social support. Preventive strategies that focus on decreasing traumatic events and improving resilience are important.

Severe mental disorders: Preventive strategies also exist for severe mental disorders like psychotic disorders. Risk factors for psychotic disorders include obstetric complications, childhood trauma, migration, socioeconomic disadvantage, urban birth and use of cannabis. Improving mental health literacy, early recognition, help-seeking and treatment are important preventive strategies for psychotic disorders.

Substance use disorders: These are also associated with a substantial burden. Taxation, restrictions on the availability and a total ban on direct and indirect advertising are effective regulatory interventions. School-based prevention programs are helpful in improving knowledge and attitudes toward addictive substances. A brief intervention in the form of advice from a general practitioner routinely given to all patients who smoke and drink is an effective intervention.

Suicide: It is one of the important causes of mortality due to mental disorders. Risk factors for suicide include mental illnesses like schizophrenia, depression and bipolar disorder, past or recent stressors, family history of suicide, poor availability of psychological help and easy access to means for committing suicide. Some of the most effective strategies to prevent suicide are the treatment of depression, reduction of access to means for committing suicide and a multicomponent school-based approach for young persons.

Preventive Strategies for Improving Mental Health of Persons with Mental Illness

Evidence-based and disorder-specific preventive strategies have been developed for mental disorders. It is possible to apply principles of primary, secondary and tertiary prevention for the management of mental illness both before and after it has occurred. The strategies are aimed at early identification and treatment, reducing time spent being ill, preventing relapse and complications and optimizing functioning.

In India, most patients with mental illness stay at home with their families. The family caregivers of patients with mental illness play an important role in the identification, treatment and management of the illness. Therefore, preventive efforts have to be directed at both the patients and their family caregivers. Sometimes, these can be directed at other significant persons, like teachers or employers.

Early identification and initiation of treatment of a mental illness are the two important steps in implementing secondary and tertiary preventive strategies. Early signs of mental illness and from whom and where to seek help have been discussed in the chapter on 'Recognizing Mental Illness'.

For implementing preventive strategies for patients with mental illness and their caregivers, it is important to gather important information about the mental illness, a person has. This information empowers both patients and their families to deal with their illness.

It is important to know how common the illness is. For example, if the prevalence of depression is about 5%, it implies that out of 100 persons, five will have depression. This means that one individual is not alone in having this illness and many others have also gone through similar experiences.

Knowing the symptoms of one's mental illness is important as symptoms may vary from individual to individual. Having a mental illness is a bewildering experience and may be very confusing at the beginning for both patients and their caregivers. When the illness recurs, the symptoms will usually be those seen at the time of initial or first presentation. So, knowledge of symptoms during the initial phase of illness helps in identifying the relapse.

There are multiple treatment options available. Usually, people are aware of medications as treatment options but are not aware of psychological treatments. Specific medications and psychological treatments exist for most mental illnesses. It is important to know the correct dose, timing of medication/s intake and their side effects.

The patient and the family members also need to be aware whether the illness is of episodic or continuous nature, how long it will last and what are the chances of its recurrence. It is important to identify difficult situations and likely solutions for those.

One of the important criteria for diagnosing mental illness is impaired functioning. Persons with mental illness may neglect personal care and social relationships and may not be able to study or work as per the assigned role. Therefore, it is also important to be aware of the changes in a patient's functioning.

Another important but neglected part is the assessment of the impact of mental illness on significant others like family members. Stigma and discrimination faced by patients and their family caregivers is also an important issue that should be acknowledged, assessed and handled.

It is also important to know what kind of functioning, coping and personality a person had before experiencing the illness. So, when a person recovers from the mental illness, he/she is expected to resume his/her previous levels of functioning.

It is a common observation that while seeking and receiving treatment for mental illness, the focus of mental health professionals as well as the patients and their families is on improvement in symptoms. This emphasis on symptom improvement results in the neglect of adequate information collection by mental health professionals and information seeking by patients and their caregivers. It is important to state here that research- and evidence-based information exists for most mental illnesses on each of the questions listed above. This information can help in the future planning not only in terms of treatment but also in the course of illness and restoration of recovery.

Therefore, it is important for the patients with mental illness and their caregivers to be ready with the list of questions to be asked from the treating physicians. They should actively engage in interaction with the physician.

In absence of a clear etiology, it may not be possible to prevent new cases of mental illness. However, primary prevention can be practiced by encouraging everyone to focus on having a healthy lifestyle – adequate sleep, balanced diet, physical exercise and avoidance of addictive substances like smoking, alcohol, cannabis, etc. Therapeutic engagement not only with patients but also with their family caregivers, especially providing information about the patient's illness on the points listed above, can empower them in planning care and reducing their stress, as family members of the patients with mental illness face significant financial and emotional burden. They may have to give up on their leisure and social activities. Therefore, the family members also need to be screened for the presence of mental health issues, and if present, they should be offered treatment for the same.

Secondary prevention in persons with mental illness is ensured by early identification and treatment that results in reducing the duration of the illness. Prevention of a relapse or recurrence is also important as it has been seen that many patients experience a relapse as they discontinue their medications due to many factors, like stigma, fear of the mind being controlled by medicines or dependence on medicines, resulting in myths regarding psychiatric medications, ignorance about the need to continue medications or their non-availability. It is important to ask questions from the treating physician about the chances of relapse and how to prevent it. Also, it is important to ensure taking the adequate dosage of the medications. The concentration of some of the drugs like lithium and valproate can be monitored in the blood.

Tertiary prevention is implemented by restoration of functioning that is disrupted due to illness. The restoration of functioning is usually gradual and should be started with simple steps. It is important to consider the pre-disease level of functioning, age, sex, occupation, marital status, financial status, type of family and residence while setting the expected goals of restoration of functioning. Patients may develop other mental and physical illnesses for which routine screening should be done. Also, it is important for patients and their families to continue normal social and pleasurable activities, as this helps reduce stress as well as stigma.

Simple Preventive Strategies for Improving Mental Health in Persons with No Mental Disorder

As we had discussed in earlier chapters, a person's activities in a day are broadly carried out in five domains: personal care, social relationships, occupation or work, pleasurable activities and biological activities, like sleep and appetite. Spiritual/religious activities belong to the sixth domain that many people carry out. All these activities play an important part in maintaining mental health and no activity is less important than the other. Neglecting or over-performing one activity at the cost of another may lead to mental distress. Therefore, it is important to balance time for all the activities.

Remaining physically and mentally active helps maintain good mental health. One can do brisk walking or mild exercise or yoga. Sometimes, it is not possible to find time for even a simple physical activity like walking. In that case, brisk walking multiple times for periods as short as ten minutes can also help

One should eat a healthy, balanced and nutritious diet. One does not need to eat fancy or costly food. A balanced diet should contain whole grain cereals, pulses, fats and oils from vegetable sources, seasonal and locally sourced fruits and vegetables, nuts, low sugar and salt – preferably iodized and dairy products. One may take an egg or other meats in moderation as per one's cultural practices.

Sleeping adequately for 8 hours is important. Sleep hygiene is a non-pharmacological strategy to improve sleep. It includes not sleeping during the daytime, avoiding caffeinated drinks or heavy exercise in the evening, keeping digital devices away at least 2 hours before sleeping, not engaging in entertaining activities at least 2 hours before sleeping and getting up at a pre-decided time.

Remaining away from addictive substances, like cannabis, alcohol and tobacco, is important. Among the youth, there is increasing acceptance of cannabis intake. Long-term use of cannabis can lead to severe mental illnesses, like psychosis, and also results in amotivation.

It is normal to feel anxious, depressed or fearful in stressful situations. It is important to acknowledge these feelings. Talking about these feelings can help reduce distress.

It is important to remain connected with family, friends and colleagues.

Conclusion

Prevention in mental health is an important sustainable strategy to improve the treatment gap for mental ill-health conditions. Reduction of risk factors and enhancing protective factors related to individuals, families and social and environmental determinants of mental health are the targets of primary intervention.

Secondary prevention targets the symptomatic population, particularly in the early stages of illness, so that time spent in illness and chances of its recurrence are reduced.

Tertiary prevention targets persons with established mental illness to reduce functional deficits.

Evidence-based preventive strategies exist for various mental disorders. It is possible to apply principles of primary, secondary and tertiary prevention in the management of mental illnesses. After an illness has occurred, the preventive efforts are aimed at early identification and treatment, reducing time spent being ill, preventing relapse and complications and optimizing functioning. Remaining physically and mentally active, regular exercise, adequate sleep, limiting time on digital devices and connecting with significant others are important for improving mental health.

KEY POINTS

➢ Prevention in health is a public health approach to any disease, which comprises the prevention of ill health and promotion of health.

➢ In the last several decades, the concept of prevention has been applied to mental health. It has been proposed to be an important sustainable strategy to improve the treatment gap for mental ill-health conditions.

➢ Preventive efforts in mental health have been divided into primary, secondary or tertiary prevention based on the targeted population and the expected outcome.

➢ Reduction of risk and enhancing protective factors related to individuals, families and social and environmental determinants of mental health are the targets of primary intervention.

➢ Secondary prevention interventions target persons with a known mental illness to decrease its duration and prevent relapse.

➢ Tertiary prevention targets the consequences of mental illness to improve functional outcomes in persons with the illness.

➢ Remaining physically and mentally active, regular exercise, adequate sleep, limiting time on digital devices and connecting with significant others is important to improve mental health.

REFERENCES

1. World Health Organization. Prevention of Mental Disorders: Effective Interventions and Policy Options – Summary Report. Geneva: World Health Organization; 2004.

CHAPTER 33

Mental Health Issues in Workplace

Rakesh K. Chadda

Introduction

Workplace is one of the most important parts of life that can influence a person's health, especially mental health since it constitutes a key component of one's psychosocial environment. We all spend a lot of our time at our workplace or place of employment. Work and employment are also important from the health promotion aspects, since these give an individual a sense of belonging to the society, and are important for self-esteem and bring satisfaction with life. However, every job is associated with some work demands along with targets of achievement. Hence, psychosocial stress in a job situation, and related health issues, including mental health problems, are not uncommon.

An individual is rarely exposed to psychosocial influences from the working environment in isolation. The influences are often a combination of multiple factors, including home situation (marital or family related issues, financial concerns, etc.), social environment (social relationship, neigbourhood, etc.) and individual characteristics (personality, coping strengths, etc.). Stress or support from any of these domains impacts the functioning at workplace. Since a rise in job ladder at a workplace would be determined by individual achievements, it brings competitiveness amongst the employees, and hence, increases work pressure and stress. In many countries like India, a large section of the workforce functions in unorganized or informal sector and is devoid of many work-related benefits available in the Western countries,

giving rise to higher risk of workplace pressure and stress, and related mental health issues. It is important to manage work-related stress and mental ill health since it can affect the workers' motivation and productivity. This chapter discusses mental health and stress related issues occurring in workplace settings, and how to identify such problems and manage them.

Mental Health Issues at Workplace

There can be a range of mental health problems that can occur in the background of workplace settings. Stress related to work or job can be considered the commonest mental health issue often called work or job stress. Work stress is a result of interactions between demands and opportunities at the work, and the individual's needs, aspirations and abilities. When one's expectations from the job are not realized, or one feels under or overtaxed at job for various reasons, it may lead to work stress, which may get expressed in different forms in cognitive, behavioral, emotional or physiological spheres. One may lose concentration at work, get irritated and lose temper, feel sad or start getting nervous. Such a problem, if not remedied, can result in mental illnesses, such as, anxiety disorder, depression, adjustment disorder, or psychosomatic illnesses, like hypertension, peptic ulcer, indigestion, etc.

Work stress has now been recognized as a major challenge to workers' health all over the world. A continued stress can also lead to burnout, which can affect the employee's productivity to a great extent. It is difficult to say what percentage of the workforce would feel stressed and develop mental health problems, since this would vary depending on the work environment, including working hours; wages; kind of work support from colleagues, seniors and the management; and an individual employee's personality, family support and personal life.

Causes of Work Stress

Work-related stress and mental health problems can result from several factors, such as factors intrinsic to job, one's role in organization, opportunities for career development, relationships at work, changes at the work environment with scientific and technological advances, organizational structure and atmosphere, work-home interface and person-specific issues. A simple example is computerization and digitalization of workplaces in the last 2 decades, which many senior employees find difficult to adjust to. In Box 1, causes of job stress are listed.

Certain jobs have an inherent stress, for example the job of a firefighter, police officer, bus driver, airplane pilot, a surgeon, etc. There may be jobs with too much work or work that may be considered as difficult. Fast work pace and time pressures add to the work-related stress. Limited opportunities for growth, job insecurity, long working hours and remuneration not being

---

Box 1. Causes of Job Stress

- Factors intrinsic to job
- Role in organization
- Career development
- Relationships at work
- Changes in scientific and technological advances
- Organizational structure and atmosphere

---

considered adequate for workload are associated with higher work stress and mental health issues. If there is sexual or psychological harassment, it further adds to the work stress.

Here, it is important to mention that an individual's vulnerability and ability also matter a lot in such situations. For example, a feeling of workload refers to an individual's capacity to manage it and the degree of difficulty of a work might relate to one's ability to do it. A feeling of overload and work being considered difficult are likely to affect job satisfaction and can lead to continuing stress and mental health issues.

A person's role in an organization also determines work-related stress. Ambiguity about one's role or unrealistic expectations from the job add to low job satisfaction and job-related tension, and one may start losing self-confidence. Sometimes, there are conflicting job demands and an employee may get unclear instructions from the authorities or may be asked to do things that one does not want to do or does not think is a part of his/her job or is not capable of doing. Degree of responsibility in job situation is also important since it helps in nurturing self-esteem. On the other hand, too much responsibility, beyond one's capability, adds to the stress. It is important to mention here that an upward growth in the job ladder is also not without stress since this will come with added responsibility and could be more stressful if one's abilities don't match with the responsibilities associated with the career rise.

Relationships at workplace are also a key factor affecting work-related stress. This would include quality of relationship with peers, subordinates, superiors and the management. If the relationship is not healthy, it adds to work stress. A trusting relationship at work adds to job performance and brings a sense of subjective well-being.

The rapid scientific and technological advances have brought about many changes in business and industrial sectors, which can add to work-related stress since these often require upgrading of skills and change in work set ups. Learning new skills, need to adopt to new ways of working, pressure for higher productivity, job competition and time pressures - all add to the work stress.

It is important to add here that work stress and mental health issues at workplace are also affected by home situation. This may be especially important for women when there are conflicts related to the family responsibility and role at workplace. This is likely to be more common when one is working from home, which has become much more common in the pandemic situation. Problems at family level, marital discord and domestic violence can further add to the work stress.

There are also person-specific issues, such as an individual's own capabilities and qualifications, personality, self-confidence, and commitment for the job. Lack of capability and commitment are likely to affect work performance and lead to work stress and mental health problems.

Impact of work stress: A continuing work stress affects the body as well as the mind, and thus, would affect both physical and mental health. The effects of work stress can be grouped under five categories: physiological, emotional, cognitive, behavioral and physical reactions.

Physiological reactions: Stress is associated with increased sympathetic nervous system activity, leading to increase in heart rate and blood pressure, and the person may start having palpitations. Stress also leads to increase in muscle tension, which can manifest in form of headache, pain chest, backache or pain in legs and general fatigue. Some people might develop excessive sweating because of stress and anxiety.

Emotional reactions: Work stress may lead to irritability both at work and at home. A person may feel anxious, tense or low (sad), and start losing interest in work and lose motivation in work.

Cognitive reactions: A person under work stress may have difficulty in attention and concentration and complain forgetfulness. This is likely to further affect performance at work, adding to the work stress.

Behavioral reactions: Some people, when stressed, may start smoking or drinking. Sometimes, the person starts taking unnecessary leaves or starts being absent from the job, further increasing the work-related problems. This might affect work performance and even lead to interpersonal quarrels or fights at workplace.

Effects on physical health: With continued work stress, a person is at risk of developing many physical problems, such as high blood pressure (hypertension); pain chest; musculoskeletal disorders like backache, peptic ulcer, etc.

Box 2 summarises the impact of work stress on a person's health.

Management of Work-Related Stress and Mental Health Problems

Management of work-related stress and mental health problems includes identification of the problem and then implementing suitable

---

Box 2. Impact of Job Stress

Physiological Reactions: Increase in heart rate, high blood pressure, palpitations, backache, headache

Emotional Reactions: Irritability, anxiety, low mood, losing interest in work

Cognitive Reactions: Lack of attention in work, forgetfulness

Behavioural Reactions: Resorting to smoking, drinking

Effects on Physical Health: Psychosomatic illness like peptic ulcer, high blood pressure

interventions. It is also important to identify risk factors for work-related stress and mental health issues so that early steps can be taken for their management.

Identification of work-related stress: The first step in identification of work-related stress or mental health issues is to sensitize everyone at workplace about work stress and related mental health issues. The management, administrative staff and employees need to be informed about the early identifiable signs of work-related stress and mental ill health. Since sometimes the manifestations of work-related stress may not be confined to the workplace and also occur in home atmosphere, for early detection, the family members also need to be sensitized and enquired about it.

Some pointers towards stress at a specific workplace include absenteeism, increasing staff turnover, decrease in commitment to work amongst the employees, effects on productivity of the organization, increasing accidents at workplace and a fall in applications for recruitment. These are listed in Box 3. Such signs should warn the management for taking necessary steps at correcting workplace stress.

Action plan: Employees can be directly asked certain questions, such as:

Box 3. Pointers towards Stress at Workplace

- Absenteeism
- Increasing staff turnover
- Reduced commitment by the employees
- Decrease in productivity of the organization
- Increasing accidents
- Incidents of violence
- Fall in applications for recruitment

- Are you feeling stressed?
- What do you think is leading to stress?
- How can it be resolved?
- Is your health being adversely affected by your work?
- Tell three best and three worst aspects of your job.

Management needs to monitor sick leaves, staff turnover, performance of the employees and accidents at workplace, if any.

Introduction of regular stress management programs or yoga sessions at workplace can help reduce stress at workplace and ameliorate the adverse effects of any such stress. Both these techniques are effective in reducing muscular tension and autonomic arousal and can bring about a feeling of well-being. This further helps reduce anxiety and stress and related problems. Some basic skills for mental health promotion need to be taught and inculcated amongst the employees. Such information could also be displayed at important locations at the workplace. The information may include some screening questions and useful advice.

Some basic screening questions:

- Are you feeling stressed?
- Are you eating well?
- Do you feel irritated often?
- Are you sleeping adequately?
- Are you feeling troubled at home?
- Are you losing interest in work, meeting friends or attending family functions?
- Are you having some trouble at work?

Some basic advice for lowering work stress:

- Go to bed and wake up in morning at regular hours.
- Sleep for 7-8 hours.

- Do some exercise daily for 40-45 minutes in the form of brisk walk, stretching exercises or yoga.
- Stay away from alcohol, tobacco and drugs.
- Limit your time on virtual media.
- Discuss about your problems with your family, friends and colleagues. Maintain healthy communication.

Conclusion

Stress at workplace is a common phenomenon. It is important to identify and manage it at the earliest. Otherwise, it can have adverse impact on the employees' mental health and performance. The employers, employee welfare agencies and the local government need to be aware of it and take proactive steps to manage such a problem.

KEY POINTS

➢ Mental health issues at workplace are common.

➢ It is both the factors related to the work atmosphere as well as the individual's personality, family support and personal strengths, which determine incidence of work stress.

➢ It is the responsibility of both the employees and the management to be aware of work stress and introduce steps to reduce it.

REFERENCES

1. Work Organization and Stress: Systematic Problem Approaches for Employers, Managers and Trade Union Representatives. Eds. Stavroula Leka, Pr Amanda Griffiths, Tom Cox. World Health Organization 2003.

2. Raising Awareness of Stress at Work in Developing Countries: Advice to Employers and Worker Representatives. Irene Houtman, Karin Jettinghoff and Leonar Cedillo. World Health Organization 2007.

CHAPTER 34

Role of Information Technology in Mental Health

Preethy K and Koushik Sinha Deb

Introduction

Information Technology (IT) is the science that deals with the collection, storage, processing and presentation of data. From earlier days, when IT predominantly referred to computer software and hardware, it has now moved far beyond mobile phones and even wearable devices like smartwatches, which has made the technology easily available and accessible to a greater number of people. This wide access to IT has made it a very important tool for accessing health-related information and monitoring.

Spread of IT:

As per the latest available data from Statista, the maximum number of internet users across the world in December 2019 were located in China (854 million), followed by India (560 million) and USA (313.2 million). However, according to Internet World Stats, internet penetration (proportion of the population having access to the internet) is higher in North America (93.9%) and Europe (88.4%). India is now a global hub in the field.

The spread of IT-enabled services among the common people, while initially slow, has shown rapid growth in recent years. The reports from the Telecom Regulatory Authority of India (TRAI) show that the number of broadband subscribers (both wireless and wired) in India increased from 151 million in 2016 to 802 million by January 2022. While broadband penetration in the country

is around 46%, mobile internet has seen a greater acceptance, with penetration being as high as 76% in urban as well as rural areas. According to the National Statistics Organization Survey on Digital Education Divide, only one in ten households in India have a computer (Desktop or laptop or tablet), whereas 79% of households have at least one mobile device.

Figure 1 summarizes the growth of telecommunication services in India.

The Digital India Program was launched in 2015 with the aim to increase digital literacy among the people and to improve online services for citizens. This increase in the use of the internet among the general population, along with the various other digital initiatives of the Government of India (GoI), such as the introduction of e-governance initiatives, hospital management information systems (e-hospital), various health-related apps as well as digital payment systems, have been helpful in increasing the accessibility and availability of different services for the general population. As of March 2022, the GoI has launched National Digital Health Ecosystem and the National Tele-Mental Health Programme, with the aim to use IT to expand health services across the country.

Scope of IT in Mental Health

In India, there is a huge shortage of mental health professionals, with only 0.75 psychiatrists per 100,000 population, which is far less than the minimum desired number of 3 per 100,000

Telecommunication & Internet Services - India

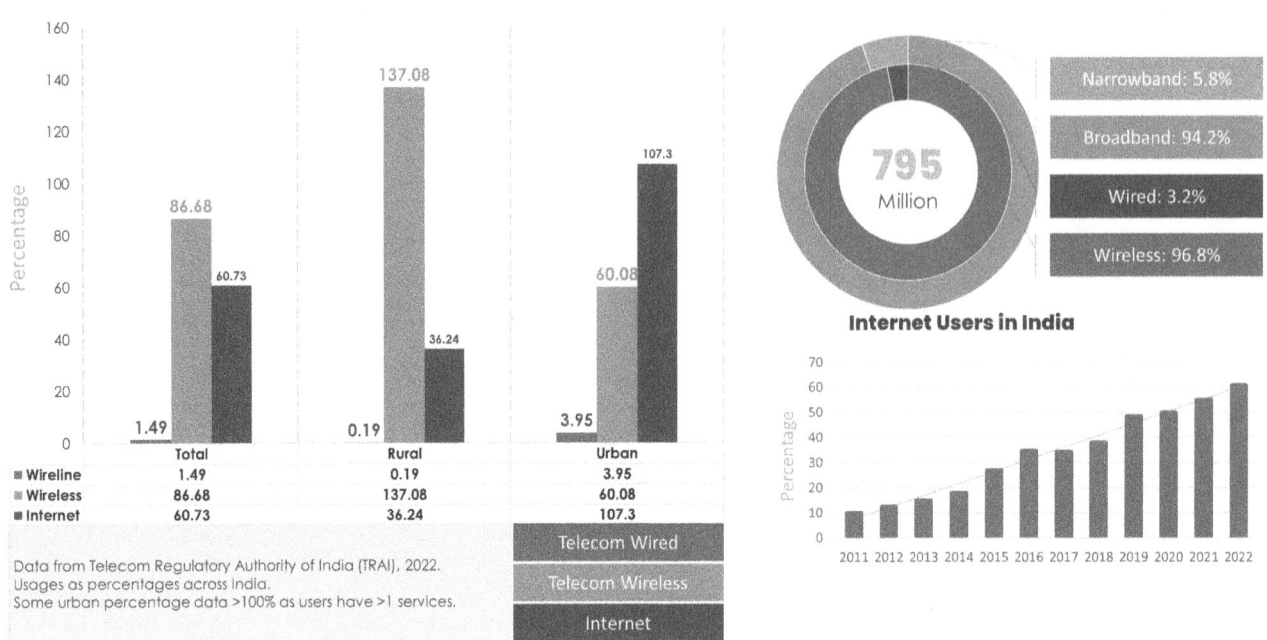

Figure 1. *Growth of Telecommunication Services in India*

population as recommended by the WHO (Interestingly, in the Western world, the number of psychiatrists is more than 1 per 10,000). This has resulted in a huge treatment gap, where 70% to 92% of patients with even common mental disorders do not receive any medical care. Adding to the difficulty is the fact that 80% of available doctors are present in urban areas only. For people living in rural areas, the time required for travel, the absenteeism from work to seek medical care and travel expenses act as significant hindrances for patients seeking medical care. Health information technologies (HITs) have enormous potential to reduce several of these barriers, with their wider geographic reach, reduced cost of implementation and efficient time management.

IT can also be used to promote positive mental health and resilience. It has the potential to disseminate universal preventive interventions to a larger population in a shorter duration of time.

IT can also identify individuals at risk of mental illness through mobile apps, mobile sensor

data and health tracking. This, in turn, can be used to alert individuals about the need to take help to prevent the development of mental illness.

Social-media groups, video call apps and mobile social games allow people to remain connected with each other, even when they are at a distance and prevent loneliness. Exchange of user-created content within a few seconds and real-time status updates have been used extensively during the COVID-19 pandemic to access medical help of various kinds. Table 1 depicts a few of the ways in which IT is changing the face of mental healthcare.

Application of Information Technology (IT) in Mental Health

Mental health is influenced by biological, social as well as environmental factors. Hence, the symptoms can vary at different times of the day or depending on the specific situation. IT offers an advantage in its ability to capture these variations objectively. For example, anxiety symptoms in

Table 1. *Role of Information Technology (IT) in Mental Health Care*

Area	Role of IT
Research	Data collection through: • Online surveys/text messages/voice call/video calls • Monitoring devices like 24-h heart rate monitor • Hospital information management system or national database
Clinical Care	• Online appointments and digital health records • Automatic or self-guided screening for illness • Aid in management – Reminders for pills, reminders for appointments, memory aid in patients with dementia • As treatment: Telemedicine, online psychotherapy • Contact with self-help groups and support for caregivers
Public Health	• Raising awareness about symptoms of mental illness and treatment by providing information through videos or text • Information about treatment facilities available nearby • Promote positive psychological wellness by providing necessary information

phobic or social anxiety disorder will be more prominent in certain situations, while cravings in patients with substance use disorder would be more prominent in certain situations or timings of a day. Due to the availability of small and easily portable devices, like mobile phones, tablets and connected wearable devices like smartphones, it is possible nowadays to collect real-time self-assessments. Also, capturing the behavior and physiological response of an individual at a relevant moment (e.g. avoidance of crowded places in agoraphobia or approaching a place like an alcohol shop) using GPS or biosensors (to get real-time physiological data, like pulse, galvanic skin conductance, etc.) can help in objectively assessing the extent of problem behavior. Apart from this, call and text logs, the proximity of a person to another person (analyzed using Bluetooth) and the extent of use of social media apps can help guide the extent of social interaction of the person. This type of assessment is called 'Digital Phenotyping'. Multiple studies have found this type of data collection to be feasible and convenient for patients.

In patients suffering from dementia, research has found a good association between the degree of cognitive impairment and digital measures like walking speed and time spent outside the home. Research in patients with bipolar disorder has reported that an artificial intelligence-based approach can help achieve fair to excellent identification of mood states, types and symptoms. Digital phenotyping has also been useful in predicting the symptoms of depression and anxiety. In psychosis, rehabilitation activities and family support have been successfully provided through mobile apps. Self-assessment at different time points has also been found to be useful in preventing relapse in patients with major depressive disorder.

Most screening and diagnostic instruments have also been applied digitally, which are useful in the clinics as well as in research for faster capture of data and analysis. These measures also confer the advantage of self-screening by an individual. During the COVID-19 pandemic, a large number of studies have been conducted through online surveys, making it possible to assess the mental health impact of the pandemic in times when the whole country was in a lockdown.

Assessment of brain structure and function using neuroimaging modalities, like magnetic resonance imaging (MRI), functional magnetic resonance imaging (fMRI), diffusion tensor imaging (DTI), single photon emission computed tomography (SPECT) and positron emission tomography (PET), and electrophysiological techniques, like electroencephalography (EEG), have led to significant advancements in understanding the neurobiological basis of mental illnesses. It has also led to the development of novel neuromodulation methods, like repetitive trans magnetic stimulation (rTMS) and transcranial direct current stimulation (tDCS), targeting the specific brain regions non-invasively. Without IT, it would be impossible to analyze the enormous data generated and give useful clinical information on neuroimaging and neuromodulation. Studies are emerging that are trying to utilize the neuroimaging data as well as other biological data, like genetics, to improve the understanding of many psychiatric disorders.

Exposure to age-appropriate media content under supervision can help improve speech and language among toddlers. Media intervention has also been found to be effective among patients with autism by improving facial recognition. A number of computer-based and internet-based psychotherapy modules have been developed for mental illnesses, like depression, anxiety disorders, obsessive compulsive disorder, post-traumatic stress disorder (PTSD), etc., which have been found to be effective and cost-saving. Mobile apps have been approved by the US FDA for the management of substance use disorders as an adjunct to conventional in-person treatment. The use of artificial intelligence to provide fully automated conversation in text-message format with the use of 'chatbots' has been found to lead to a significant decrease in depressive symptoms. Digital interventions in the form of video games have been found to improve attention and executive function among children, with US FDA approving EndeavorRx, a video game for the improvement of attention for children with attention deficit hyperactivity disorder. Apart from these, other newer technologies like virtual

reality are being explored for the management of symptoms of different mental illnesses. It has been used as a simulation tool in patients with dementia, as a distraction tool for relaxation in patients with anxiety disorders, as an interaction tool for exposure and reducing symptoms of PTSD and craving in substance use disorders, social phobia, as well as other types of phobias. Avatar therapy is another treatment modality developed using IT to cope with auditory hallucinations in patients with psychosis, where patients create and interact with virtual avatars who take on the role of the voices.

Telemedicine is a cost-effective solution to provide services to people suffering from mental illness in far-off locations, saving on travel and time. The COVID-19 pandemic and associated lockdown provided an opportunity to expand the use of IT for the treatment of people with mental illnesses. With the introduction of telemedicine and telepsychiatry guidelines, there has been a rapid expansion of the use of telepsychiatry in the country. Service delivery through telepsychiatry has been reported to be highly efficacious in treating all age groups while decreasing cost and reducing stigma.

Health informatics can analyze the data of a large number of individuals within very short duration of time, providing trends on the changing scenario in the country. Health Information Systems (HIS) enable patients and clinicians to access the requisite patient data as and when required, without the patient having to always carry large heavy documents.

Specific Benefits of Information Technology for a Person with Mental Health Issues

For any person with mental health issues, IT can be advantageous in a variety of ways.

To gain knowledge and information about symptoms of mental illness and its treatment: IT can help provide easy access to the requisite knowledge and information about the symptoms of mental illness, availability and modality of treatments, and the places where treatment is available. IT also provides information about various crisis helpline numbers that a person can access in times of need. However, as with all information, one must exercise caution and not fall a victim to internet misinformation. Similar to charlatans of the past selling amulets and herbs with a magical cure for illnesses, the online world is also filled with false narratives. One must understand that technology is a tool, neither good nor bad, with its outcome depending on the mode of use. The reputation of a website or an app should always be considered while accepting recommendations. Reliable sources of such information would include organizations like the WHO, the Department of Health of the Government or the professional organizations of psychiatrists, clinical psychologists, etc.

As an aid in screening for mental illness symptoms: IT can help an individual with mental health issues to screen self for the presence or absence of mental illness using computerized tools or software and take the decision for treatment accordingly. Although there are currently more than 2000 apps on mental health on the Google App store and Apple store, any mood diary app might be beneficial in tracking mood fluctuations over time. Apps that chart mood or anxiety over time can even be useful to your treating clinician in understanding your pattern of illness. Apps that allow you to associate events with anxiety or drug use are of significant help to therapists and clinicians.

As an aid in the monitoring of symptoms and instantaneous feedback: As mentioned earlier, with the advent of various technologies, which have made ecological momentary assessment and digital phenotyping easier, it is now possible for individuals to easily monitor their symptoms.

Certain apps that use 'Chatbots' are able to respond to voice or text-based conversations based on artificial intelligence or in a pre-programmed manner. These have been found to be beneficial for individuals who suffer from depressive or anxiety symptoms by providing them with a constant source of support.

As a tool to seek therapy and for crisis intervention: Helplines for mental illness are provided by many organizations across the country. Day care centers, where patients may be sent for skill development can be of great help to caregivers. Helplines that provide information about various disability benefits and the process of disability certification increase awareness and provide access to government support. Some apps provide help in quitting drugs. These apps provide distraction during periods of severe craving and can help associate patterns of behavior with drug use. The record of such apps might be beneficial in treatment as doctors can then devise ways to avoid these triggers. Apps for crisis interventions go beyond suicide helpline numbers. These apps generally have trusted contacts to whom SOS-SMS can be sent, video calls can be made and even alert the treating clinician to initiate emergency intervention. Telepsychiatry services, web-based interventions and digitally delivered psychotherapy have all been found to be beneficial to a certain extent, as mentioned in previous sections.

It is important to note that in the current state of technological progress, these apps and IT interventions are best used as an adjunct to in-person clinical treatment, which still remains the gold standard for mental health diagnosis and treatment.

As an assistive support tool: IT can provide an assistive role in giving reminders for pills, appointment scheduling and stimulation in

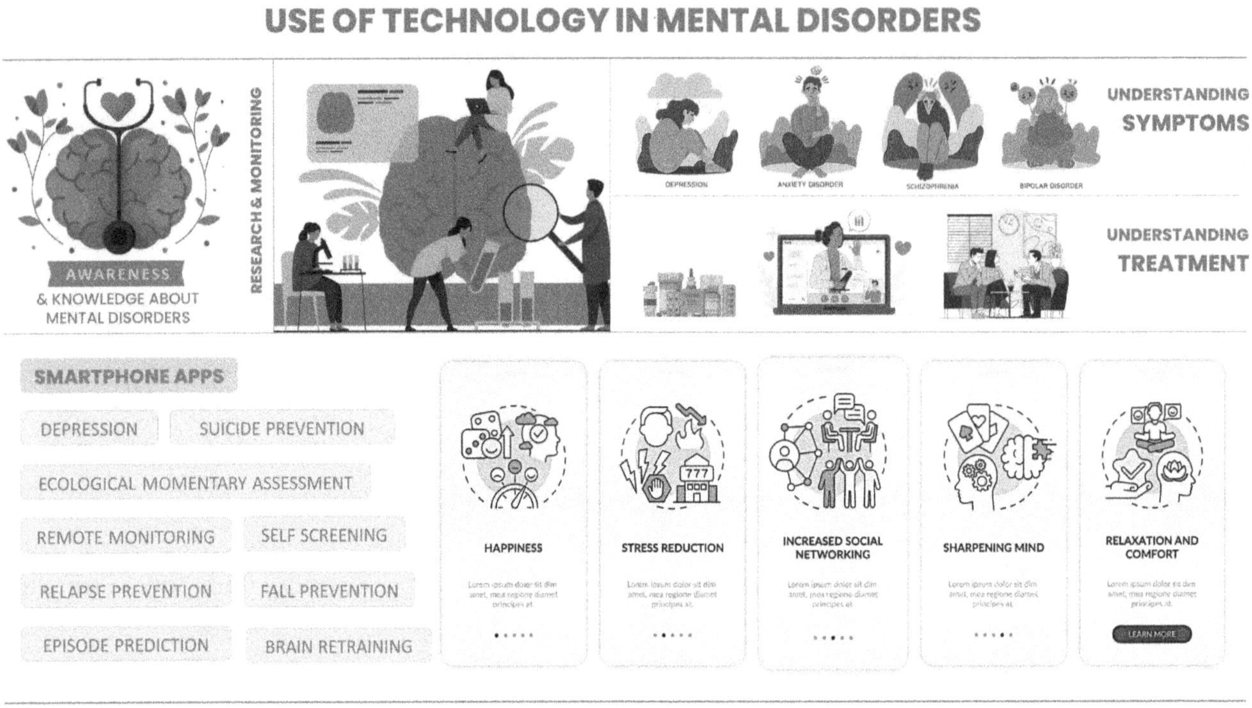

Figure 2. *Use of Information Technology in Mental Health*

patients with autism spectrum disorder, dementia, etc. Wearable devices have been used to prevent and inform about falls in the geriatric population and in helping dementia patients find a way home, in case of losing their way. Some robots are also being developed to assist elderly patients with small tasks and providing support.

To join self-help groups: IT also provides an opportunity for people with mental health issues to join support groups, where they can get into contact with people with similar mental health issues, thus supporting each other.

Figure 2 summarizes the uses of IT in mental health.

Limitations of IT

While there are a lot of advantages of using IT like being relatively cheap, easily available and easily accessible, there are certain disadvantages too. It requires language literacy and, often,

understanding of the English language, as most content on the internet and in apps is still not available in vernacular languages. This leads to a huge divide, as only persons with knowledge of English have easy access to services. Usage of apps also requires digital literacy. Additionally, preoccupation with mobile phones or computers can lead to addiction to screens, poor parenting through distraction and even accidents. There is also a risk of breach of privacy, cyberbullying, exposure to age-inappropriate content and a reduction in in-person communication.

Improvements in data privacy with further advances in technology may help improve the uptake and harness the benefits of the same.

Conclusion

IT can help increase the access to quality mental health services to a larger population in a shorter duration of time. It can also help improve the awareness of mental health among the general public and promote positive mental health. It also provides an easy, fast and cost-effective way to assess the mental health symptoms of an individual at different time points and acts as a medium through which interventions can be provided at the time of crisis. However, it also has its own limitations and risks, and hence, needs to be used with appropriate caution.

KEY POINTS

➤ IT is the science that deals with the collection, storage, processing and presentation of data.

➤ IT has enormous potential to increase the outreach of psychiatric services.

➤ IT also plays a major role in research, clinical care as well as in public health aspects of mental health.

➤ IT can help individuals with mental illness in various aspects – in gaining knowledge about mental illness and its treatment, as an aid in screening as well as monitoring for mental health symptoms and as a tool to seek treatment or join self-help support groups.

➤ People using IT should also be mindful of its limitations, like the risk of addiction to screening, exposure to age-inappropriate content or cyberbullying, and hence, should use it with appropriate caution.

REFERENCES

1. Magnavita JJ (Ed). Using Technology in Mental Health Practice, 1st edition. ed. American Psychological Association, 2018.

2. Goldberg SB, Lam SU, Simonsson O, et al. Mobile phone-based interventions for mental health: A systematic meta-review of 14 meta-analyses of randomized controlled trials. PLOS Digit. Health 2022, 1, e0000002. https://doi.org/10.1371/journal.pdig.0000002

3. National Drug Dependence Treatment Center, AIIMS New Delhi, 2021. NAAT – In collaboration with MSJE [WWW Document]. URL https://naat.co.in/ Last accessed 14th March 2022

4. Department of Psychiatry, AIIMS New Delhi, 2021. Psychiatry Publications [WWW Document]. URL https://www.aiims.edu/en/2014-12-12-06-39-37/psychiatry_publication.html Last accessed 14th March 2022

5. Technology and the future of mental health treatment | National Institute of Mental Health. URL https://www.nimh.nih.gov/health/topics/technology-and-the-future-of-mental-health-treatment#:~:text=Technology%20has%20opened%20a%20new,increase%20understanding%20of%20mental%20wellbeing. Last accessed 14th March 2022

Index

F

Fetishism 119

Fluoxetine 36, 54, 112, 119, 167

Forgetfulness 9, 32, 40, 43, 141, 168, 256

Free-floating 31

Freud 176, 231

G

Gambling 73–75, 77

Gaming 73–74, 76–77

Ganja 13, 65

Gastrointestinal 36, 109–110

Gender-dysphoria 121

Grandiosity 41, 58

Grief 195, 224, 234

Guardianship 195, 197, 217–218

H

Hallucination 9, 141

Hallucinogens 64, 66–67

Haloperidol 144, 165–166

Handicap 214–215

Handwashing 50, 54

Headache 4, 32, 34, 36, 43, 75, 125, 133, 142, 166–167, 169–171, 256

Histrionic 58

Hyperactivity 13, 74, 110, 133, 138, 156, 168, 262

Hypersomnia 125, 127–128

Hypnosis 176

Hypomania 41, 49

Hysteria 27, 231

I

Idiopathic 127

Imipramine 36, 164, 167

Impairment 8, 31, 40–41, 57, 98, 122, 141, 214–216, 261

Impulse 54, 60

Insight 9, 12–13, 15, 92, 174, 184, 225, 229

Insomnia 31, 36, 65, 74, 125–126, 128, 148, 164, 166–167, 169

Intellectual disability 17, 19–20, 132, 136, 138, 216, 219

Internet Addiction 73–74, 77

Intoxication 66, 69–70, 81

J

Judgment 9, 12, 15, 40, 85, 93, 141, 143, 230

Juvenile 85

K

Koro 27

L

Libido 10, 109, 117

Lithium 101, 164, 168–169, 251

Loneliness 59, 134, 140, 143, 178, 182, 186, 260

Long-stay 192, 199

Lorazepam 36, 144, 168

M

Mania 12, 28, 40–41, 49, 98, 100, 168

Masturbation 116, 118

Media xiii, 5, 22, 28–30, 73–74, 77, 81, 84–88, 90, 94, 101, 107, 110, 113, 123, 140, 146, 154, 203, 205, 258, 260–262

Meditation 5, 61, 104–105, 195, 223–227, 230–233

Melatonin 123–124, 128, 167

Memantine 144, 169

Menopause 148

Menstruation 147, 152

Metabolic Syndrome 92, 101, 124, 192

Methadone 170

Methylphenidate 136, 168–169

MHCA 192, 197, 217

Migraine 81, 150

Migrants 83, 244

Mind-body 224

Mindfulness 104, 230–231, 233

Mind-Reading 179

Mirtazapine 36, 112, 167

Modeling 178, 188

Mood 8–9, 11–13, 31, 37, 39, 41, 45–46, 48–49, 53, 58–59, 61–62, 74–76, 81, 90, 98, 101, 104, 118, 125, 133, 136, 141, 147–150, 164, 168–169, 174–175, 186, 201, 205, 232, 256, 261, 263

Mood-stabilizers 168

Morbidity 8, 17, 38, 62, 98, 141, 145, 150, 162, 241, 244

Mortality 17, 62, 81, 98, 100, 112, 143, 231, 244, 250